Social Public Health System and Sustainability

Social Public Health System and Sustainability

Editors

Quan-Hoang Vuong
Khuat Thu Hong

MDPI • Basel • Beijing • Wuhan • Barcelona • Belgrade • Manchester • Tokyo • Cluj • Tianjin

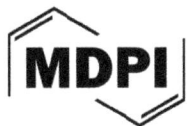

Editors
Quan-Hoang Vuong
ISR
Phenikaa University
Hanoi
Vietnam

Khuat Thu Hong
Research
ISDS
Hanoi
Vietnam

Editorial Office
MDPI
St. Alban-Anlage 66
4052 Basel, Switzerland

This is a reprint of articles from the Special Issue published online in the open access journal *Sustainability* (ISSN 2071-1050) (available at: www.mdpi.com/journal/sustainability/special_issues/public_health_system).

For citation purposes, cite each article independently as indicated on the article page online and as indicated below:

LastName, A.A.; LastName, B.B.; LastName, C.C. Article Title. *Journal Name* **Year**, *Volume Number*, Page Range.

ISBN 978-3-0365-5328-3 (Hbk)
ISBN 978-3-0365-5327-6 (PDF)

© 2022 by the authors. Articles in this book are Open Access and distributed under the Creative Commons Attribution (CC BY) license, which allows users to download, copy and build upon published articles, as long as the author and publisher are properly credited, which ensures maximum dissemination and a wider impact of our publications.

The book as a whole is distributed by MDPI under the terms and conditions of the Creative Commons license CC BY-NC-ND.

Contents

Preface to "Social Public Health System and Sustainability" vii

Danielle Resiak, Elias Mpofu and Rodd Rothwell
Sustainable Harm Reduction Needle and Syringe Programs for People Who Inject Drugs:
A Scoping Review of Their Implementation Qualities
Reprinted from: *Sustainability* **2021**, *13*, 2834, doi:10.3390/su13052834 1

Mariana Cernicova-Buca and Adina Palea
An Appraisal of Communication Practices Demonstrated by Romanian District Public Health
Authorities at the Outbreak of the COVID-19 Pandemic
Reprinted from: *Sustainability* **2021**, *13*, 2500, doi:10.3390/su13052500 13

Gema Gutierrez-Romero, Antonio Blanco-Oliver, Mª Teresa Montero-Romero and Mariano Carbonero-Ruz
The Impact of CEOs' Gender on Organisational Efficiency in the Public Sector: Evidence from
the English NHS
Reprinted from: *Sustainability* **2021**, *13*, 2188, doi:10.3390/su13042188 33

Tatjana Fischer
Understanding the Spatial-Related Abstraction of Public Health Impact Goals and Measures:
Illustrated by the Example of the Austrian Action Plan on Women's Health
Reprinted from: *Sustainability* **2021**, *13*, 773, doi:10.3390/su13020773 49

Quang "Neo" Bui and Emi Moriuchi
Economic and Social Factors That Predict Readmission for Mental Health and Drug
Abuse Patients
Reprinted from: *Sustainability* **2021**, *13*, 531, doi:10.3390/su13020531 69

Raúl Payá Castiblanque and Pere J. Beneyto Calatayud
Inequalities and the Impact of Job Insecurity on Health Indicators in the Spanish Workforce
Reprinted from: *Sustainability* **2020**, *12*, 6425, doi:10.3390/su12166425 81

Thanh-Long Giang, Dinh-Tri Vo and Quan-Hoang Vuong
COVID-19: A Relook at Healthcare Systems and Aged Populations
Reprinted from: *Sustainability* **2020**, *12*, 4200, doi:10.3390/su12104200 103

Viet-Phuong La, Thanh-Hang Pham, Manh-Toan Ho, Minh-Hoang Nguyen, Khanh-Linh P. Nguyen, Thu-Trang Vuong, Hong-Kong T. Nguyen, Trung Tran, Quy Khuc, Manh-Tung Ho and Quan-Hoang Vuong
Policy Response, Social Media and Science Journalism for the Sustainability of the Public Health
System Amid the COVID-19 Outbreak: The Vietnam Lessons
Reprinted from: *Sustainability* **2020**, *12*, 2931, doi:10.3390/su12072931 113

Minh-Hoang Nguyen, Manh-Tung Ho, Viet-Phuong La, Quynh-Yen Thi. Nguyen, Manh-Toan Ho, Thu-Trang Vuong, Tam-Tri Le, Manh-Cuong Nguyen and Quan-Hoang Vuong
A Scientometric Study on Depression among University Students in East Asia: Research and
System Insufficiencies?
Reprinted from: *Sustainability* **2020**, *12*, 1498, doi:10.3390/su12041498 141

Dominika Głąbska, Valentina Rahelić, Dominika Guzek, Kamila Jaworska, Sandra Bival, Zlatko Giljević and Eva Pavić
Dietary Health-Related Risk Factors for Women in the Polish and Croatian Population Based on the Nutritional Behaviors of Junior Health Professionals
Reprinted from: *Sustainability* **2019**, *11*, 5073, doi:10.3390/su11185073 167

Mengying Wang and Chunhai Tao
Research on the Efficiency of Local Government Health Expenditure in China and Its Spatial Spillover Effect
Reprinted from: *Sustainability* **2019**, *11*, 2469, doi:10.3390/su11092469 183

Minh Hoang Nguyen, Tam Tri Le and Serik Meirmanov
Depression, Acculturative Stress, and Social Connectedness among International University Students in Japan: A Statistical Investigation
Reprinted from: *Sustainability* **2019**, *11*, 878, doi:10.3390/su11030878 201

Quan-Hoang Vuong, Kien-Cuong P. Nghiem, Viet-Phuong La, Thu-Trang Vuong, Hong-Kong T. Nguyen, Manh-Toan Ho, Kien Tran, Thu-Hong Khuat and Manh-Tung Ho
Sex Differences and Psychological Factors Associated with General Health Examinations Participation: Results from a Vietnamese Cross-Section Dataset
Reprinted from: *Sustainability* **2019**, *11*, 514, doi:10.3390/su11020514 221

Lovro Štefan, Vlatko Vučetić, Goran Vrgoč and Goran Sporiš
Sleep Duration and Sleep Quality as Predictors of Health in Elderly Individuals
Reprinted from: *Sustainability* **2018**, *10*, 3918, doi:10.3390/su10113918 235

Quan-Hoang Vuong, Anh-Duc Hoang, Thu-Trang Vuong, Viet-Phuong La, Hong Kong T. Nguyen and Manh-Tung Ho
Factors Associated with the Regularity of Physical Exercises as a Means of Improving the Public Health System in Vietnam
Reprinted from: *Sustainability* **2018**, *10*, 3828, doi:10.3390/su10113828 243

Jiaping Zhang, Mingwang Cheng, Xinyu Wei and Xiaomei Gong
Does Mobile Phone Penetration Affect Divorce Rate? Evidence from China
Reprinted from: *Sustainability* **2018**, *10*, 3701, doi:10.3390/su10103701 259

Agnieszka Bem, Rafał Siedlecki, Paweł Prędkiewicz, Patrizia Gazzola, Bożena Ryszawska and Paulina Ucieklak-Jeż
Hospitals' Financial Health in Rural and Urban Areas in Poland: Does It Ensure Sustainability?
Reprinted from: *Sustainability* **2019**, *11*, 1932, doi:10.3390/su11071932 279

Heyeon Park, Hyunjin Oh and Sunjoo Boo
The Role of Occupational Stress in the Association between Emotional Labor and Mental Health: A Moderated Mediation Model
Reprinted from: *Sustainability* **2019**, *11*, 1886, doi:10.3390/su11071886 297

Preface to "Social Public Health System and Sustainability"

This Special Issue reprint contains 18 articles published in *Sustainability* from late 2018 to early 2021. During that time, the world faced the fatal and widespread health crisis, COVID-19, which had threatened the social and public health systems at every corner for quite some time.

As the Guest-Editors and also a contributing authors, we are glad that the academic contents from the Special Issue will now be put together in this reprint, making the authors' hard work and efforts accessible to the larger audience.

We would like to thank the authors for spending time and effort contributing to the Special Issue. My appreciation also goes on to MDPI for organizing and supporting this SI volume.

Quan-Hoang Vuong and Khuat Thu Hong
Editors

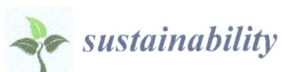

Review

Sustainable Harm Reduction Needle and Syringe Programs for People Who Inject Drugs: A Scoping Review of Their Implementation Qualities

Danielle Resiak [1,*], Elias Mpofu [1,2,3,*] and Rodd Rothwell [1]

[1] Faculty of Medicine and Health, The University of Sydney, Sydney 2006, Australia; rod.rothwell@sydney.edu.au
[2] Rehabilitation and Health Services, University of North Texas, Denton, TX 26203, USA
[3] Educational Psychology Department, University of Johannesburg, Johannesburg 2092, South Africa
* Correspondence: dres2715@uni.sydney.edu.au (D.R.); elias.mpofu@sydney.edu.au (E.M.)

Citation: Resiak, D.; Mpofu, E.; Rothwell, R. Sustainable Harm Reduction Needle and Syringe Programs for People Who Inject Drugs: A Scoping Review of Their Implementation Qualities. *Sustainability* **2021**, *13*, 2834. https://doi.org/10.3390/su13052834

Academic Editor:
Quan-Hoang Vuong

Received: 29 December 2020
Accepted: 26 February 2021
Published: 5 March 2021

Publisher's Note: MDPI stays neutral with regard to jurisdictional claims in published maps and institutional affiliations.

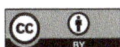

Copyright: © 2021 by the authors. Licensee MDPI, Basel, Switzerland. This article is an open access article distributed under the terms and conditions of the Creative Commons Attribution (CC BY) license (https://creativecommons.org/licenses/by/4.0/).

Abstract: While substance use disorders (SUD) continue to be a global concern, harm reduction approaches can provide sustainable harm minimization to people who inject drugs (PWID) without requiring abstinence. Yet, the evidence for the sustainable implementation of harm reduction approaches is newly emerging. This scoping review sought to map the evidence on implementation qualities of sustainable harm reduction needle and syringe programs (NSPs). We searched the Cochrane Database of Systematic Reviews, PubMed, ProQuest Central, and Directory of Open Access Journals for empirical studies (a) with an explicit focus on harm minimization NSPs, (b) with a clearly identified study population, (c) that described the specific NSP implementation protocol, (d) that provided information on accessibility, affordability, and feasibility, and (e) were published in English between 2000–2020. Following narrative qualitative synthesis, the evidence suggests individual implementer characteristics directly influenced sustainable availability and scope of NSP provision while implementation processes explained the predictability and continuity of service provision across services. External factors including community perceptions of NSPs and policing activity influenced the sustainability of NSP implementation. The emerging evidence suggests that sustainable NSP programs for PWID require provider, consumer, and community engagement, supported by enabling health policies.

Keywords: NSP; harm reduction; harm minimization; low threshold settings; PWID; sustainable implementation qualities

1. Introduction

Substance misuse remains an ongoing health crisis affecting every region of the world, increasing the burden of disease globally [1]. Across the globe, approximately 250 million people use addictive substances every year of which 63.5 million have a substance use disorder (SUD) [2]. Despite substance use disorder mitigation efforts [3], relapse rates remain high at 40–60% [3], with mortality from drug and alcohol use disorders at 6.9 deaths per 100,000 globally [4]. Harm minimization approaches appear to hold promise for those with a history of addiction or dependence not wishing to obtain abstinence [5,6]. Harm reduction approaches that support people with a poor prognosis for abstinence-based treatment would make for sustainable needle and syringe program (NSP) practices [5]. Sustainable NSPs are human-centered, cost-effective, socially embedded, aligned to the health policies of jurisdictions [6], and offered at sufficient intensity to achieve program goals and population outcomes in the long-term [7].

While, harm reduction approaches to substance use dependency and addiction are increasingly being adopted, a paucity of research exists pertaining to the sustainability of their implementation protocols across service types [8]. More specifically, emerging evidence as to the sustainable implementation qualities of NSPs is yet to be aggregated. As such, we aimed to scope the evidence for implementation qualities of sustainable harm reduction NSPs. Such evidence would inform NSP services for those with a history of addiction or dependence for which abstinence would be less successful.

1.1. Harm Reduction Approaches: Sustainable Implementation Considerations

In the context of drug treatment policy, harm reduction refers to minimizing the health, social and economic costs of drug use to both individuals with addiction or dependency and the communities in which they participate [9]. Early adopters of harm reduction approaches included Australia, Canada, Portugal, Switzerland, the United Kingdom, and The Netherlands, and have since spread through Asia, Latin America, and Central Eastern Europe [10]. The sustainability of harm reduction policies and programs would greatly depend on their implementation design, responsiveness, and resourcing, alongside financial longevity, social acceptance, and accessibility. We aim to review the evidence on implementation design, responsiveness, and resourcing of harm reduction focused NSP.

Needle and syringe programs are low threshold services for people who inject drugs characterized by few to no access obstacles [11]. They comprise of primary, secondary, mobile and outreach services, syringe vending machines and pharmacies that sell or provide injecting equipment free of charge, predominately run within publicly funded health services [12]. The primary goal of an NSP is the distribution of sufficient injecting equipment, supported by educational interventions to reduce or eliminate the reuse of injecting equipment among people who inject drugs (PWID) [13]. Needle and syringe programs are proven to reduce the risks of blood borne virus transmission through the provision of sterile injecting equipment to people who inject drugs (PWID) [14] and come at comparatively lower cost than alternative approaches [15]. Despite their relative cost-effectiveness, NSP implementation is largely shaped by a country or regions philosophical approach to drug treatment [16], often with little research evidence on implementation guidelines. Furthermore, while NSPs continue to operate funded through public health agencies, political, media or community campaigns mean they remain vulnerable to closure in the absence of the evidence for their sustainability [13].

1.2. Health Policy Frameworks

Health policy frameworks provide the context for implementation of programs aimed at aligning a country's priorities with its populations health needs, in partnership with government, health and development partners, civil society and the private sector for improved use of available resources [17]. Consensus building across multiple stakeholders in health policy framing slows the implementation of NSPs, given the politics of drug policy and stigmatization of people who inject drugs [18]. Moreover, policy framing and planning that occurs at all levels of a countries health care system can support sustainable NSP implementation due to increased public buy in [19]. Partners in sustainable NSP implementation would commit, if they perceived evidence of quality, affordability, acceptability, and accessibility [6]. We aim to apply a theory driven framework to aggregate the emerging research evidence on NSP program implementation qualities with PWID using the Consolidated Framework for Implementation Research (CFIR) [20].

1.3. Implementation Study Framework

The CFIR defines five implementation determinants: (1) individuals involved in service delivery (e.g., their knowledge and beliefs about the intervention), (2) the internal organization setting (e.g., leadership engagement), (3) the implementation processes (e.g., executing the innovation), (4) the program/intervention characteristics (e.g., complexity, accessibility, quality, affordability and acceptability) and (5) the external setting (client needs and resources). We expect sustainable NSPs would be designed to these qualities, yet the evidence is unclear as to how the interactions among these determinants would influence implementation outcomes. For instance, trust building among potential service users would be influenced by implementation processes, particularly given that social stigma has been linked to the mis-trust of health services experienced by people who inject drugs (PWID) [13]. Similarly, the context of service provision by organizational, geographical, political, and cultural factors would influence the resourcing of NSPs [21], while acceptability of NSP services is dependent upon how much they are trusted by prospective adopters [13]. For those with a substance use disorder, social stigma is behind the mistrust of health services and therefore detracts from service engagement [13].

Legalization of NSPs increased their visibility which in some contexts, resulted in client arrests [22]. Noted as a structural barrier to the sustainability of an NSP is police arrest and prosecution activity. Arrest or prosecution of NSP clients when accessing a legal NSP undermines the trust PWID have in the inclusiveness of public health laws [23] and compounds the risk of unsafe drug injecting [22] while also deterring NSP service uptake. This in turn places PWID at a greater risk of blood borne virus transmission and overdose [23]. User-oriented NSP implementation can reduce stigma as it is mutually understood that PWID may not require assistance beyond the provision of clean injecting equipment and associated paraphernalia (tourniquets, alcohol wipes and so forth) [13]. There is no expectation from staff that PWID will require, nor want assistance for their drug use [13].

1.4. Goal of the Review

We aimed to conduct an exploratory scoping systematic review [24,25] to identify both gaps and trends in literature, clarifying definitions, and report practices that can inform future research and practice. A scoping systematic review is appropriate for summarizing the emerging evidence on sustainable NSP health interventions.

Objectives

This scoping review aims to map evidence for the sustainability of NSPs defined by the CFIR framework of implementation determinants inclusive of; program implementers and internal setting, implementation process and characteristics, and external factors. Our specific research question was: What is the emerging evidence pertaining to sustainable NSP implementation qualities including implementers, internal setting, implementation process and characteristics, and external factors?

Findings would be important for the sustainability of NSPs framed on implementation qualities evidence in harm reduction studies considering the perspective of those who are most directly affected by their operation. Moreover, the evidence would inform future studies on NSP implementation, providing benchmarks for evaluation and improvement at both an individual, program, and systems level.

2. Materials and Methods

2.1. Search Strategy for Identification of Studies

We searched the Cochrane Database of Systematic Reviews for previous reviews on the sustainable implementation of NSPs and yielded a null result, which justifies this systematic scoping review. We then searched electronic databases including PubMed, ProQuest Central and the Directory of Open Access Journals for peer-reviewed studies pertaining to NSP implementation, restricting our search to the period 2000 to 2020. Our selection of databases prioritized studies that described implementation protocols at a sufficient level of detail to allow for determination of their relevance to the study aims. Moreover, we searched field specific journals inclusive of *Substance Use and Misuse*, *Addiction*, *Aids and Behaviour*, *Harm Reduction Journal* and *The International Journal of Drug Policy* for relevant studies. We searched each database and journal using a combination of search terms inclusive of needle and syringe program implementation, implementation science, addiction, and NSPs (see Table 1).

Table 1. Overview of search procedure key topics, terms and criteria.

Topic	Key Words/Phrases Searched	CFIR Criteria
Needle and syringe program/Syringe (exchange program implementation)	Needle and syringe program, AND implementation, AND people who inject drugs, OR implementation science, addiction, dependence OR sustainable needle and syringe, program characteristics, AND community, health policy, accessibility, feasibility, affordability, cost evaluation.	(1) Service delivery (e.g., their knowledge and beliefs about the intervention), (2) Internal organization setting (e.g., leadership engagement), (3) Implementation processes (e.g., executing the innovation), (4) Program/intervention characteristics (e.g., complexity, accessibility, quality, affordability and acceptability) (5) the external setting (client needs and resources).
Needle and Syringe program/Syringe protocols.	Harm minimization, OR harm reduction, dependency, addiction, substance use disorder, AND individual characteristics, long-term, adherence, fidelity, AND regulations, providers, sites.	

2.1.1. Eligibility Criteria

We included for review empirical studies that (a) were published in English, and (b) had an explicit focus on harm minimization needle and syringe program implementation. To be eligible, studies were (i) case studies, cross-sectional, or longitudinal studies, (ii) on a clearly identified study population, (ii) with description of their specific harm reduction/NSP implementation procedure or protocol and (iv) with information on sustainability characteristics of user involvement in design accessibility, affordability, and feasibility. In doing so, we prioritized studies that included a process and/outcome evaluation of the harm reduction/NSP implementation protocol by users and/or providers as well as how program characteristics aligned with health care policy. We excluded studies that were in languages other than English and did not describe the harm reduction/NSP implementation protocol they used in a manner that enabled determination of their sustainability. See Table 2 for variable inclusion and exclusion criteria.

Table 2. Study variable inclusion and exclusion criteria.

Variable	Inclusion Criteria	Exclusion Criteria
Study Design	Empirical studies.	Literature reviews and studies that were not peer-reviewed.
Publication Years	2000—present.	Published prior to the year 2000.
Participants	People who inject drugs, needle and syringe service providers and related stakeholders inclusive of community members, policymakers, and police.	Participants who could not be identified as either a needle and syringe program implementer, member of an NSP internal setting or external setting.
Intervention	Needle and syringe program/syringe exchange program implementation and evaluation.	Other harm reduction programs inclusive of; opioid substitution treatments and medically supervised injecting centers/drug consumption rooms.
Process	Description of implementation protocol, process evaluation procedure.	Missing details on implementation protocol.
Outcomes	Sustainable needle and syringe program implementation characteristics relating to implementers, inner setting, implementation process, intervention characteristics or outer setting.	Sustainable implementation characteristics not relating to the implementation of needle and syringe programs.

2.1.2. Search Tree Procedure and Outcomes

We retrieved a total of 722 articles for screening (see Figure 1), and screened the articles by titles and abstracts, excluding a total of 652 at this stage. Our selection process yielded a preliminary list of 70 articles for further scrutiny against inclusion criteria, excluding 42 that did not meet the inclusion criteria. The first and second listed authors then accessed the full text of the 28 articles, applying the pre-determined eligibility criteria. We excluded 23 articles at this stage leaving five articles. To optimize our search yield, we browsed the reference lists of each of the articles that met the inclusion criteria for any additional articles of relevance. From this manual search, we found an additional study, resulting in six articles for this study. Final study inclusion was by consensus between the first two listed authors, moderated by the third listed author as needed.

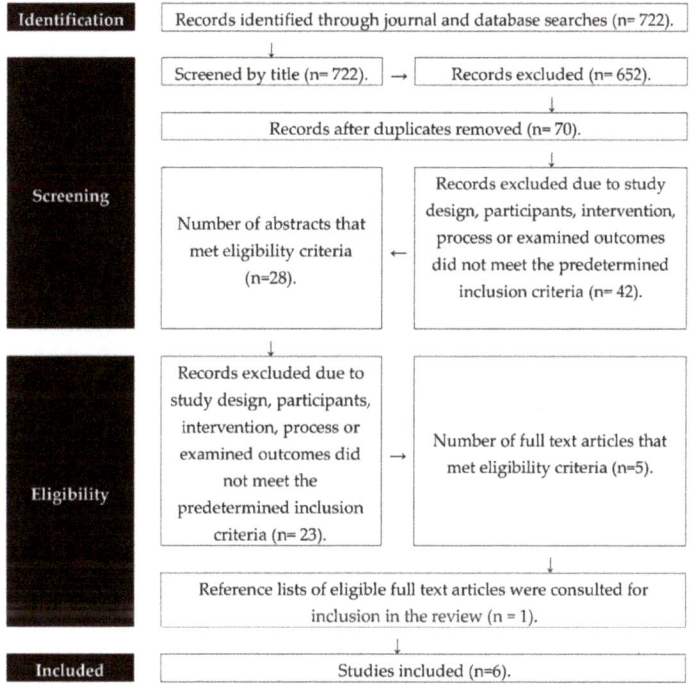

Figure 1. Search strategy.

2.2. Data Extraction and Management

For the data capture and organization relevant to the research aim, we utilized a modified version of Arksey and O'Malley [24] data extraction tool. This tool organizes according to the following categories: (1) author/year, (2) study design, (3) methods and recruitment, (4) description of study objectives, and (5) outcomes or findings [24]. Our modification was to include an implementation protocol description and evaluation. This method modification allowed for data mapping identifying both implementation approach and NSP outcomes. Table 3 presents the studies included from our search procedure.

Table 3. Studies included in the review.

Authorship	Study Design and Objectives	Participants and Context	Implementers and Inner Setting	Implementation Process and Characteristics	External Setting
				Sustainability of Implementation Qualities	
[18]	In-depth qualitative interviews examining the historical, social, political, and scientific contexts for the implementation of publicly funded NSPs.	Key stakeholders (policy makers, community stakeholders and advocates) from three US cities; Baltimore, Philadelphia, and Washington.	Sustainable Needle and Syringe program implementation is supported by an implementation willingness of policy makers based on community sentiment.	Community implementation models top down versus community activist impact program sustainability.	Empirical research evidence has a fear and concern mitigating role in driving policy change for the sustainable implementation of NSPs.
[26]	Electronic Survey to assess community pharmacists' willingness to participate in one harm reduction initiative: syringe/needle exchange.	Kentucky community pharmacists with active licenses (n = 827) for NSP services.	Pharmacists were willing to provide NSP services although fewer were willing to dispose of needles/syringes. Agreement with the public health impact of NSPs impacted pharmacist's willingness for service provision.	Barriers to the sustainable implementation of an NSP were reported to include clientele, ethics surrounding supply of materials for abuse or illegitimate use, company policy conflict, legal concerns, record keeping, time, reputation, supply problems and finding/handling needles.	None identified.
[27]	Qualitative study to assesses barriers and effectiveness of NSP's, effectiveness and barriers across Vietnam.	Key informant interviews (n = 23), focus group discussions (n = 6-8 participants per group) Peer Educators (8 groups) IDU's (5 groups) Local residents (7 groups), in-depth interviews (n = 8).	Peer Educator led NSP would be more sustainable with higher literacy and retention with NSP programs.	Sterile water ampules were not provided at NSPs due to concerns from implementing partners. Trust building would therefore contribute to sustainable NSP implementation that fosters adequate equipment provision.	Implementation sustainability is improved with law enforcement support and intensive advocacy with community stakeholders, local government, mass organizations and local residents.
[28]	Face-to-face survey to examine community-level support for a newly implemented ADM in an inner-city Sydney area known for high levels of drug use.	Local area residents (n = 118) and businesses (n = 35) located within the vicinity of needle and syringe program (NSP) services including the ADM.	Business entities showed greater support for fixed-site NSP's in general comparatively to those situated locally.	Offering extended hours for NSP via ADM would be cost effective. Anonymity for clients may increase sterile injecting equipment use.	Community member support would be important for the sustainability of NSPs.
[29]	Qualitative (interviews) to identify factors and conditions that facilitated or deterred the adoption of NSPs.	Key informants (n = 17) from nine U.S. cities.	Program leadership a key facilitator to sustainable implementation of NSPs, and when leaders with access to local power and resources.	NSP program processes that (a) respectful of political and cultural norm sensitivities, and (b) prioritized coalition building and community involvement, would be sustainable.	NSPs would be more successful aligned to community values and public policy.

2.3. Data Analysis and Synthesis

We summarized findings from the studies using narrative qualitative synthesis [30]. This data synthesis approach allowed for identifying NSP implementation determinants framed on the CRFI according to implementers and their inner setting, the implementation process, and its characteristics (e.g., quality, complexity, affordability, accessibility, and acceptability) and community based external factors.

3. Results and Discussion

Findings from our scoping review indicate the importance of implementer qualities (willingness and beliefs), implementation process factors (inclusion of PWID), program intervention characteristics (accessibility and acceptability) and external factors (policy, community acceptance and policing) for improved NSP sustainability. Above all, the evidence suggests sustainable harm reduction NSPs require support from multiple stakeholders, given the multifaceted requirements of their implementation [31], and interactions among each of the implementation determinants. The specific findings of each are discussed below.

3.1. Implementers and Internal Setting Factors of Sustainable NSPs

Implementer willingness and self-efficacy or beliefs about NSP feasibility would enhance sustainability [18], as would leadership resourcing [26,29]. For instance, pharmacists who agreed with the public health impact of NSPs were more likely to provide clean needles and syringes to PWID and dispose of used needles and syringes within the pharmacy [26]. Kentucky community pharmacists expressed 3.56 times more willingness to provide clean needles. However, the perceived barriers to selling needles and syringes without a prescription differed between Kentucky independent and chain/supermarket pharmacists with independent pharmacists reporting workflow barriers contrary to chain/supermarket pharmacists who reported clientele safety concerns as a barrier to selling needles and syringes without a prescription.

Local business support for NSPs influenced implementation feasibility in that they might show token support for NSPs at fixed sites as opposed to widespread automatic dispensing machines (ADM) [28]. Automatic dispensing machines are a sustainable and inexpensive method of increasing needle and syringe distribution to PWID. In Australia, although general support for harm reduction programs was high among survey business leaders, their awareness of such services operating in the immediate vicinity was less so. For instance, significantly lower proportions of businesses indicated awareness of fixed-site NSPs generally (63% vs. 83%, $p = 0.01$), the existence of pharmacy NSP (29% vs. 50%, $p = 0.03$) and an ADM (31% vs. 53%) ($p = 0.03$) in the local area comparatively to residents [28].

Peer implementers of NSPs with high literacy demonstrate service provision aligned to community sentiment and are more likely to remain engaged with NSP service provision then those less literate. As such, supporting improved literacy and employment retention could benefit the sustainability of peer led NSPs [27], suggesting both an education and internal program function.

3.2. Sustainable Implementation Process and Characteristics

NSP implementation process and characteristics of (a) community coalitions, (b) community activists or (c) bottom-up approaches enhanced NSP sustainability [18], as did implementers flexibility to adopt emerging empirically based interventions [28]. This could be explained by the fact that grassroots based approaches have user buy-in, and flexible hours are a well-known low threshold service access quality. Evidence-based practices are important for legitimizing NSPs [29]. For instance, Strike, Watson, Lavigne, Hopkins, Shore, Young, Leonard and Millson [15] reported implementation success of the Ontario Needle Exchange Best Practice that followed evidence-based needle and syringe recommendations, including distribution of sterile water ampoules and safer inhalation equipment. NSP processes that (a) are respectful of political and cultural norm sensitivities, and (b) prioritized coalition building and community involvement, would be more sustainable than those lacking in these qualities [29]. Greater community support for NSPs would enhance sustainability of implementation [18], so too would long-term financial commitment [8] minimizing risk for rapid depletion of the pool of available resources [29].

3.3. Sustainable NSP External Setting Characteristics

The study by Ngo, Schmich, Higgs and Fischer [27] conducted in Northern Vietnam found community support was a critical component of NSP implementation. A finding consistent with that of Downing, Riess, Vernon, Mulia, Hollinquest, McKnight, Jarlais and Edlin [29] whereby coalition building, and community consultation were deemed critical steps required for acceptability and sustainability of NSPs. To obtain community support required intensive advocacy with community stakeholders including local government, mass organizations, local residents, PWID and their families with the acquisition of law enforcement officials [27]. As an example, White, Haber and Day [28] reported on community attitudes to harm reduction and automatic dispensing machines (ADMs) in Sydney, Australia. ADMs are a sustainable and inexpensive method of increasing needle and syringe distribution to people who inject drugs. They reported local community opposition to ADMs despite national Australian data indicating support for harm reduction. Respondents to the study had concerns about possible increases in drug related crime. However, the majority of business leader participants were in support for NSP services in general (fixed-site NSPs (83%), pharmacy NSP (82%), and to a lesser extent, ADMs (67%)). Conversely, local businesses' support was slightly lower (fixed-site NSPs (77%); pharmacy NSP (80%), ADMs (60%)) [28].

External NSP setting characteristics such as partnerships between health, law enforcement, PWID, clinicians, researchers and government officials are essential for sustainable NSP implementation [8]. Furthermore, Downing, Riess, Vernon, Mulia, Hollinquest, McKnight, Jarlais and Edlin [29] suggest community NSP support is highest in places where HIV transmission presentation is a predominant community concern.

3.4. Implementation Determinants Interaction Factors

Implementer and internal setting factors at the policy level would influence the sustainable implementation of NSPs. For instance, Clark [32] suggests that drug treatment policies are influenced by national or regional prerogatives, perhaps more so than documented evidence for NSP programs. Yet, while the provision of research evidence does not guarantee policy change, it is a necessary step for sustainable implementation [18]. Moreover, policymakers may have varying opinions on the merits and moral obligations of expanding services to meet the needs of PWID [18]. Such merit and moral obligations result in policymakers struggling to implement evidence-based policies while simultaneously addressing electorate priorities [18].

Allen, Ruiz and O'Rourke [18] examined the role of research evidence in policy change processes for the sustainable implementation of publicly funded syringe exchange services in three US cities: Baltimore, MD, Philadelphia, PA, and Washington, DC. Results indicated sustainable implementation of NSPs in Baltimore and Philadelphia were dependent on research evidence application to secure policy change, conversely policy change discussions in DC were influenced by community and stakeholder fears and concerns that NSPs would increase both substance use related crime and the number of discarded syringes found in public locations. White, Haber and Day [28], also reported perceived increases in drug related crime and drug use a barrier to sustainable implementation, despite there being no empirical evidence to support such perceptions [8].

3.5. Implications for NSP Implementation Sustainability Research and Practice

In efforts to confront the health disparities among an estimated 15.9 million people who inject drugs globally [33] NSPs have been implemented. However, sustainable access to such services is not equal across the globe, with low and middle-income countries implementing NSPs at coverage levels below that required to stabilize and reverse HIV epidemics among PWID [18]. Commonly cited implementation barriers included funding, senior management, and decision-making. The primary weakness of government-initiated implementation models includes bureaucratic systems and susceptibility to pressure from community criticism creating an inability to respond quickly or flexibly change [29]. Our findings suggest that empirically based best practice recommendations are implemented successfully within NSPs when available. Additionally, community consultation at the design stage of protocol implementation, improves community acceptance.

Needle and syringe program's sustainability is dependent upon both their accessibility and continued utilization among the population base they aim to serve [34]. The World Health Organization [35] recommends NSPs distribute 200+ needles per PWID annually for their sustainable use [35]. However, substantial variability in NSP service provision, utilization, coverage, range, needle and syringe distribution and program reach are obstacles to their sustainable implementation [14]. Moreover, provider, structural, and societal barriers to NSP access for PWID [36], alongside communities lack of knowledge surrounding NSP objectives, policies, laws, regulations, locations and stigma hinder their sustainable implementation [34].

A longstanding societal value to prevent drug misuse rather than safer use of a person's substance of choice continues to run counter to NSP implementation [14]. This is despite NSPs being a proven health intervention for reducing the transmission of blood borne viruses among PWID [37]. For NSPs to be sustainable, they need to be feasible within the intended context [31]. Essential for improved health outcomes of PWID is mutual trust and communication with NSP providers. Vuong, et al. [38] suggest that when service providers are perceived not to have a genuine interest in a client's views an asymmetrical relationship presents placing the client in a vulnerable position. Furthermore, medical distrust results in reduced service engagement [38] which in turn affects its sustainability.

3.6. Limitations of the Applicability of Evidence

Few of the studies provided descriptions of their implementation protocols, and even fewer reported on their implementation process evaluation. This limited our ability to map the implementation protocols for sustainability qualities. We synthesized the data applying the CRFI framework, which is not exhaustive. Other studies may find a different profile from using alternative criteria. Furthermore, with very few studies that met our inclusion criteria, we could not determine the influence of publication bias, the tendency for statistically significant positive results to be published in greater proportions than those of statistically significant negative or null results [39]. An included study reported an attempted contact with opponents of NSPs that was not successful. As such, the perspectives of those prospective participants were not captured in the study results [29]. Furthermore, while we were able to capture results from studies conducted in Australia, Canada, the USA and Vietnam paucity of available literature addressing implementation qualities of sustainable NSPs impacts the scope of comparison between countries. Additionally, not all countries with a harm reduction drug treatment policy were represented in the findings further justifying the need to aggregate sustainable implementation qualities as they emerge.

4. Conclusions

We found evidence to suggest the importance of implementer resourcing, engagement, and willingness on the design and implementation of sustainable NSPs. Such factors would veritably translate across diverse implementer communities inclusive of program managers, peer educators, pharmacists, and NSP providers. Sustainable implementation process factors aim to build ownership and trust of NSPs, as measured by relevance and accessibility to PWID. External factors such as NSP user-friendly law-enforcement, community support and cost-containment improve NSP sustainability. Overall, there is more literature evaluating specific areas of policy or practice, comparatively to NSP provider engagement and consumer responsive sustainable implementation. Similarly, the mapped evidence trends toward implementer process characteristics and external policy frameworks. Such findings could guide both new and existing NSP provision, evaluation, and adaptation to be more consumer responsive.

Author Contributions: D.R., conceptualized the study, wrote the initial draft, completed the data curation and implemented the methodology; D.R. and E.M., carried out the formal analysis of data; E.M., the project's primary supervisor, guided the research, writing—review and editing; R.R., the project's auxiliary supervisor, provided further review and ongoing writing review. All authors have read and agreed to the published version of the manuscript.

Funding: This research received no external funding.

Institutional Review Board Statement: Not applicable.

Informed Consent Statement: Not applicable.

Data Availability Statement: Not applicable.

Acknowledgments: The article is work in partial fulfillment of a PhD thesis within the Faculty of Medicine and Health, Rehabilitation Counseling Discipline at the University of Sydney.

Conflicts of Interest: The authors declare no conflict of interest.

References

1. Peacock, A.; Leung, J.; Larney, S.; Colledge, S.; Hickman, M.; Rehm, J.; Giovino, G.A.; West, R.; Hall, W.; Griffiths, P.; et al. Global statistics on alcohol, tobacco and illicit drug use: 2017 status report. *Addiction* **2018**, *113*, 1905–1926. [CrossRef] [PubMed]
2. United Nations Office on Drugs and Crime. *World Drug Report 2016*; United Nations: New York, NY, USA, 2016; ISBN 978-92-1-148286-7.
3. Brandon, T.H.; Vidrine, J.I.; Litvin, E.B. Relapse and Relapse Prevention. *Annu. Rev. Clin. Psychol.* **2007**, *3*, 257–284. [CrossRef] [PubMed]
4. Tran, B.X.; Moir, M.; Latkin, C.A.; Hall, B.J.; Nguyen, C.T.; Ha, G.H.; Nguyen, N.B.; Ho, C.S.H.; Ho, R.C.M. Global research mapping of substance use disorder and treatment 1971–2017: Implications for priority setting. *Subst. Abus. Treat. Prev. Policy* **2019**, *14*, 1–14. [CrossRef] [PubMed]
5. Watts, J.; MacDaniels, B.; Rivera, S.; Resiak, D.; Mpofu, E.; Redwine, S. *Community Substance Use Safety*; Mpofu, E., Ed.; Palgrave/Macmillan: New York, NY, USA, 2020.
6. *Toward Sustainable Transitions in Healthcare Systems*; Routledge: London, UK, 2017.
7. Shelton, R.C.; Cooper, B.R.; Stirman, S.W. The sustainability of evidence-based interventions and practices in public health and health care. *Annu. Rev. Public Health* **2018**, *39*, 55–76. [CrossRef]
8. Wodak, A.; McLeod, L. The role of harm reduction in controlling HIV among injecting drug users. *AIDS* **2008**, *22*, S81. [CrossRef] [PubMed]
9. Rhodes, T.; Hedrich, D. Harm reduction and the mainstream. In *Harm Reduction: Evidence, Impacts and Challenges*; Rhodes, T., Hedrich, D., Eds.; MONOGRAPHS: Lisbon, Portugal, 2010.
10. Ritter, A.; Cameron, J. A review of the efficacy and effectiveness of harm reduction strategies for alcohol, tobacco and illicit drugs. *Drug Alcohol Rev.* **2006**, *25*, 611–624. [CrossRef]
11. Edland-Gryt, M.; Skatvedt, A.H. Thresholds in a low-threshold setting: An empirical study of barriers in a centre for people with drug problems and mental health disorders. *Int. J. Drug Policy* **2012**, *24*, 257–264. [CrossRef]
12. Kwon, A.J.; Anderson, C.J.; Kerr, J.C.; Thein, M.H.-H.; Zhang, G.L.; Iversen, P.J.; Dore, P.G.; Kaldor, P.J.; Law, P.M.; Maher, P.L.; et al. Estimating the cost-effectiveness of needle-syringe programs in Australia. *AIDS* **2012**, *26*, 2201–2210. [CrossRef] [PubMed]
13. Treloar, C.; Rance, J.; Yates, K.; Mao, L. Trust and people who inject drugs: The perspectives of clients and staff of Needle Syringe Programs. *Int. J. Drug Policy* **2016**, *27*, 138–145. [CrossRef] [PubMed]
14. Somlai, A.M.; Kelly, J.A.; Otto-Salaj, L.; Nelson, D. "Lifepoint": A case study in using social science community identification data to guide the implementation of a needle exchange program. *AIDS Educ. Prev.* **1999**, *11*, 187.
15. Strike, C.; Watson, T.M.; Lavigne, P.; Hopkins, S.; Shore, R.; Young, D.; Leonard, L.; Millson, P. Guidelines for better harm reduction: Evaluating implementation of best practice recommendations for needle and syringe programs (NSPs). *Int. J. Drug Policy* **2010**, *22*, 34–40. [CrossRef]

16. Resiak, D.; Mpofu, E.; Athanasou, J. Drug Treatment Policy in the Criminal Justice System: A Scoping Literature Review. *Am. J. Crim. Justice* **2016**, *41*, 3–13. [CrossRef]
17. World Health Organisation. National Health Policies, Strategies and Plans. Available online: http://www.who.int/nationalpolicies/about/en/ (accessed on 27 February 2017).
18. Allen, S.T.; Ruiz, M.S.; O'Rourke, A. The evidence does not speak for itself: The role of research evidence in shaping policy change for the implementation of publicly funded syringe exchange programs in three US cities. *Int. J. Drug Policy* **2015**, *26*, 688–695. [CrossRef]
19. World Health Organisation. National Health Policies, Strategies, and Plans: From Vision to Operation. Available online: http://www.who.int/nationalpolicies/processes/operational/en/ (accessed on 27 February 2017).
20. Wallace, B.; van Roode, T.; Pagan, F.; Phillips, P.; Wagner, H.; Calder, S.; Aasen, J.; Pauly, B.; Hore, D. What is needed for implementing drug checking services in the context of the overdose crisis? A qualitative study to explore perspectives of potential service users. *Harm Reduct. J.* **2020**, *17*, 29. [CrossRef] [PubMed]
21. Demiris, G.; Parker Oliver, D.; Capurro, D.; Wittenberg-Lyles, E. Implementation science: Implications for intervention research in hospice and palliative care. *Gerontologist* **2014**, *54*, 163–171. [CrossRef] [PubMed]
22. Bluthenthal, R.N.; Heinzerling, K.G.; Anderson, R.; Flynn, N.M.; Kral, A.H. Approval of Syringe Exchange Programs in California: Results From a Local Approach to HIV Prevention. *Am. J. Public Health* **2008**, *98*, 278–283. [CrossRef]
23. Silverman, B.; Davis, C.S.; Graff, J.; Bhatti, U.; Santos, M.; Beletsky, L. Harmonizing disease prevention and police practice in the implementation of HIV prevention programs: Up-stream strategies from Wilmington, Delaware. *Harm Reduct. J.* **2012**, *9*, 17. [CrossRef]
24. Arksey, H.; O'Malley, L. Scoping studies: Towards a methodological framework. *Int. J. Soc. Res. Methodol.* **2005**, *8*, 19–32. [CrossRef]
25. Peters, M.D.; Godfrey, C.M.; Khalil, H.; McInerney, P.; Parker, D.; Soares, C.B. Guidance for conducting systematic scoping reviews. *Int. J. Evid. Based Healthc.* **2015**, *13*, 141–146. [CrossRef]
26. Goodin, A.; Fallin-Bennett, A.; Green, T.; Freeman, P.R. Pharmacists' role in harm reduction: A survey assessment of Kentucky community pharmacists' willingness to participate in syringe/needle exchange. *Harm Reduct. J.* **2018**, *15*, 4. [CrossRef] [PubMed]
27. Ngo, A.D.; Schmich, L.; Higgs, P.; Fischer, A. Qualitative evaluation of a peer-based needle syringe programme in Vietnam. *Int. J. Drug Policy* **2007**, *20*, 179–182. [CrossRef] [PubMed]
28. White, B.; Haber, P.S.; Day, C.A. Community attitudes towards harm reduction services and a newly established needle and syringe automatic dispensing machine in an inner-city area of Sydney, Australia. *Int. J. Drug Policy* **2015**, *27*, 121–126. [CrossRef]
29. Downing, M.; Riess, T.H.; Vernon, K.; Mulia, N.; Hollinquest, M.; McKnight, C.; Jarlais, D.C.D.; Edlin, B.R. What's Community Got to Do with It? Implementation Models of Syringe Exchange Programs. *AIDS Educ. Prev.* **2005**, *17*, 68–78. [CrossRef] [PubMed]
30. Saso, S.; Panesar, S.S.; Siow, W.; Athanasiou, T. Systematic Review and Meta-analysis in Clinical Practice. In *Evidence Synthesis in Healthcare: A Practical Handbook for Clinicians*; Darzi, A., Athanasiou, T., Eds.; Springer: London, UK, 2011; pp. 67–113.
31. Louie, E.; Barrett, E.L.; Baillie, A.; Haber, P.; Morley, K.C. Implementation of evidence-based practice for alcohol and substance use disorders: Protocol for systematic review. *Syst. Rev.* **2020**, *9*, 25–26. [CrossRef] [PubMed]
32. Clark, F. Global drug policy fuels hepatitis C epidemic, report warns. *Lancet* **2013**, *381*, 1891. [CrossRef]
33. Mathers, B.M.; Degenhardt, L.; Phillips, B.; Wiessing, L.; Hickman, M.; Strathdee, S.A.; Wodak, A.; Panda, S.; Tyndall, M.; Toufik, A.; et al. Global epidemiology of injecting drug use and HIV among people who inject drugs: A systematic review. *Lancet* **2008**, *372*, 1733–1745. [CrossRef]
34. Naserirad, M.; Beulaygue, I.C. Accessibility of Needle and Syringe Programs and Injecting and Sharing Risk Behaviors in High Hepatitis C Virus Prevalence Settings. *Subst. Use Misuse* **2020**, *55*, 1–9. [CrossRef]
35. World Health Organization. *WHO, UNODC, UNAIDS Technical Guide for Countries to Set Targets for Universal Access to HIV Prevention, Treatment and Care for Injecting Drug Users–2012 Revision*; World Health Organization: Geneva, Switzerland, 2012.
36. Iversen, J.; Grebely, J.; Topp, L.; Wand, H.; Dore, G.; Maher, L. Uptake of hepatitis C treatment among people who inject drugs attending Needle and Syringe Programs in Australia, 1999–2011. *J. Viral Hepat.* **2014**, *21*, 198–207. [CrossRef] [PubMed]
37. Aspinall, E.J.; Nambiar, D.; Goldberg, D.J.; Hickman, M.; Weir, A.; Van Velzen, E.; Palmateer, N.; Doyle, J.S.; Hellard, M.E.; Hutchinson, S.J. Are needle and syringe programmes associated with a reduction in HIV transmission among people who inject drugs: A systematic review and meta-analysis. *Int. J. Epidemiol.* **2014**, *43*, 235–248. [CrossRef] [PubMed]
38. Vuong, Q.-H.; Ho, T.-M.; Nguyen, H.-K.; Vuong, T.-T. Healthcare consumers' sensitivity to costs: A reflection on behavioural economics from an emerging market. *Palgrave Commun.* **2018**, *4*, 1–10. [CrossRef]
39. Torgerson, C.J. Publication Bias: The achilles' heel of systematic reviews? *Br. J. Educ. Stud.* **2006**, *54*, 89–102. [CrossRef]

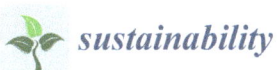

Article

An Appraisal of Communication Practices Demonstrated by Romanian District Public Health Authorities at the Outbreak of the COVID-19 Pandemic

Mariana Cernicova-Buca * and Adina Palea *

Department of Communication and Foreign Languages, Politehnica University Timisoara, 300006 Timisoara, Romania
* Correspondence: mariana.cernicova@upt.ro (M.C.-B.); adina.palea@upt.ro (A.P.)

Abstract: Communication during an ongoing crisis is a challenging task that becomes even more demanding during a public health crisis. Early in the start of the pandemic, global leaders called upon the public to reject infodemics and access official sources. This article focuses on the communicative aspects of health services management, with a particular focus on the communication strategy of the Romanian district public health authorities during the COVID-19 lockdown, as seen on official websites and social networks. The 15 most affected districts were selected, according to the officially reported health cases. The issued press releases and the posts on Facebook pages show an uneven experience on the part of district authorities in dealing with public information campaigns. In addition, the results of the study indicate a lack of sustainable communication approaches as well as the need of professional training and strategy in dealing with the public health crisis. From a communication point of view, a strategic approach on behalf of the public health sector is crucial to enhance the preparedness of appropriate institutions to act during emergencies and to respond to the needs of the media and the public with timely, correct, and meaningful information.

Keywords: public health; public health authorities; public communication; risk communication; social networks; lockdown; crisis; COVID-19 pandemic; sustainability

Citation: Cernicova-Buca, M.; Palea, A. An Appraisal of Communication Practices Demonstrated by Romanian District Public Health Authorities at the Outbreak of the COVID-19 Pandemic. *Sustainability* **2021**, *13*, 2500. https://doi.org/10.3390/su13052500

Academic Editors: Quan-Hoang Vuong and Khuat Thu Hong

Received: 26 December 2020
Accepted: 22 February 2021
Published: 25 February 2021

Publisher's Note: MDPI stays neutral with regard to jurisdictional claims in published maps and institutional affiliations.

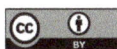

Copyright: © 2021 by the authors. Licensee MDPI, Basel, Switzerland. This article is an open access article distributed under the terms and conditions of the Creative Commons Attribution (CC BY) license (https://creativecommons.org/licenses/by/4.0/).

1. Introduction

The ongoing public health threat posed by the COVID-19 pandemic challenged the modus operandi of public health authorities, governments, and even international organizations, due to the length and intensity of the crisis. Health is a fundamental right of every human being, as stated in the Constitution of the World Health Organization since 1946. It is also understood as a major element of sustainability; the United Nations 2030 Agenda for Sustainable Development included health distinctively as a goal (SG3), with actions being necessary to "strengthen the capacity of all countries (. . .), for early warning, risk reduction and management of national and global health risks" [1]. However, the year 2020 made the international community aware that the sustainability goals—SG3 included—need rethinking and that addressing the weaknesses of domestic and global governance is a matter of utmost priority. [2]. As Miriam Bodenheimer and Jacob Leidenberger bluntly put it, the lack of ecological sustainability contributed to the coronavirus outbreak, the lack of economic sustainability to its rapid and global spread, and the lack of social sustainability to its severity [3]. The international community tried to make sense of and contain the pandemic, find the appropriate responses, and mobilize all forces to overcome the effects of the multi-level crisis brought on by COVID-19. As the World Health Organization (WHO) acknowledged "humbly", the fast-evolving situation made it difficult to anticipate the evolution of the situation. The organization also recognized that "there is no one-size-fits-all approach to managing cases and outbreaks of COVID-19" and advised the public to stay informed and follow the lead of healthcare providers as well as national and local public health authorities [4]. While the full impact of the pandemic on society is still difficult to evaluate, despite the massive mobilization of researchers in all domains to offer responses to the multiple challenges encountered throughout 2020 [5–7], it seems possible to appraise the communication efforts undertaken by public health authorities in keeping the public informed and fostering compliance with the cascading measures adopted to limit the spread of COVID-19. It is important to reflect on the capitalization of this knowledge towards improving health risk communication and ensuring social sustainability in the post-crisis period [3,8]. The lessons learned from prior global security risks show that getting information out to the public in a timely manner is a must, "but so are adequate framings of the illness, stories of the heroic efforts of those on the front line, and galvanizing metaphors that can bind the community together even when the illness is unpredictable and the chances of scientific success are uncertain" [9] (p. 10).

As Jan Servaes highlights [10] (p. 1472), "communication and information play a strategic and fundamental role by (a) contributing to the interplay of different development factors, (b) improving the sharing of knowledge and information, and (c) encouraging the participation of all concerned". In all areas of sustainable development, including the case of sustainability in the health sector, this works by "facilitating participation: giving a voice to different stakeholders to engage in the decision-making process; making information understandable and meaningful. It includes explaining and conveying information for the purpose of training, exchange of experience, and sharing of know-how and technology; fostering policy acceptance: enacting and promoting policies that increase people's access to services and resources" [10].

The United Nations and the World Health Organization alike called upon member states to communicate intensively, consistently, and in a timely fashion with the public [11] to fight an infodemic, described as "an over-abundance of information—some accurate and some not—that makes it hard for people to find trustworthy sources and reliable guidance when they need it" [12] and to counter misinformation.

Therefore, our research aimed to identify the amount and type of communication efforts undertaken by the district health authorities to manage the ongoing public health crisis and contain the effects of the pandemic on the district community, while maintaining a meaningful and relevant dialogue with the public via technologically mediated channels.

The communication management of the risk communication of the COVID-19 pandemic is a rich field for understanding the interaction between public relations, health communication, journalism and the public. According to J. Barry, for the influenza pandemic, "the single most important weapon against the disease will be a vaccine. The next important weapon will be communication" [13]. COVID-19, due to the magnitude of the pandemic, already had all the features of a newsworthy event, with intense local implications. It dominated the public agenda, and people all over the world tried to make sense of their lives through the lenses of available information on the measures undertaken to contain the disease. For authorities, as sources of information, leadership and action, it was crucial to make information available both to the public and to journalists, as disseminators of information and partners in shaping the public agenda. Here, agenda-building theory, as a new wave in understanding the shaping of public messages in society, is an appropriate scientific framework [14–16]. As McCombs convincingly states, the "basic agenda-setting role of the news media is to focus public attention on a small number of key issues and topics. Although there are dozens of issues and other aspects of the world outside competing for attention, the news media can cover only that handful deemed most newsworthy" [16]. News concerning the spread of the disease and the measures taken internationally and nationally by far dominated the news cycle at the beginning of 2020.

Information subsidies are often involved in agenda building [17]. The term "information subsidy" generously encompasses press releases, information pieces, speeches and other types of organizational communication tools used by public relations practitioners as ready-made products for the media [15,18]. Most studies focus on agenda building for traditional media, while social media has already changed the realities of the circulation of information. There is a strong expectation that members of the public have the same access to this information as members of the media, via online newsrooms [17]. This necessity is acknowledged also by the WHO in their insistence regarding the use of all communication channels, including social media sites, to fight the pandemic and bring relevant and correct information to the public [12,19]. Our research aims to enhance knowledge about agenda building through information subsidies like press releases and posts on social media platforms as made available by the Romanian public health authorities during the hottest period of the COVID-19 pandemic, i.e., in the early stages of the crisis in 2020. It fills gaps in the literature and aims at enhancing the body of knowledge regarding crisis and risk communication. We look only at the communication efforts undertaken by the public health authorities, as official sources of information that have the possibility to shape and set the agenda by providing timely, accurate and relevant information.

In the analyzed case of COVID-19, a spatial–temporal contextualization is needed to understand the specificity of public communication outcomes. The disease began as an outbreak in the Wuhan province of China, but it spread rapidly around the globe. The COVID-19 outbreak at the beginning of 2020 took Romania by surprise. Prior global health emergencies of the 21st century, such as the Ebola virus in 2014, H1N1 (Swine Flu) in 2009 and SARS in 2003, although creating public awareness that they lurked in the world, did not affect Romania. As in other societies where large-scale disasters were absent for decades, which is the case in many countries since World War II [20], the communication of risk mitigation measures during a major crisis adds significant challenges. The severe acute respiratory syndrome Coronavirus 2, known as SARS-Cov-2 or Novel Coronavirus 2, and ultimately referred to as COVID-19, is the first major health challenge for Romanian public life. The World Health Organization (WHO) declared COVID-19 a Public Health Emergency of International Concern on 30 January 2020 [4].

On 21 February, the Romanian government took its first COVID-19-related measures, announcing a 14-day quarantine for persons coming to Romania from disease-stricken regions. The first documented case in Romania occurred on 26 February 2020, but it did not stir public concern at the time [21]. However, it soon became obvious that the novel coronavirus had the features of a pandemic, as WHO reluctantly recognized 11 March 2020. On 14 March, after over 100 people had been diagnosed with the coronavirus, Romania had enough reasons for public health concern. On 16 March, President Klaus Iohannis announced his decision to decree a state of emergency for a 30-day period, which was prolonged until 14 May. After that date, Romania entered a state of alert, which meant the relaxation of some of the measures [22].

According to the principle of subsidiarity, the district (judet) level is immediately under the national one. It organizes all public life in the territory from an administrative point of view, including health issues. In Romania, there are 42 district public health authorities (DPHAs), 41 representing districts and one for the national capital, Bucharest. They represent the Ministry of Health at the local level and are responsible for the provision of public health services locally. DPHAs are responsible for the collection of data from the territory, the monitoring of the health of the population and health determinants and the identification of public health needs of communities [23]. The reform of public services in Romania, carried out in the post-communist period, shifted competencies from the central government towards local/regional bodies, but studies show that the burden is perceived at times as overwhelming [24,25].

In times of crisis, public authorities are expected to share knowledge, communicate with relevant audiences, find alliances in society and build confidence [8]. The WHO placed special emphasis on risk communication and community engagement as one of the eight pillars of successfully managing a health crisis [11]. The newly created "Risk Communication and Community Engagement" division of the WHO recommended authorities in all countries to "implement and monitor an effective action plan for communicating effectively with the public, engaging with communities, local partners and other stakeholders to help prepare and protect individuals, families and the public's health during early response to COVID-19". The advice was unequivocal: "Make sure that this happens through diverse channels, at all levels and throughout the response" [26] (p. 3). Such channels, beyond discussion, are represented by social media owned by the appropriate authorities. In addition, as activities were now organized remotely and carried out through digital tools, many Romanians used their social media accounts, previously employed mainly for private purposes, to access services, information and labor from home [27].

The challenges brought about by the COVID-19 pandemic have underlined the importance of professional public communication based on correct, timely, comprehensive and accessible information. Social distancing was one of the measures recommended internationally [28] as an effective (though insufficient) means of preventing the spread of the virus. Face-to-face events were reduced to a minimum, and the classical press conferences, a preferred media event in the toolkit of authorities in dealing with journalists to disseminate information, were put to a halt. Only press releases posted on the authorities' websites remained as tools pertaining to the habitual media relations strategy.

This study reports on these aspects, as seen from the institutional websites and from the social media accounts of Romanian DPHAs, from the point of view of the amount and type of content posted to meet the expectations of the general public during the COVID-19 lockdown. The following research objectives were defined:

RO_1: To determine whether there is a correlation between the number of health incidents and information subsidies made available to the public by relevant authorities.

RO_2: To evaluate the communication efforts of DPHAs, expressed by the information subsidies (number of press releases on website and number of posts on social media platforms), from the point of view of timeliness and rhythmicity.

RO_3: To examine the type of content disseminated by DPHAs via social media, from the point of view of ownership (produced in-house vs. share of content produced by other institutions) and triggered engagement (comments, shares).

2. Materials and Methods

The findings of this paper are based essentially on a qualitative research approach, i.e., on content data analysis, although quantitative indicators were used to enhance the results. Data collection took place at the beginning of the pandemic and covered the 2 months of total lockdown in Romania: 16 March–14 May 2020. Our strategy was to analyze the communication efforts of the District Public Health Authorities of the most affected regions. Considering the official information at the time, we selected a sample of 15 regions where the number of patients with specific COVID-19 symptoms kept the attention of authorities and the media (14 districts and the national capital, Bucharest). Drawing inspiration from the occurrence of national media reports in the regions, we switched to the data provided by the National Institute for Public Health for a final selection [29]. The order of presentation herein is based on the number of COVID-19 cases registered in the analyzed region in the first two weeks after the outbreak of the disease: Suceava, Bucharest, Timis, Neamt, Arad, Hunedoara, Brasov, Galati, Cluj, Constanta, Ilfov, Iasi, Mures, Botosani and Vrancea. The order changed in time, with the national capital being at the top, but we maintained the initial choice of presentation in order to follow through with the data in a coherent manner.

As formulated in the research objectives, we monitored the frequency of press releases throughout the sample. For the analysis of website traffic, we chose a popular content marketing platform—SEMrush. It is among the most used platforms of its kind and has a friendly interface that allows for in-depth data collection [30]. The SEMrush dashboard enabled us to gather information about organic traffic, organic key words, the source of visitors on DPHA websites, etc., all of which helped us draw conclusions on the impact of the information posted on their webpages.

Moreover, we identified the existence of Facebook, Twitter, Instagram and YouTube accounts and examined the communication behavior of DPHAs in the social media world. We gathered a corpus of 412 Facebook posts, which was analyzed from the point of view of engagement, focusing on the number of shares and comments per post. Monitoring of the websites and social media accounts curated by DPHAs was followed by an analysis of the type of content related to COVID-19. Experts acknowledge that "failing to engage users equates with (...) no transmission of information from a Web site; people go elsewhere to perform their tasks and communicate with colleagues and friends" [31]. Thus, we also traced the capacity of the analyzed public health authorities to trigger shares, comments, or other types of reaction as a sign of community engagement.

We also compared the communication behavior displayed by the analyzed institutions with the principles of risk communication, as described in relevant professional literature, to draw lessons from a crisis that affected all strata of society, i.e., global, continental, national and local.

3. Results and Discussion
3.1. The COVID-19 Outbreak in Romania

In the first two months of 2020, Romania was only mildly aware of the danger posed by COVID-19. Information in the media appeared in the external news section, and in February some measures were taken to monitor incoming persons from regions already facing the health crisis. The outbreak of the disease in March brought the lockdown, and the communication space was completely dominated by the topic of the pandemic [32].

At the national level, Romania followed the pattern against which the WHO had warned; avalanches of messages concerning public health issues poured out via all available channels. Following the recommendations of the WHO, on 17 March the Romanian Government launched an online platform, www.stirioficiale.ro [33], to channel trustworthy, quality information to whomever sought information beyond issues discussed in traditional or social media. Nationally, the voices during the lockdown (coinciding with the state of emergency period) were those of top officials in the country, i.e., the President, Klaus Iohannis, the Prime Minister, Ludovic Orban, the Health Minister, Victor Costache/Nelu Tataru, and the Secretary of State at the Ministry of Internal Affairs, head of the Department for Emergency Situations, Raed Arafat. Occasionally, other ministers came to the fore to comment on topics from their area of competence (public order, education, foreign policy, labor, economy, etc.), and health experts were called upon to offer clarification regarding the evolution of the disease and the steering of public life. Because face-to-face activities were not allowed during the lockdown, the population switched to remote labor and TV watching. Media consumption grew exponentially, with the press conference organized by national authorities in the first week of the lockdown being watched by almost 6 million Romanians [34]. National media monitoring showed that Romanians started watching TV more than 6 h per day, being exposed to 4000 h of breaking news and 84,000 h of informative TV spots during the lockdown. As for sources of information, half of the Romanian population actively watched news on TV channels, and 47% gathered news from social media sources [34].

Taking the rules of crisis communication as mandatory [35], the central government took upon itself the task of coordinating and filtering communication. Thus, in the first weeks of the lockdown, only central authorities released information on the crisis, to the great surprise and dissatisfaction of other voices in society. Seventeen civic organizations, many of which dealt with journalism, public communication, and information, signed a manifesto in March 2020 to restore access to regional/local information; they succeeded in their endeavors some weeks later [36]. Local voices also took an active part in informing the public, based on official information. For instance, in Timis county, the AntiCovidTM platform was developed, at the initiative of several non-governmental organizations with a civic vocation, to create a partnership dedicated to supporting the efforts of active humanitarian initiatives/campaigns in the region and increasing the degree of public information on health issues [37].

According to Malikhao [38] (p. 99), the sustainability of health is a process of social mobilization empowered by both stakeholders (some of whom can be health communicators) and health communicators from outside, who have empathy toward the stakeholders, to achieve two goals: first, to engage the people in the community in upgrading their health and media literacy status so that they can make an informed choice on their body, health and health care; second, to build up community capacity and networking with other communities so that people can solve problems related to community health, achieve social justice in health, prevent diseases, maintain well-being, and cultivate health knowledge, good attitude, ethical values, a cosmopolitan worldview, and health behaviors, including advocating for structural change for a local commitment to healthy lifestyle and an accommodating environment.

3.2. The Public Health System in Romania and Its Reaction to the COVID-19 Pandemic—An Overview

The pandemic of 2020 put a serious damper on these two goals, testing the capacity of countries to communicate strategically [39] (p. 14) and of the WHO to effectively manage the COVID-19 health risk.

In Romania, public health is defined by Law 95/2006 as "the organized effort of the society towards the protection and promotion of population health" [40]. Public health services include health promotion, disease prevention and improving quality of life and comprise the following activities: immunization; control and surveillance of diseases and risk factors; monitoring population health and health determinants; measuring the efficiency and effectiveness of health care; the assessment of population needs; health promotion and health education campaigns; occupational health; and environmental health, among others. The National Health Strategy 2014–2020 is still in use, and it includes public health as one of the three main priority areas [23] (p. 93). The coordination for the provision of public health services is the responsibility of the Ministry of Health, which is also responsible for the strategic planning and organization of public health services. Other institutions with responsibilities in public health are the National Centre for Environmental Monitoring of Risks in the Community, the National Centre for Communicable Diseases Surveillance and Control (NCCDSC), the National Centre for Methodological Coordination and Information on Occupational Diseases and the National Centre for Health Status Evaluation and Health Promotion. In addition, six regional public health centers, which are located in Bucharest, Cluj, Iași, Sibiu, Târgu Mureș and Timișoara, function as the regional branches of the National Institute of Public Health (NIPH). The regional centers have mainly methodological and technical roles. At the local level, the Ministry of Health is represented by 42 DPHAs. Their responsibilities include [41] monitoring the health of the population and health determinants; identification of public health needs of communities; performing controls of health institutions; coordinating the implementation of national public health programs at the local level; carrying out sanitary inspection and health promotion activities, etc.

European and international reports on the Romanian health system describe it as hyper-centralized, antiquated, and failing to ensure communication between health information system players [42–45].

These features had an impact on the public communication effort during the COVID-19 lockdown. Duplicated information appeared on websites and communication projects developed by each player, most of the time without ensuring interoperability or cross-fertilization of the initiatives. Traditional media monitoring showed that the main voices in television were President Klaus Iohannis, Prime Minister Ludovic Orban (who went through a period of self-isolation due to exposure to a risk population), Health Minister Viorel Costache, replaced in the middle of the crisis by Nelu Tataru, and the Head of the Department for Emergency Situations Raed Arafat, the four officials whom the population trusted most during the lockdown [46]. Other ministers or top health experts were also invited to the fore, to offer stewardship and guidance for different aspects of life, from individual behaviors to work, leisure and faith-related activities. At times, these voices did not form a coherent view, a feature identified in other countries as well, despite the warning of experts that "any conflicting information carries a risk of harm, but unfortunately it abounds"; the response to the crisis was addressed mainly at national levels in a variety of ways. Those who analyzed the situation concluded that "the European approach has not prevailed", but that communication efforts should be consistent and coherent to build public trust as well as to maintain the response capacity of the healthcare system to react: "Where communication is well-structured, staff is more engaged and motivated to work for the sake of better healthcare, and this raises the quality of healthcare as a whole and may improve patient outcomes" [47].

In evaluating Romania's response to the crisis in its early stages, experts consider that the country "has one of the highest levels of poverty, social exclusion, and restricted access to education in the EU, and any public information campaigns would have needed to consider these aspects" [48] (p. 5). In addition, despite demonstrating an initially strong capacity to contain the COVID-19 pandemic, the Romanian healthcare system showed areas in need of improvement, among which was the "best use of the available resources and channels of communication during an ongoing health crisis' [48] (p. 5).

A terminological clarification is appropriate at this point. Although the COVID-19 pandemic is treated and discussed in terms of crisis, the communication related to the effort of limiting the spread of the disease belongs to risk communication. The terms do not overlap entirely and need clarification. The WHO framed the issue in terms of "risk communication" and announced that it was making 24/7 efforts to provide "public health information and advice on the 2019-nCoV, including myth busters, available on its social media channels (including Weibo, Twitter, Facebook, Instagram, LinkedIn, Pinterest) and website" [12] (p. 2). In this paper, social media is defined as "Internet based applications that allow users to create, exchange, or simply consume user-generated content—that is, content created, developed, and shared by individuals" [49] (p. 173). Examples of social media include, but are not limited to, collaborative projects (e.g., Wikipedia), weblogs (e.g., online diaries), microblogs (e.g., Twitter), video/photo sharing (e.g., YouTube, Instagram), social networking sites (e.g., Facebook), virtual game worlds, and virtual social worlds.

Dennis Wilcox specifies the difference between risk communication and crisis communication, with the first category being applied (explicitly) to (public) health outbreaks or other risk-related topics, and the latter being specific to organizations shaken by events that may threaten the very existence of the organization [50]. His strong advice is that, for risk communication, emphasis should be placed on the "dissemination of accurate information. The communicator must begin early, identify and address the public's concerns, recognize the public as a legitimate partner, anticipate hostility, respond to the needs of the news media, and always be honest" [50] (p. 300). For crisis communication, the crisis management plan needs activation, and reparatory measures should be part of the lessons learned from the whole process [50] (p. 300). Other authors [51,52] do not make the distinction using such nuances, including risk communication under the broader umbrella of crisis communication. The lessons Mats Eriksson draws from practice, for instance, put together risk and crisis communication and assess that "despite the powerful digitization of society in recent years, the development of social media, and the fast-growing body of research concerning social media crisis communication, the overall lessons identified here still primarily seem to be about actions like the need for pre-event planning, partnerships with the public, listening to the public's concerns, and understanding the audience's need for credible sources" [51] (p. 541). Ruhert Genc, in a recent paper, highlights the fact that "in any sustainable plan or strategy communication plays a vital role" [53] (p. 511), while Ericsson, based on American experiences and calling for more studies in other geographic regions, states that the "new social media landscape for crisis communications seems to work much like that of the old media society". His recommendation, among others, is to bridge the gap between research and practice and enhance organizations' reaction capacity to crises on the basis of evidence-based lessons and/or advice that would deal with all channels of communication. A much-quoted researcher for crisis communication, Timothy Coombs, sets forth theoretical clarifications for the stages and typology of crises, advising professionals to be present, timely and polite in communicating with the media and the public. He warns that "the Internet is many communication channels, not just one. These channels include websites, discussion boards, blogs, microblogs, chat rooms, Listservs, image sharing, and social networking sites, to name but a few. Internet communication channels emphasize the interactive and interconnected nature of the Internet" [52] (p. 34). As opposed to private sector services, where these media are already heavily used, "social media are evidently underused by audit institutions as public service providers, both on general and on specific topics" as revealed by a recent study on European institutions [54].

Our study also gathered information about the variety of channels used for communication with the public by the relevant authorities involved in crisis management at a national level. The analysis of social media buttons displayed on their websites revealed a lack of coordination. Our conclusion is backed by the following data:

- The Romanian presidency has on the website buttons for Facebook and Twitter.
- The Romanian Government has only a Facebook button.
- The Health Ministry is present on Facebook and YouTube.
- The Department for Emergency Situations has the largest number of social media channels: Twitter, Facebook, Instagram, YouTube and Google Groups.
- The Ministry of Interior has accounts on Facebook, Twitter, Instagram, YouTube and Flickr.
- The National Center for Surveillance and Control of Communicable Diseases has no social media channels.

The online platform, www.stirioficiale.ro, (accessed during our research from March 2020 throughout the lockdown period, up to May 2020) towards which national authorities guide the public for verifiable, correct information, has buttons to help the public sort out fake news, but has no associated Facebook, Twitter or YouTube page. They only invite visitors to subscribe to their newsletter. We find this insufficient, as we consider that a Facebook page with posts conveying official messages would have helped the spread of correct and useful information.

Such a variety of styles and channels fails "to make the communication more sustainable" [54] (p. 2500), does not serve the interconnectedness of Internet resources, and fails to capitalize on existing resources and messages and help keep the public informed and trusting of authorities' capacity to contain the health risk situation. In addition, in the analyzed period, three top government positions had a change of occupant, due to resignation or being removed, mainly for failure of properly communicating the measures undertaken to limit the spread of COVID-19. Thus, the Health Minister, Viorel Costache, lost his portfolio exactly one month after the declaration of the state of emergency. The same happened to Dr. Adrian Streinu-Cercel, who chaired a special committee created at the level of the Health Ministry, though his removal occurred shortly after the state of emergency ended. In the monitored period, six of the directors of DHAs resigned or were removed from their position, all of this resulting in uneven efforts to communicate on COVID-19 measures. Against this background, we carried out our research. The presentation of the national level is necessary for understanding some issues at the district level, where the highly centralized system functions with constant reference to the leadership provided from the top of the authoritative pyramid, as observed also by other researchers who deal with Romanian health system topics [25] (pp. 331–359).

3.3. District Public Health Authorities and Their Communication Behavior during the COVID-19 Lockdown

At the district level as analyzed in this paper, research indicates that the information posted on the websites of the District Public Health Authorities (DPHAs) was mainly top-down, based on the official press releases provided by the Ministry of Health, the Ministry of Internal Affairs through the Strategic Communication Group, and the National Institute of Public Health (NIPH) through the National Center for Surveillance and Control of Communicable Diseases (NCCDSC).

3.3.1. Correlation between the Number of Health Incidents and Information Subsidies

Our research aimed to determine whether there was a correlation between the number of health incidents and the amount of information communicated on the media section of institutional websites and/or disseminated via social media channels. Figure 1 highlights the fact that no such correlations can be traced, and that in some cases exactly the opposite behavior can be seen. For example, the most problematic districts—Suceava and the national capital, Bucharest—had no Facebook page during the analyzed period and posted only a couple of press releases. Furthermore, the highest number of press releases was published on the webpage of the DPHA for Botosani, which was the least infected at the beginning of the lockdown period. Therefore, our assumption that the efforts to keep the community informed would be enhanced in the most affected regions was partially invalidated. Further findings point to a reluctance to communicate.

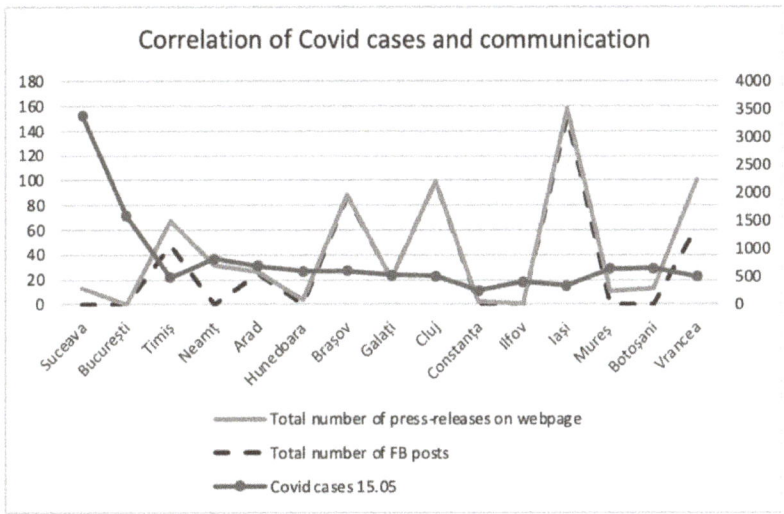

Figure 1. Reported COVID-19 cases vs. number of information subsidies (press releases and social media posts). Note: FB = Facebook.

It is worth mentioning that the DPHA webpage for Bucharest was very new and had no press releases available prior to 18 May, which was outside the state of emergency period analyzed. Thus, there was no traceability regarding the issued press releases or public announcements made in the timespan between 16 March and 14 May 2020. The fact that the Facebook page of the District Public Health Authority in Bucharest was created on 16 May also does not give tangible evidence regarding the way communication was handled throughout the ongoing crisis. The results, however, pointed us towards further analyzing the communication instances produced by these DPHAs.

The literature review and WHO recommendations highlighted the importance of communication for risk management and the positive impact triggered by the use of various platforms in public communication. Experts point to the fact that "it is getting difficult to be transparent, engaging and satisfying other stakeholders without digital platforms, artificial intelligence, innovative software, mobile applications, and video advertising. Moreover, the society and key strategic partners bit by bit set higher communication standards as well as expectations towards civil service experts and their communication style" [55]. Capitalizing on the above, and given the data available for the study, we took a closer look at the webpages of the 15 DHAs analyzed and aimed to identify the following:

- the number of press releases published throughout the lockdown period;
- the number of COVID-19-related press releases from the total amount of issued press releases;
- other means of helping the public access the correct (official) information;
- the importance given to social media, i.e., the presence of social media buttons on websites and platforms, towards which the public was directed;
- the changes in user behavior regarding the use of DPHA websites, i.e., an increase in traffic, as reflected by online analytics tools.

The number and type of press releases is addressed in Figure 2. It shows that, throughout the analyzed period, most press releases issued tackle the problem of COVID-19.

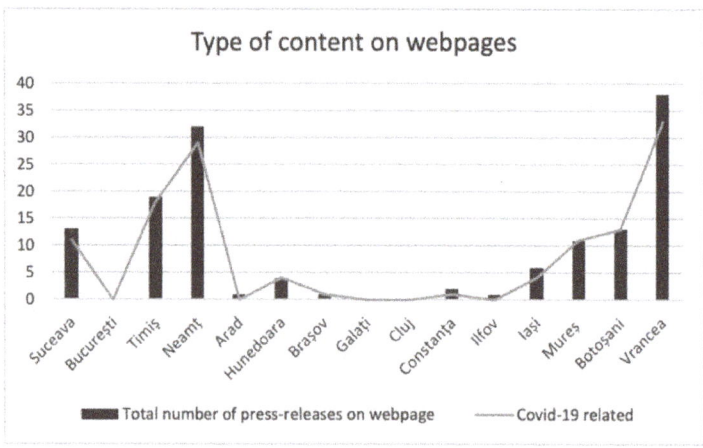

Figure 2. Number of press releases on DPHA webpages.

3.3.2. Assessment of Rhythmicity in the Communication Effort of DPHAs

When verifying whether the district authorities sought other means of informing the public, we were interested in finding out if essential information about COVID-19 was visible and accessible in other forms, like dedicated sections on the website or easy-to-understand infographics.

The webpage of the DPHA in Hunedoara drew our attention. Even if the number of press releases issued in the state-of-emergency months (March, April, May) was small (four), we could not ignore the structure of the homepage, which was well adapted to answer most questions about COVID-19 (self-isolation, quarantine and isolation, protection, myths, shopping, public transport, etc.). Furthermore, the website had in its main menu a button labelled "COVID-19", which gathered all official statements on the pandemic as published by the district authority. Unfortunately, our research could not determine the time at which that information was published on the website and whether it was available to the public before 14 May.

We discuss distinctively the webpage of DPHA Cluj, a multi-ethnic district, which mentions the possibility of accessing the information in English and French (however, the buttons failed to provide information in these languages). We found this example interesting as, on the one side, it showed the vision of the team that created the website, but on the other side, revealed the poor implementation of the project and, we dare say, a limited interest in addressing the needs of that particular community, despite the WHO recommendation to address the communication information needs of minorities (for instance [56], expats and other groups of stakeholders).

Concerning the importance given to social media by the 15 analyzed DPHAs, the research revealed the following:

- Nine out of the 15 webpages did not display any social media button.
- Three of the pages had a Facebook button, but it was not active, so the visitor of the website was not redirected to the Facebook page.
- Only three webpages had an active Facebook button.

The results of the analysis are presented in Figure 3 below.

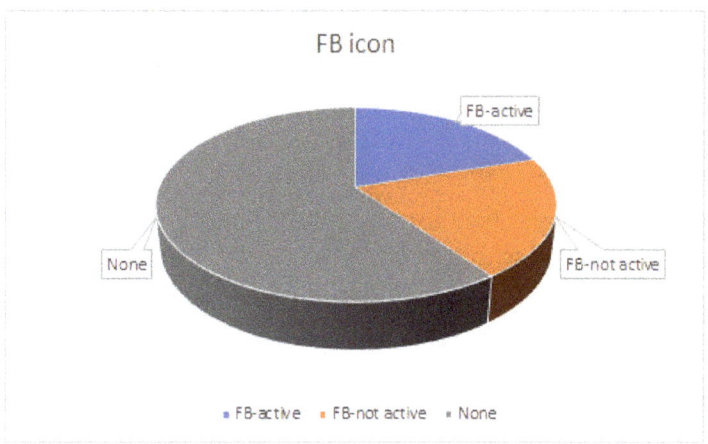

Figure 3. Signs of social media channels on institutional websites.

The case of the Brasov, Cluj and Iasi districts was interesting, as the DPHAs in these districts had the three most active Facebook (FB) pages (as can be seen in Figure 4), but there was no FB icon on their website. This raises the question of in-house coordination of communication efforts.

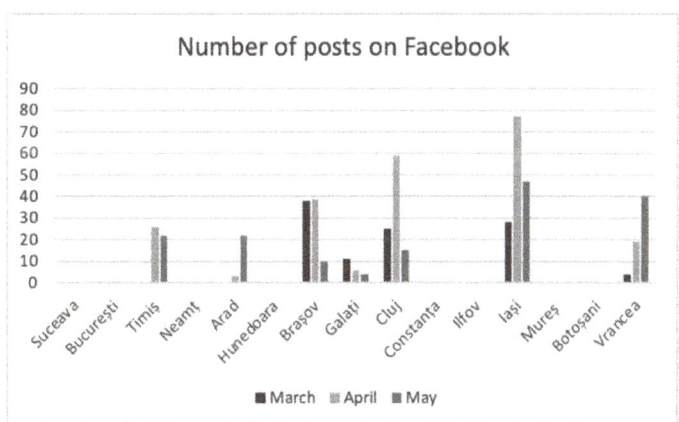

Figure 4. Number of COVID-19-related posts during the monitored months.

On the other hand, DPHAs from Constanta and Botosani districts integrated a Facebook button on their websites, even though no such Facebook page existed. Bucharest is the only case in which the Facebook button and the Facebook page existed but were not linked. The website of the DPHA in Bucharest also had an inactive Twitter icon.

Since Facebook proved to be the social media channel of choice, we present the results of the communication effort of DPHAs via this type of page in Figure 4.

We want to highlight the fact that the Facebook page of DPHA Arad was created on 30 April, and throughout the rest of the 16 lockdown days, it showed an intensive communication effort, with more than one post per day. The Timis DPHA displayed a similar pattern, with a Facebook page created 16 days earlier than Arad, on 14 April. As mentioned before, DPHA Bucharest also made the decision to create a Facebook page, but it was operationalized on 16 May (a day after the end of the state of emergency). Therefore, its activity was not relevant for the current research.

The changes regarding the traffic on DPHA websites were analyzed with the help of SEMrush, an online visibility management and content marketing platform [30]. The results showed that nearly all web traffic was organic and generated by search engines (more than 95%), which was not surprising as DPHA websites were not very well known before the pandemic. However, our research revealed an unexpected trend in users' behavior, as in all analyzed cases we found little or no relevant increase in traffic on the websites of District Public Health Authorities between 16 March and 14 May. An increase in traffic could be seen only towards the end of the lockdown period, and it continued to grow, with a peak in June and another in October–November, as can be seen in Figures 5 and 6.

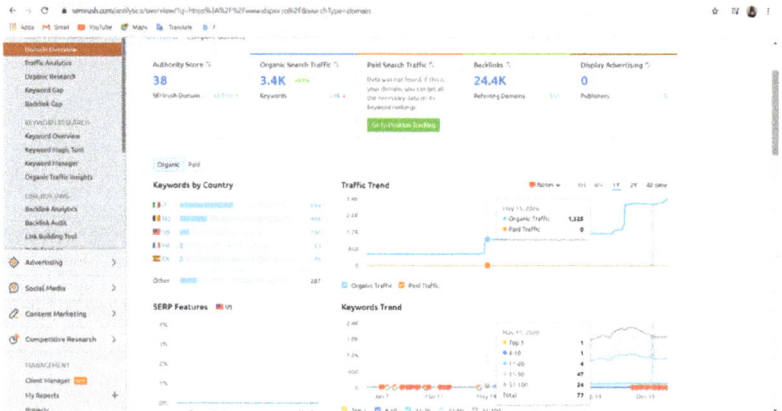

Figure 5. Traffic on District Public Health Authority (DPHA) Vrancea website.

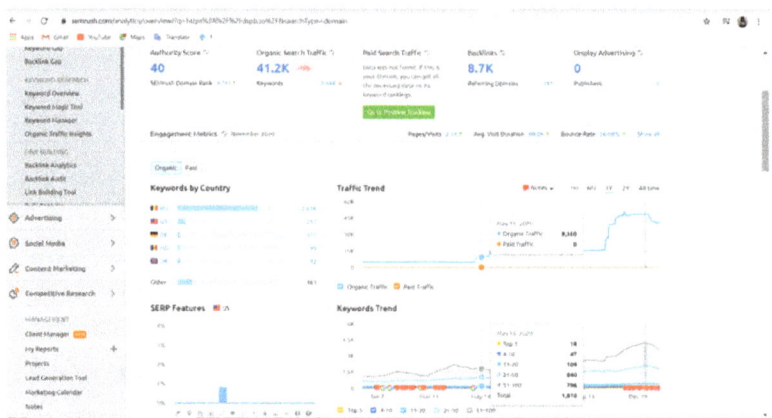

Figure 6. Traffic on DPHA Bucharest website.

We believe that the results are an indicator of media usage habits, and that Romanians still show a preference for television and centralized official communication. It may also mean that the information needed was available on other websites, which are not subject of this research.

3.3.3. Type of Content Disseminated by DPHAs via Social Media Accounts

Our third research objective was to examine the type of content disseminated by DPHAs via social media, from the point of view of ownership (produced in-house vs. share of content produced by other institutions) and engagement (comments, shares). Figure 7 sums up the results of our analysis concerning the type of content posted on DPHA Facebook pages.

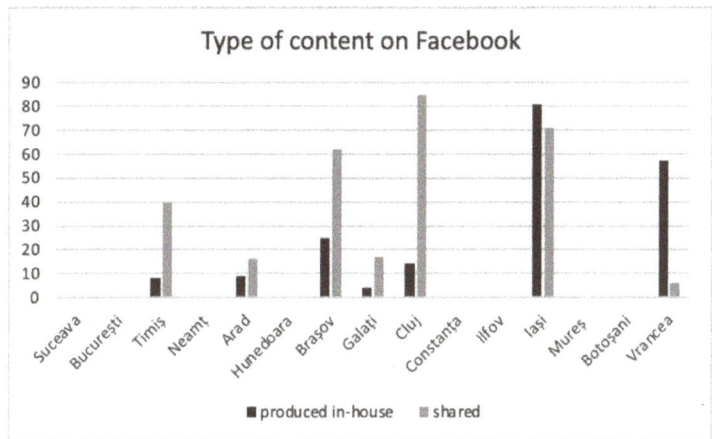

Figure 7. Type of content posted.

Additionally, we found a tendency of local authorities to share the data communicated by the Strategic Communication Group and the Ministry of Health, without disseminating local data, in five out of the seven active Facebook pages.

In addition, we highlight the Vrancea DPHA Facebook page, which displayed a communication approach totally different from the rest in the sample. Almost all the posts were adapted for local audiences, and besides the essential press releases, they referred to decisions made by Vrancea Prefecture, promoted local COVID-19 initiatives, presented the way in which lockdown regulations were implemented, etc.

The most active Facebook page analyzed was that of the District Public Health Authority in Iasi, with a total of 152 posts between 16 March–14 May 2020. As in the case of the Vrancea district, the amount of content produced in-house surpassed the shared content. Particularly impressive was the attention given to design, not only to content. For example, they published data about the evolution of COVID-19 cases in the format illustrated by the infographic bellow (Figure 8), or they illustrated relevant collaboration with original photos, proving a professional approach aligned to web 2.0 affordances.

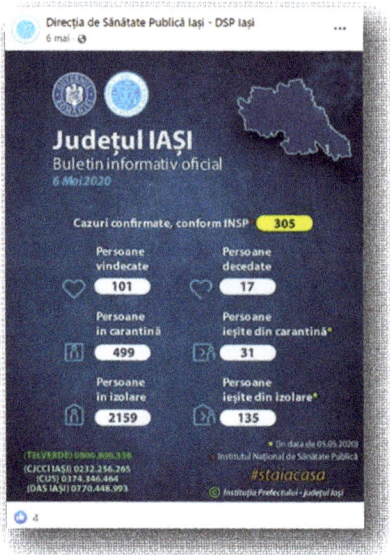

Figure 8. Example of use of infographic on Facebook page of DPHA Iasi.

Such an approach to information is rare, even among the national authorities in charge of public health responsibilities. In the example above, the post even includes the hashtag #staiacasa (#stayathome), a rather popular hashtag at the time [57], and other useful information.

Beyond monitoring the number of posts on the DPHA Facebook pages, we analyzed the engagement displayed by the followers. The results are presented in Figure 9.

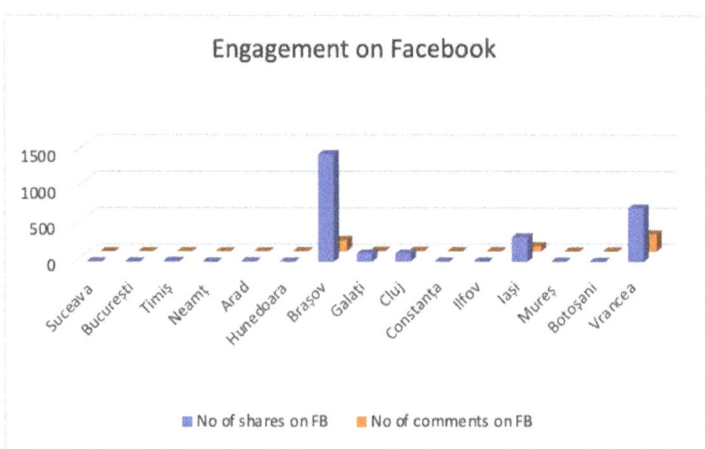

Figure 9. Engagement of Facebook pages' followers.

The behavior of Facebook users was very uneven. In most cases there were no or few reactions to the posts. However, we encountered a few exceptions.

For example, DPHA Brasov held the record for the most shared post. As can be seen in Figure 10, the information posted at the beginning of the lockdown (18 March) was shared 871 times. It contained contact information that people lacked at the beginning of the pandemic.

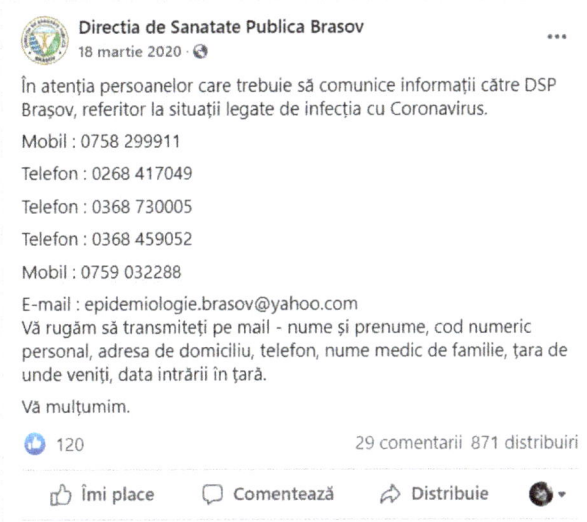

Figure 10. The most shared post from a DPHA Facebook page.

The next most shared post was one from Vrancea's Facebook page (16 April, 135 shares), and it contained information about the fact that testing with an RT-PCR device had begun within DPHA Vrancea.

We would also like to point out that, in the case of DPHA Iasi, almost all posts were shared by a person called "Madalina M.H". In about half of the posts, she was the only one sharing the information. This practice is not unknown and helps boost the impact of the main Facebook page, but it is not an indicator of real engagement. Most probably, once that person changes his/her job, (s)he will no longer share the content posted on that particular Facebook page.

Another indicator of engagement lays with the comments received for the published information. Our research showed that the majority of posts received no reaction, and when comments were made, they were mostly negative, relating to negative experiences regarding communication with or by the District Public Health Authorities.

Again, we identified an exception to the general behavior: the post from 17 April by DPHA Vrancea received a total number of 116 comments and 84 shares. Almost all followers wrote negative comments to the information posted, with some being impolite and even furious ("You really are not ashamed?", "Who should we trust in, when everything is done on political criteria?? All thieves!!", etc.). The post provided details about the way in which the newly acquired testing equipment was proposed to be used, and thus showed that it was really difficult for common people to gain access to the services.

4. Conclusions and Lessons Learned

We resonate with the conclusions of Woulter Jong that healthcare organizations and institutes need to establish trust and engage actively and positively with stakeholders [58]. Once the crisis is over, the quality of the response and the management need to be discussed [19,58]. Our research is an attempt to offer an evaluation of the healthcare authorities at an intermediate stage, while the crisis is still unfolding.

The COVID-19 pandemic put a stress on all walks of life and on all types of organizations. The Romanian DPHAs, as part of the public sector at an intermediate level, are faced with multiple challenges and expectations. It falls on them to respond in a timely and massive manner to public concerns. However, the assumption on which we based our first research objective was partially invalidated by the analysis. The fact that there is no correlation between the severity of the crisis and the information subsidies could lead us to state that efforts to address the situation were not taken locally. Yet, the fact that two Facebook pages were created in the middle of the lockdown period (Timis, Arad), and one immediately after (Bucharest), suggests that local teams were aware of their responsibility and tried to get closer to the public via social media. It was "on-the-job" training and "learning by doing".

The type of content posted on Facebook is also an indicator of strategic communication with the public. Roughly one third of the content was produced in-house, with only two districts having more in-house content than shared content. An in-depth analysis showed that the "courage" to put a mark on the posts grew with experience, as most FB pages were no older than one year, except for Iasi and Vrancea, which were created in 2017 (31 August and 6 November, respectively).

We can conclude that there was no clear communication strategy valid for all DPHAs and implemented at a national level. In addition, there were also no clear risk management and crisis communication procedures shared among public authorities. The spokespersons of the District Public Health Authorities analyzed were not visible during the crisis, despite handbook recommendations for crisis and/or risk periods. The task of communicating with the public was assumed by often underprepared directors, taking the stand and generating additional communication crises, a situation that in many cases cost them their positions. Romanian public health officials failed to use the situation of "lockdown and standstill as a window of opportunity to change direction and prevent future crises" and thus failed to turn towards sustainable communication strategies [3]. While communication efforts were not negligible, a certain hesitation and lack of mastering the rules of risk/crisis communication were encountered in the analyzed sample [3,52]. Not only were the content and timeliness of communications important, but also the formats and design.

In accordance with the literature review, social media platforms emphasize the importance of design in rendering the message. Considering the data collected, we assume that older Facebook pages mean better communication skills and exercise for those involved. However, examples of digital skills and organic integration of available tools were rarely identified in the analyzed Facebook pages.

For an emerging infectious disease such as COVID-19, various forces involved in the interactions between the public authority bodies, society, and the news media could lead to strengthening the fabric of society, building unity and solidarity. This study does not examine all the intertwined factors and relationships mentioned above. The study shows, however, that communication efforts were rather chaotic and lacked coherence and coordination, despite apparent efforts to channel the public opinion towards a unified reaction to the rising risk of spreading disease. Despite WHO recommendations [11], the regional level authorities were entrusted to communicate with the public late in the game [36] and when given the chance, they lacked the exercise and the courage to mount an energetic response to the many questions posed by citizens concerning their well-being, recommended courses of action and possibilities to control their own health issues, as seen from the comments to the posts on the Facebook pages under DPHA authority.

COVID-19 had, in the context of this study, at least two major effects. First, it made the international and the local communities aware that the natural world can take everyone by surprise, and that in envisaging a (better) future, a "stop and go" strategy can be the answer to the many challenges posed by the (current) crisis [8]. Second, it tested the reaction capacity of public systems to address major crises on many levels, the communication level included. For the Romanian health system, the initial communicative response was confusing and timid. Public health authorities at the national level dealt with global information, while locally, where incidents of disease spreading were reported, the relevant authorities failed to provide their share of information and take part in agenda building. Post-lockdown, the communication improved, proving that lessons were learned, and that reaction capacity is growing [7].

5. Limitations of the Study

This study has several potential weaknesses. First, the analyzed institutional websites do not present strategic plans for communication issues related to risk communication in general, and to the 2020 pandemic as a distinct case. Interviewing media officers or spokespersons did not prove to be a successful enterprise; thus, there is a necessity to supplement data with comments from the people in charge of communication, but only when the crisis lessens in power. Second, we analyzed only 15 out of the total number of DPHAs, based on the early-stage situation of the pandemic outbreak. No centralized data are provided on the official websites of central authorities. Even the Health Ministry, which presents the table with the DPHAs, does not allow landing on the respective webpages. In addition, the crisis is ongoing, leaving appreciations on the success or failure of communication strategies to a post-crisis period, when reflection will be welcomed and possible. Further research should also be oriented towards analyzing the communication style of the posts, visibility in the media, changes in communication approaches, etc., thus exploring the behavior of media, the major partner in building the communication agenda for the COVID-19 pandemic.

Author Contributions: Conceptualization, M.C.-B. and A.P.; writing—original draft preparation, M.C.-B. and A.P.; writing—review and editing, M.C.-B. and A.P. All authors have read and agreed to the published version of the manuscript.

Funding: This research received no external funding.

Conflicts of Interest: The authors declare no conflict of interest.

References

1. United Nations. Transforming Our World: The 2030 Agenda for Sustainable Development. Available online: https://sustainabledevelopment.un.org/post2015/transformingourworld (accessed on 5 June 2020).
2. Santos-Carrillo, F.; Fernández-Portillo, L.A.; Sianes, A. Rethinking the governance of the 2030 agenda for sustainable development in the COVID-19 Era. *Sustainability* **2020**, *12*, 7680. [CrossRef]
3. Bodenheimer, M.; Leidenberger, J. COVID-19 as a window of opportunity for sustainability transitions? Narratives and communication strategies beyond the pandemic. *Sustain. Sci. Pract. Policy* **2020**, *16*, 61–66. [CrossRef]
4. World Health Organization. WHO Announces COVID-19 Outbreak a Pandemic. Available online: https://www.euro.who.int/en/health-topics/health-emergencies/coronavirus-covid-19/news/news/2020/3/who-announces-covid-19-outbreak-a-pandemic (accessed on 1 July 2020).
5. Cell Press. Analysis of COVID-19 Publications Identifies Research Gaps. Available online: https://www.sciencedaily.com/releases/2020/09/200917105411.htm (accessed on 12 November 2020).
6. Zhang, H.; Shaw, R. Identifying research trends and gaps in the context of COVID-19. *Int. J. Environ. Res. Public Health* **2020**, *17*, 3370. [CrossRef] [PubMed]
7. De Roodenbeke, E. Filling the Gaps: Learning from each other during the COVID-19 Pandemic. *Health Manag.* **2020**, *20*, 258–259. Available online: https://healthmanagement.org/uploads/article_attachment/hm3-v20-5may-filling-the-gaps.pdf (accessed on 12 November 2020).
8. Cori, L.; Bianchi, F.; Cadum, E.; Anthonj, C. Risk perception and COVID-19. *Int. J. Environ. Res. Public Health* **2020**, *17*, 3114. [CrossRef]
9. Powers, J.H.; Xiao, X. (Eds.) *The Social Construction of SARS. Studies of a Health Communication Crisis*; John Benjamins Publishing Company: Amsterdam, The Netherlands; Philadelphia, PA, USA, 2008. [CrossRef]
10. Servaes, J. *Handbook of Communication for Development and Social Change*; Springer: Singapore, 2020; pp. 1471–1482. [CrossRef]
11. World Health Organization. COVID-19 Strategic Preparedness and Response Plan Operational Planning Guidelines to Support Country Preparedness. Available online: https://digitallibrary.un.org/record/3859863?ln=en (accessed on 7 June 2020).
12. World Health Organization. 1st WHO Infodemiology Conference. How Infodemics Affect the World & How They Can Be Managed. Available online: https://www.who.int/news-room/events/detail/2020/06/30/default-calendar/1st-who-infodemiology-conference (accessed on 12 October 2020).
13. Barry, J. Pandemics: Avoiding the mistakes of 1918. *Nature* **2009**, *459*, 324–325. [CrossRef] [PubMed]

14. Turk, J.V. Information subsidies and influence. *Public Relat. Rev.* **1985**, *11*, 114. [CrossRef]
15. Turk, J.V.S.; Franklin, B. Information subsidies: Agenda-setting traditions. *Public Relat. Rev.* **1987**, *13*, 29–41. [CrossRef]
16. McCombs, M.A. Look at Agenda-setting: Past, present and future. *J. Stud.* **2005**, *6*, 543–557. [CrossRef]
17. Carroll Craig, E. *The Handbook of Communication and Corporate Reputation*; Wiley Blackwell: Hoboken, NJ, USA, 2013.
18. Berkowitz, D.; Adams, D.B. Information subsidy and agenda-building in local television news. *J. Mass Commun. Q.* **1990**, *67*, 723–731. [CrossRef]
19. La, V.-P.; Pham, T.-H.; Ho, M.-T.; Nguyen, M.-H.P.; Nguyen, K.-L.; Vuong, T.-T.; Nguyen, H.-K.T.; Tran, T.; Khuc, Q.; Ho, M.-T.; et al. Policy response, social media and science journalism for the sustainability of the public health system amid the COVID-19 outbreak: The vietnam lessons. *Sustainability* **2020**, *12*, 2931. [CrossRef]
20. Bruinen de Bruin, Y.; Lequarre, A.S.; McCourt, J.; Clevestig, P.; Pigazzani., F. Initial impacts of global risk mitigation measures taken during the combatting of the COVID-19 pandemic. *Saf. Sci.* **2020**, *28*, 104773. [CrossRef] [PubMed]
21. Marin, A.; Vasilescu, L.; Marin, G.G.; Tudosie, V.G.; Baicus, C.A. Retrospective of the first 3 weeks of infection with SARS-CoV-2 in Romania. *Mod. Med.* **2020**, *27*, 79–82. Available online: https://medicinamoderna.ro/a-retrospective-of-the-first-3-weeks-of-infection-with-sars-cov-2-in-romania/ (accessed on 27 June 2020).
22. Presidency.Ro. Available online: https://www.presidency.ro/ro/media/comunicate-de-presa (accessed on 22 May 2020).
23. Vladescu, C.; Scîntee, S.G.; Olsavszky, V.; Hernández-Quevedo, C.; Sagan, A. *Health Systems in Transition: Romania*; WHO Regional Office for Europe: Copenhagen, Denmark, 2016; Volume 18, Number 4. Available online: https://www.euro.who.int/__data/assets/pdf_file/0017/317240/Hit-Romania.pdf?ua=1 (accessed on 30 June 2020).
24. Cernicova, M. Reforming public services in Romania. In *REFORMS of Public Services: Experiences of Municipalities and Regions in South-East Europe*; Friedrich Ebert Stiftung: Zagreb, Croatia, 2003; pp. 65–71. Available online: https://library.fes.de/pdf-files/bueros/kroatien/50253.pdf (accessed on 20 May 2020).
25. Popa, A.E. Implementing a social policy in the health care sector: The media construction of the process. In *Mapping Heterogeneity: Qualitative Research in Communication*; Ivan, L., Daba-Buzoianu, C., Gray, B., Eds.; Tritonic: Bucharest, Romania, 2014; pp. 331–359.
26. World Health Organization. Risk Communication and Community Engagement (RCCE) Action Plan Guidance COVID-19 Preparedness and Response. Available online: https://www.who.int/publications/i/item/risk-communication-and-community-engagement-(rcce)-action-plan-guidance (accessed on 22 June 2020).
27. Survey: 2 in 3 Romanian Consumers Now Use at Least One Digital Service. Available online: https://www.romaniajournal.ro/business/survey-2-in-3-romanian-consumers-now-use-at-least-one-digital-service/ (accessed on 20 June 2020).
28. ECDC Report. Guidance for Social Distancing Measures Aimed at Minimising the Spread of SARS-CoV-2. p. 6. Available online: https://www.ecdc.europa.eu/sites/default/files/documents/covid-19-social-distancing-measuresg-guide-second-update.pdf (accessed on 22 November 2020).
29. Analiza Evolutiei Epidemiei Covid-19 in Romania Pentru Perioada 18.03–27.06.2020 Efectuata in Cadrul INSP-CNEPSS [Analysis of the Evolution of the Covid-19 Epidemic in Romania for the Period 18.03-27.06.2020 Performed Within INSP-CNEPSS]. Available online: https://insp.gov.ro/sites/cnepss/wp-content/uploads/2020/07/Analiza-evolutiei-epidemiei-Covid-19-in-Romania-Final-13-iulie.pdf (accessed on 20 July 2020).
30. Semrush. Available online: https://www.semrush.com/company/ (accessed on 15 June 2020).
31. O'Brien, H.L.; Toms, E.G. What is user engagement? A conceptual framework for defining user engagement with technology. *J. Assoc. Inf. Sci. Technol.* **2008**. [CrossRef]
32. Foarfecă, E. România Intră în Scenariul 3, După Cazul 100 de Coronavirus. Ce Presupune Acesta [Romania Enters Scenario 3, after Coronavirus Case Number 100. What Does This Entail]. Mediafax. Available online: https://www.mediafax.ro/coronavirus/romania-intra-in-scenariul-3-dupa-cazul-100-de-coronavirus-ce-presupune-acesta-18985736 (accessed on 20 May 2020).
33. Covid-19 Official News Online Platform Has Been Launched. Available online: https://www.mediafax.ro/english/covid-19-official-news-online-platform-has-been-launched-18994384 (accessed on 15 June 2020).
34. Telespectator în Vremea Covid-19 [TV Viewer in the Time of Covid-19]. Available online: https://www.arma.org.ro/stiri/telespectator-in-vremea-covid-19/ (accessed on 15 November 2020).
35. Wingen, K. Der Krise Kommunizieren: Zehn Tipps Fur das, was Jetzt Wichtig Ist (Communicating in a Crisis: Ten Tips for what is Important Now). 2019. Available online: https://www.wissenschaftskommunikation.de/in-der-krise-kommunizieren-zehn-tipps-fuer-das-was-jetzt-wichtig-ist-23541/ (accessed on 15 June 2020).
36. Manifest Pentru Publicarea Completă a Datelor Privind Evoluția Pandemiei Covid-19 pe Teritoriul României [Manifesto for the Complete Publication of Data on the Evolution of the Covid-19 Pandemic on the Romanian Territory]. Available online: https://covid19.geo-spatial.org/manifest (accessed on 5 June 2020).
37. AntiCovidTM. Available online: https://anticovidtm.ro/despre-noi/ (accessed on 15 November 2020).
38. Malikhao, P. *Effective Health Communication for Sustainable Development*; NOVA Publishers: New York, NY, USA, 2016.
39. Servaes, J.; Patchanee, M. Communication and sustainable development. In *Selected Papers from the 9th UN Roundtable on Communication for Development*; FAO: Roma, Italy, 2007; pp. 1–38. Available online: http://www.fao.org/3/a1476e/a1476e01.pdf (accessed on 15 June 2020).
40. Law 95/2006. Available online: http://legislatie.just.ro/Public/DetaliiDocument/71139 (accessed on 19 June 2020).

41. Regulamentul de Organizare și Funcționare a Direcțiilor de Sănătate Publică Județene și a Municipiului București din 27 July 2010 [Regulation of Organization and Functioning of the County and Bucharest City Public Health Authorities of 27 July 2010]. Available online: https://lege5.ro/Gratuit/geztmnbsgu/regulamentul-de-organizare-si-functionare-a-directiilor-de-sanatate-publica-judetene-si-a-municipiului-bucuresti-din-27072010 (accessed on 7 May 2020).
42. OECD/European Observatory on Health Systems and Policies. *Romania: Country Health Profile 2019*; State of Health in the EU, OECD Publishing; Paris/European Observatory on Health Systems and Policies: Brussels, Belgium. Available online: https://www.oecd-ilibrary.org/docserver/f345b1db-en.pdf?expires=1614244349&id=id&accname=guest&checksum=230AB3255906B447894DC03D8E0A50F0 (accessed on 22 June 2020).
43. Lozan, O.; Zile, I.; Malkevica, I.; Bogaert, P.; Calleja, N. Health Information System in Romania 2019. Available online: https://insp.gov.ro/sites/cnepss/wp-content/uploads/2019/10/HIS_Romania_Final.pdf (accessed on 1 June 2020).
44. Björnberg, A.; Phang, A.Y. The Euro Health Consumer Index 2018 Report. Available online: https://healthpowerhouse.com/ (accessed on 23 June 2020).
45. Voicu, M. *Pandemia COVID19 din Perspectivă Demografică. Raport Social al ICCV 2020*; [COVID 19 pandemics from a demographic perspective. Social report of the Institute for Life Quality]; Institutul de Cercetare a Calității Vieții: București, Romania, 2020. Available online: http://www.iccv.ro/wp-content/uploads/2020/05/Raport-social-COVID-din-perspectiva-demografica-200518.pdf (accessed on 5 June 2020).
46. Survey: Head of Emergency Service, the Leader Romanians Admire most during Coronavirus Crisis. Available online: https://www.romania-insider.com/unlock-survey-arafat-leader-may-2020 (accessed on 23 November 2020).
47. Vermeir, P. Crisis Communication: Challenges, Priorities and Perspectives. *Health Manag.* 2020, 20, pp. 239–242. Available online: https://www.researchgate.net/publication/341735090_Crisis_Communication_Challenges_Priorities_and_Perspectives (accessed on 23 July 2020).
48. Dascalu, S. The successes and failures of the initial COVID-19 pandemic response in Romania. *Front. Public Health* **2020**, *8*, 344. [CrossRef] [PubMed]
49. Valentini, C. Is using social media "good" for the public relations profession? A critical reflection. *Public Relat. Rev.* **2015**, *41*, 170–177. [CrossRef]
50. Wilcox, D.L.; Cameron, G.T.; Reber, B.H. *Public Relations: Strategies and Tactics*; Global Edition; Pearson Higher Education & Professional Group: London, UK, 2014.
51. Eriksson, M. Lessons for crisis communication on social media: A systematic review of what research tells the practice. *Int. J. Strateg. Commun.* **2018**, *12*, 526–551. [CrossRef]
52. Coombs, W.T. *Ongoing Crisis Communication*; SAGE Publications: Thousand Oaks, CA, USA, 2014.
53. Genc, R. The importance of communication in sustainability & sustainable strategies. *Procedia Manuf.* **2017**, *8*, 511–516. [CrossRef]
54. Hancu-Budui, A.; Zorio-Grima, A.; Blanco-Vega, J. Audit institutions in the European Union: Public service promotion, environmental engagement and COVID crisis communication through social media. *Sustainability* **2020**, *12*, 9816. [CrossRef]
55. Laužikas, M.; Miliūtė, A. Impacts of modern technologies on sustainable communication of civil service organizations. *Entrep. Sustain. Issues* **2020**, *7*, 2494–2509. [CrossRef]
56. World Health Organization Europe. How Health Systems Can Address Health Inequities Linked to Migration and Ethnicity. Available online: https://www.euro.who.int/__data/assets/pdf_file/0005/127526/e94497.pdf (accessed on 1 July 2020).
57. Hashtags of Month April-#Respect, #Staiacasa, #Covid19. Available online: https://www.zelist.ro/blog/hashtag-urile-lunii-aprilie-2020-respect-stamacasa-covid19/ (accessed on 22 June 2020).
58. Jong, W. Evaluating crisis communication. A 30-item checklist for assessing performance during COVID-19 and other pandemics. *J. Health Commun.* **2021**, 1–9. [CrossRef] [PubMed]

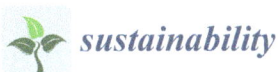

Article

The Impact of CEOs' Gender on Organisational Efficiency in the Public Sector: Evidence from the English NHS

Gema Gutierrez-Romero [1,*], Antonio Blanco-Oliver [2], Mª Teresa Montero-Romero [1] and Mariano Carbonero-Ruz [1]

[1] Financial Economics and Accounting, Universidad Loyola Andalucía, Dos Hermanas, 41704 Seville, Spain; tmontero@uloyola.es (M.T.M.-R.); mcarbonero@uloyola.es (M.C.-R.)
[2] Financial Economics and Operations Management, University of Seville, 41018 Seville, Spain; aj_blanco@us.es
* Correspondence: ggutierrez@uloyola.es; Tel.: +34-607093294

Abstract: Increasing operational efficiency is an objective relevant for all institutions, but it is essential in public entities and even more in public health systems because of the number of resources they consume and their impact on general welfare. This research analyses the effect that CEOs' gender has on the operational efficiency of the entities they manage. Despite the impact that the management team and notably the CEO have on the development of institutions, studies on their effect on performance are practically non-existent, especially for public organisations. We have used data from acute care hospital trusts belonging to the English National Health System (NHS) concerning its development. The results were obtained from a two-stage analysis. First, the entities' economic efficiency and health/social efficiency (two operational efficiency measures) were evaluated using two data envelopment analysis (DEA) models. Secondly, the results have been regressed with the CEOs' gender. The results obtained are robust and consistent, revealing that male CEOs have greater performance than female CEOs. This result provides insight into determining features that relate to operational efficiency, which it is of interest to the research and policymakers.

Keywords: efficiency; gender; CEO; top management team (TMT); data envelopment analysis (DEA); truncated regression; bootstrap; upper echelon theory

1. Introduction

The analysis of efficient management in the public sector and the key factors that determine it are of great interest to researchers [1,2], especially in public health systems [3]. The analysis of efficiency in the public health sector takes on even greater importance in the context of COVID-19, which has highlighted the limitations of the health system. While recent studies have analysed the health system's present and future challenges [4], concerns about efficient management in the public sector are not new. They have been the basis for policies known as New Public Management (NPM) [5]. Public health system concern regarding efficiencies is not only to do with the impact on public opinion and the welfare of society but also due to the large volume of economic resources consumed by health systems, which on average in the EU amounts to 9.9% of a nation's GDP [6]. Since the mid-1980s, public system management and practice theories have shifted towards implementing NPM [7], whose central hypothesis is to manage public systems more similarly to the private sector to make government entities more efficient [8]. Within these management policies related to NPM, the literature pays particular attention to the upper echelon theory (UET) [9]. This theory posits that the performance of the senior management team (TMT) is one of the factors that most affects the operational efficiency of an institution, since they are the ones who carry out most of the strategic decisions [10,11]. According to the UET, the management team members' previous experience, values, and personalities influence their decision-making and, therefore, the performance of the entities for which they make such decisions [12] (p. 334).

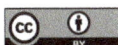

Provided that something improves the TMT's performance, this would also enhance the firm's performance [13]. Traditionally, previous research has focused on the effects of TMTs as a single unit, using the same level for the chief executive officer (CEO) and the rest of the top management. However, several studies have refuted such an approach based on the particularity of the CEO's role compared with the role of the rest of the TMT [14]. Indeed, the CEO is considered to hold a strategic position to convey signals, non-quantitative information, and management styles to the organisations' stakeholders [15]. This aspect is especially relevant in public institutions, where controversial managerial topics, such as women's access to executive positions, are firstly addressed for signalling and subsequently drive private sector behaviour [16]. However, more research is needed to understand the impact of CEOs' attributes on public sector organisations [17]. The need for more research becomes more pertinent than ever in testing the effect of a CEO's gender on the performance of an organisation, since there is no agreement yet on this in the literature [18]. In this vein, the literature is still intensively debating whether higher female representation in TMTs leads to positive [13,19], negative [20,21], or no [22,23] effects on a firm's performance.

Therefore, this research's main objective is to study the effect of the CEO's gender on operational efficiency (note that operational efficiency is a measure of organisational performance and is defined as the capacity to optimise and adapt resources (inputs) to results (outputs); the present research does not measure this) in a case study of public hospitals' cost efficiency in the English National Health Service (NHS). To do so, we carried out a two-stage analysis. In the first stage, data envelopment analysis (DEA) ranked the hospitals according to their technical efficiency score, calculated assuming a constant returns to scale approach. In the second stage, since the efficiency scores were censored at the maximum value of the efficiency scores (1), we ran a panel Tobit and truncated regressions to analyse the effect of CEOs' gender on the efficiency of public hospitals. Additionally, due to the fact that the use of Tobit regression in the second stage caused explanatory variables to be correlated with the error term as inputs and outputs are correlated with explanatory variables, we ran a double bootstrapped procedure (Algorithm II) that permitted making valid inferences while simultaneously generating standard errors and confidence intervals for the efficiency estimates [24].

This study is fully justified, since women remain significantly underrepresented in hospital CEO positions [25]. Indeed, the healthcare sector has been considered a male-dominated field for decades, despite the fact that women make up most of the healthcare workforce [26]. This paper's contribution is remarkable, since we document new evidence on the role of CEOs' gender in UK public health institutions' performance. Our findings have great value for researchers, practitioners, and policymakers and provide more clarity and instruments for regulators to design policies to improve efficiency in a critical area such as public health systems.

The rest of the paper proceeds as follows. Section 2 provides an overview of the literature on the relationships between gender and firm performance and develops our hypothesis. Section 3 presents the data and describes the methodology adopted, while Section 4 summarises the main results and discusses the significance of the findings. Lastly, Section 5 concludes the paper and highlights this research's implications, including its limitations, and makes suggestions for future studies.

Review of the Literature and Hypothesis

Although research has drawn much attention to the underrepresentation of women and minorities in TMTs, the impact of gender on organisational performance is still an open research question [18]. As stated in [27], various individual, organisational, and societal factors explain the lower proportion of women in leadership positions. Regarding the impact of individual factors, including education, expertise, and family responsibilities, on progress into CEO positions, Ref. [28] shows that women fail to progress into CEO positions despite completing graduate degrees in healthcare administration and having equivalent expertise rates to men. That is, there is a gender driver that damages women's possibilities of labour promotion. Some studies assume that female labour discrimination suggests that female executives need a male mentor figure for career advancement [29]. Indeed, Ref. [30] indicate that it is not enough for women to have mentors; it is necessary for them to have sponsorship from a highly placed executive who advocates for them.

These arguments cause gender biases in favouring men in leadership positions in the healthcare industry [25]. However, there is no conclusive evidence demonstrating that women underperform compared to men in organisational management, whether public nor private. Indeed, the literature shows that women have superior management skills and capabilities in some labour contexts, such as in the green and third sectors [31] or in carrying out marketing tasks [32]. Additionally, Ref. [33] suggest that women often pursue less aggressive strategies and adopt more sustainable investment criteria because women are more risk-averse than men, especially where financial decisions are concerned [34]. Being less overconfident means that financial markets more favourably receive financial transactions made by women, since it is assumed that female CEOs exercise greater scrutiny and exhibit less hubris in strategic decisions [35]. Therefore, these arguments would positively impact the effect of female executives on organisations' economic outcomes.

As mentioned above, there is no clear evidence that women have lower performance in management positions. However, most studies on the effects on women's performance have been conducted in the context of diversity in management teams [21,36,37]. Even in this context, there is no consensus regarding the impact on institutions. Among the studies that discuss the possibility that the gender of managers affects the performance of entities, there are two main lines: *liberal feminist theory* and *social feminist theory* [38]. The liberal feminist theory holds that female-managed entities may perform worse due to systematic factors that limit the scope of relevant resources. In contrast, the social feminist theory holds that women and men are different by their very nature and will cope differently (not necessarily worse) with management, such as taking fewer risks [39]

Following this point of view of social feminism, we found that particularly for hospitals' social or healthcare outcomes, several arguments would support a positive relationship between female leadership and the performance of hospitals, measured in terms of patient well-being. Indeed, Ref. [40] show that the chief executive officer's (CEO) gender may affect patient experience. In this vein, Ref. [41] found that female CEOs improve interpersonal care experience faster than male CEOs, particularly in the most complex executive job environments. It has been noted that women seem to fit better in this particular industry due to healthcare services' relational and interpersonal nature. We can theoretically explain this from the social preference perspective, which suggests that women are more sensitive to social cues in determining appropriate behaviour [42] due to their more compassion [43] and inequality aversion [44].

Consequently, with women's social preferences being more situationally specific than those of men, they will be more likely to show respect for and be willing to help individuals with healthcare needs such as patients. As shown in [45], management styles are influenced by gender differences in relational orientation, since women CEOs are more prone to enact transformational versus transactional leadership behaviours. In summary, the literature supports the notion that female CEOs have a management style that focuses to a greater extent on the social and healthcare view in the decision-making process. Conversely, there is also opposing evidence questioning the ability of women to achieve superior performance in managerial contexts. For example, Ref. [46] point out that female CEOs' preference for more social or people-oriented decisions means that less importance is given to the financial performance of the entities they manage. This greater inclination towards social issues leads them to devote more significant resources to improving corporate social performance, leaving aside organisational performance factors [47]. Several authors also find women to be less ambitious and to exercise less power [37]. The capacity to influence subordinates has arisen as a critical success factor for CEOs, and even more so in a hospital context where highly trained -and hard-to-monitor individuals run separate but interconnected production processes [38]. This feature would imply that female CEOs may underperform compared to males in a hospital environment.

Similarly, Ref. [48] finds that females' higher risk aversion could lead to the accumulation of suboptimal decisions, which would lead to the lower performance of women-managed entities.

In the UET exposition, although [10] does not mention gender specifically, the paper presents distinctive characteristics that can predict how managers will deal with certain situations. Consequently, such features could be used to predict the level of performance of the entities they manage. In the same vein, particularly for the public sector, the Public Sector Management theory (PSM) agrees that several particular characteristics make individuals more likely to work in the public sector [29]. In this sense, feminist theories, both social and liberal, agree with the UET and PSM in the presence of a series of personal and system characteristics which would affect (not necessarily negatively) the performance of the managed entities [39].

Liberal feminist theory, for example, argues that women face systemic constraints that make it difficult for them to access the resources necessary for the better functioning of the entities they manage, which would be an obstacle to their performance compared with entities controlled by men [38]. In the same vein, Ref. [49], points out that in highly competitive markets with resource constraints, the CEO's male power has the most significant positive effect on the institutions they manage.

For instance, we found several authors who base reputation on CEOs' educational background; previous positive experiences in similar positions; and human or social capital, which translates into more significant networks, giving them access to financial and information resources [50]. Such access to resources in a competitive environment will lead to higher performance levels [51]. When we analysed these characteristics from a gender perspective and a liberal feminist perspective concerning the systematic restrains, we could see how the females have more limited access to networks than males [52]. We also found empirical evidence that creating these links or contacts is favoured by similarity between individuals [53]. This concept of "homophily" [54], explains the entry barriers specific individuals, women, and ethnic minorities [55] experience in accessing the resources provided by such social capital, limiting their possibilities to improve their performance. In a recent study on social identity theory [56], the authors found that concerning the favouritism implied by homophily, men protect the "monopoly value generated by their elite status", which limits women's access to resources.

Among the characteristics that provide access to resources is the prestige of directors. The presence of directors on several boards is directly related to these directors' perceived prestige [57]. As presented by [58,59], the male elites will block the presence of women on boards of directors to protect their distinctive effect. This has the effect of blocking access to these boards and therefore the recognition that goes with it.

In the same vein, Ref. [60] explain that females will have limited access to resources since the "old boy network" has the most to lose from women's entry.

On the other hand, and in line with women's difficulties in accessing managerial positions, evidence shows that female CEOs tend to be selected when institutions experience problems [61]. While this could be related to women's social skills that allow them to manage people in delicate situations better [62], there is extensive literature that supports the idea of the "glass cliff" [63].

The glass cliff represents the idea that females will be more likely to jump into riskier positions, such as assuming the role of CEO in a company in a difficult situation, to gain experience that otherwise is inaccessible for females [64].

For all the above reasons, we propose the following hypothesis:

Hypothesis 1 (H1). *Female CEOs have a negative impact on hospitals' operational efficiency.*

2. Materials and Methods

2.1. Data Source

To test our hypothesis, we used as a case study the public health system of the United Kingdom, belonging to the NHS. The selection of this entities is very appropriate due to several aspects. The UK's NHS was the first universal and free healthcare system. However, since its birth in 1948, it has undergone several reforms and modifications. Of particular relevance for its management is the 1990 reform. The state transferred the provision of services to NHS trusts, which are semi-independent, not-for-profit organisations. The NHS trusts act under state control but on a competitive basis—i.e., the end-user can choose the centre where he/she will be treated. NHS trusts are regulated and have specific and homogeneous reporting obligations, favouring results' reliability. In this same vein, and as the second most noteworthy aspect concerning NHS hospital management, progress has been made in public–private collaboration. The first private finance initiative (PFI) was launched in 1992. This framework has since allowed the contracting of private companies to build and operate NHS facilities through long-term contracts. The final relevant managerial transformation was the creation in 2004 of the first NHS foundation trusts (FT). NHS foundation trusts were created to devolve decision-making from central government to local organisations and communities, enabling them to respond to local people's needs and wishes. A foundation trust (FT) is publicly owned and is accountable to the local population, patients, carers, and staff through a Council of Governors. The Council of Governors is appointed from stakeholder organisations such as Local Councils or is elected by FT members.

We had access to public information for data collection, such as the individual hospital trusts' financial statements published in their annual reports. Additional information was also obtained through the Health and Social Care Information Centre (now called NHS Digital). Additionally, to improve the comparability, we limited the analysis to acute care hospital trusts (known as foundation trusts and ordinary trusts) in England. Our sample includes the entire acute care trust population in England, with 128 acute care trusts in October 2009.

2.2. Key Variables

As stated previously, this paper tests the impact of CEOs' gender on hospitals' operational efficiency. Consequently, the leading variables of our analysis were (i) efficiency, which acts as the dependent variable, and (ii) the CEO's gender, which is the independent variable. Efficiency scores were obtained using a DEA model, where the input and output factors were selected according to previous research and applying a theoretical argument. It is worth noting that there is no optimal way to select inputs and outputs to perform a DEA [65]. Nevertheless, in the healthcare literature the most typical inputs are related to each hospital's capacity to care for patients, such as the number of beds available, the total number of staff, and the number of doctors [66].

In contrast, outputs are linked to healthcare organisations' singular outcomes, such as survival rates or the number of finished consultant episodes (FCE) [67]. Table 1 shows the most common inputs and outputs used by the healthcare literature to construct efficiency DEA models. As shown in Table 1, there is no general agreement regarding the suitability of the best inputs and outputs. However, there is consensus that the input variables must be related to hospitals' (material and human) resources to serve their patients. Outputs must be aligned to the outcomes that generate a hospital, which are linked to two areas: one is focused on the economic field and other has great emphasis on the healthcare dimension.

Consequently, on the one hand the outputs of the DEA model must be related to the capacity to become a financially sustainable hospital, including the ability to govern the hospital and adapt its performance to the state budget allocations. On the other hand, the output variable must be related to the patients' healthcare quality, which is the hospital's raison d'être. In other words, the outputs used in the efficiency DEA model have to consider that hospitals are hybrid organisations, in the sense of the definition of [68], where two separate variables must be combined: the economic performance and the healthcare outcomes.

Table 1. Output Input variables.

Variables	
Outputs	Inputs
Inpatient days [69]	Doctors [69]
Clinical examinations [69]	Nurses [69]
Laboratory test [69]	Other personnel [69]
Total acute patient days [70]	Number of beds [70]
Total intensive patient days [70]	Type of ownership [70]
Number of inpatient and outpatient surgeries performed [70]	Case-mix severity [70]
Number of outpatient visits (emergency room and clinic visits delivered) [70]	Net plant assets [70]
Number of residents per attending physician [70]	Total annual expenditures [70]
General surgery [71]	Nursing [71]
General medicine [71]	Administration [71]
Maternity [71]	Ancillary [71]
A&E [71]	Specialist [71]
	Beds [71]

Based on the previous arguments, we constructed two separate operational efficiency DEA models. Both DEA models used the same input variables: (i) the number of hospital beds and (ii) the number of staff (medical and administrative personnel). These two inputs have been previously used by the literature [66,67] and are justified because they are the primary (material and human) resources that hospitals use to serve their patients.

However, these two DEA models have different outputs. Firstly, we developed a DEA model that focused more on hospitals' economic efficiency and used a more economy-oriented output. This efficiency DEA model (Model 1) employed the days of inpatient care as the output variable. The days of inpatient care variable measures the days that patients stay in the hospital receiving medical care. This variable is clearly related to the healthcare dimension and incorporates economic connotations, since the managers of a hospital can accelerate the discharge of patients to reduce the occupation rate and, thus, healthcare costs. As suggested in [72], releases are argued to be a better output measure than inpatient days because unnecessary inpatient days for a hospital episode might falsely indicate a high efficiency. To solve this problem, we constructed a further efficiency DEA model (Model 2) which emphasised the healthcare dimension of the hospitals by using the average survival rate (i.e., the inverse of the average mortality rate) as an output variable, which been widely used as an output in the literature [73–75].

On the other hand, the independent variable "CEO gender" is a dummy variable that takes a value of 1 when the CEO is a woman and 0 otherwise. According to the literature and surveys focused on healthcare systems, we observed that hospitals are male-dominated organisations in our sample. We find that in our sample, there is a substantial gender difference in the CEO position: male CEOs represent 71.88% of the total.

2.3. Controls

Several control variables were included in the regression model to separate the impact of the CEO gender from the efficiency of other statistically significant potential effects. Control variables are useful to contextualise the environment where each hospital operates and, at the same time, fit the statistical significance of the regression model better. We controlled for the size of the hospital by using the number of beds. Additionally, we used a dummy variable, "teaching status", that captured if the hospital, further than healthcare services, had learning areas. The reason behind our use of this control variable is that teaching hospitals usually deal with treatment and interventions that are more complex. Hospitals were also split into a dummy group according to their legal status. The relevance of this is that foundation trusts (FTs) are more autonomous and face more substantial external pressure to demonstrate efficiency. FT hospitals are part of the NHS and treat patients according to the NHS principles of free healthcare. Being a FT means that these institutions are better able to provide and manage its services to meet the needs and priorities of the local community, as the trust is free from central government control.

Furthermore, we used several variables that capture information related to patients that directly affect the hospitals' operational efficiency. These variables were the average age of the patients served, the length of stay, and the number of staff assigned to the hospital. Finally, we included a variable to control the hospital's outsourcing policy, which is also linked to the increase in operational efficiency, since outsourcing is often used to contract external services that are not produced efficiently internally. Therefore, we controlled our model with variables related to the efficiency of each hospital.

2.4. Methodology

2.4.1. First-Stage DEA Efficiency Estimate

Hospital efficiency scores were estimated using DEA [76]. Unlike parametric efficiency models (such as Stochastic Frontier Analysis), DEA is a non-parametric method that does not impose a specific structure on an efficient frontier shape; this is its main advantage [77]. However, a non-parametric treatment of the efficiency frontier relies on general regularity properties, such as monotonicity, convexity, and homogeneity.

DEA analysis enables assessing a hospital's performance relative to a 'best practice' frontier [76]. DEA ranks, by comparison between peers, hospitals from higher to lower efficiency scores, allowing us to define the optimal situation as a minimisation input or maximisation output problem.

The first version of DEA [78] assumes constant returns to scale (CRS)—i.e., a change in inputs is followed by a change in outputs in the same proportion. We used an input-oriented DEA model with variable returns to scale (VRS) developed by [79]. VRS relaxes the constant returns to scale assumption and allows for the possibility that the hospitals' production technology may exhibit increasing, constant, or decreasing returns to scale.

We used an input-oriented VRS model, since our presumption was that hospital managers have more control over inputs than outputs. Essentially, our model offers an efficiency score for n number of Data Management Units (DMUs) using m outputs and s inputs, as presented below:

$$\theta = max_{u,y} \frac{\sum_{r=1}^{s} \mu_r y_{ro}}{\sum_{j=1}^{m} v_j x_{jo}}. \quad (1)$$

This is subject to:

$$\frac{\sum_{r=1}^{s} \mu_r y_{ri}}{\sum_{j=1}^{m} v_j x_{ji}} \leq 1, \quad i = 1, 2, \ldots, n, \quad (2)$$

$$\mu_r > 0, \ v_j > 0, \ for \ all \ r, j, \quad (3)$$

where the *j* DMU consumes inputs to produce outputs, where the weights of the outputs and inputs, respectively, have to be > 0 [49]. The efficiency scores are ranked between 0 and 1, with the value 1 showing the most efficient observations.

2.4.2. Second-Stage Truncated Regression

Following [75], we regressed the CEO gender on the DEA models' efficiency scores. For that, we carried out a Tobit regression with the maximum likelihood estimation method for parameter estimations, since the efficiency scores from the first-stage analysis having a censored structure and ordinary least square regression makes them biased and they provide inconsistent estimations with censored dependent variables [80].

Therefore, we consider the following general Tobit model:

$$y_i^* = \beta_0 + \beta_1 CEO_i + \beta_i X_i + u_i, \qquad (4)$$

$$y_i = \begin{cases} y_i^*, & \text{if } y_{i,t}^* < 1 \\ 1, & \text{otherwise} \end{cases} \quad i = 1, \ldots, N, \qquad (5)$$

where the i subscript denotes the cross-sectional dimension. The dependent variable, y_i, is the efficiency score obtained from the DEA. CEO_i is the CEO gender, measured using a dummy variable; X_i is the vector of each hospital's control variables; u_i is the error term. As argued previously, the control variables (X_i) matrix includes variables related to the efficiency levels of each hospital (dependent variable) and other controls such as the size of the hospital or the provision of the teaching services.

Additionally, to check our analysis results we conducted a truncated regression, an alternative statistical method with which we obtained the same findings.

Finally, to confirm our findings, we implemented a robustness test using the [24] procedure. This is a two-stage DEA analysis where efficiency scores are evaluated and then regressed on potential covariates using a double-bootstrapped truncated regression. From the theoretical point of view, when Tobit regression is applied in the second stage, it provokes statistical inconsistency, since the independent variables correlate with the error term [24]. The [24] procedure allows valid inferences to be made, as well as generating standard errors and confidence intervals for the efficiency estimates.

3. Results

Table 2 contains the descriptive statistics of the variables collected for the sample of public hospitals.

Table 2. Descriptive statistics.

Variable	Mean	Sd	P50	Min	Max
N. Staff	4383.8	2192	3701	1403	11005
N. Beds	754.1	315.77	695	250	1827
FCE Bed days	2.5×10^5	1.1×10^5	2.2×10^5	81,156	5.9×10^5
DEA cor 1	0.87459	0.06085	0.87589	0.7306	1
Value	1.0043	0.10067	1.0126	0.6729	1.2141
Inverse value	1.0069	0.11462	0.98756	0.82366	1.4861
DEA cor 2	0.41956	0.19053	0.38603	0.13743	1
Teaching	0.64063	0.4817	1	0	1
Foundation T	0.53906	0.50043	1	0	1
Percentage D	0.28776	0.18762	0.30769	0	0.75
CEO Female	0.26357	0.44228	0	0	1
Board Size	10.736	4.5715	12	1	17
Turnover_000	3.1×10^5	1.7×10^5	2.6×10^5	74,969	9.9×10^5
Mean_age	51.24	4.2459	51	38	66
Mean length of stays	4.2977	0.62067	4.2	3	7.6
Contracted services	34.386	28.65	25.46	0	100
Population	4.7×10^5	3.7×10^5	3.7×10^5	1.6×10^5	3.0×10^6

Table 3 shows the results of our analysis. It can be observed in Table 2 that the gender of the CEO matters in terms of firm performance. The fact of finding influence, negative or positive, has relevance for the literature, since some studies doubt the existence of the relation between gender and firm performance (see, e.g., [18]).

Table 3. Efficiency score from DEA models.

	Dependent Variable: Efficiency Score from Model 1			Dependent Variable: Efficiency Score from Model 2		
	Tobit Regression	Truncated Regression	Simar & Wilson	Tobit Regression	Truncated Regression	Simar & Wilson
Independent variable: CEO gender (dummy)	−0.0258 *	−0.0292 **	−0.0292 **	−0.0362 **	−0.0306 **	−0.0306 **
	(0.0141)	(0.0142)	(0.0141)	(0.0144)	(0.0145)	(0.0145)
Control variables:						
% female in the board	0.0034	0.0147	0.0147	0.0375	0.0154	0.0154
	(0.0474)	(0.0487)	(0.0485)	(0.0485)	(0.0500)	(0.0499)
Board size	0.0023	0.0021	0.0021	0.0014	0.0012	0.0012
	(0.0020)	(0.0021)	(0.0021)	(0.0021)	(0.0021)	(0.0020)
Teaching (dummy)	−0.0057	−0.0054	−0.0054	−0.0009	−0.0054	−0.0054
	(0.0131)	(0.0133)	(0.0129)	(0.0134)	(0.0133)	(0.0126)
Foundation Trust (dummy)	−0.0138	−0.0123	−0.0123	−0.0215 *	−0.0119	−0.0119
	(0.0124)	(0.0126)	(0.0127)	(0.0127)	(0.0129)	(0.0130)
Number beds	0.0000519	0.0000669 *	0.0000669 *	0.0000149	0.000041	0.000041
	(0.0000355)	(0.000036)	(0.0000354)	(0.0000362)	(0.0000358)	(0.0000364)
Turnover	−1.83e07 **	−1.84e−07 **	−1.84e07 **	−1.75e07 **	−1.70e07 **	−1.70e−07 **
	(7.57e−08)	(7.71e−08)	(7.47e−08)	(7.71e−08)	(7.62e−08)	(7.75e−08)
Mean age	−0.0038 **	−0.0036 **	−0.0036 **	−0.0033 *	−0.0028	−0.0028
	(0.0017)	(0.0018)	(0.0018)	(0.0018)	(0.0018)	(0.0018)
Mean length of stay	0.0493 ***	0.0454 ***	0.0454 ***	0.0529 ***	0.0515 ***	0.0515 ***
	(0.0132)	(0.0136)	(0.0133)	(0.0135)	(0.0136)	(0.0138)
Contracted out services	0.0005 **	0.0004 *	0.0004 **	0.0005 **	0.0005 **	0.0005 **
	(0.0002)	(0.0002)	(0.0002)	(0.0002)	(0.0002)	(0.0002)
Population served	1.65e−8	8.22e−9	8.22e−9	2.04e−8	9.27e−9	9.27e−9
	(2.28e−8)	(2.34e−8)	(2.35e−8)	(2.32e−8)	(2.29e−8)	(2.45e−8)
Constant	0.8407 ***	0.8380 ***	0.8380 ***	0.8371 ***	0.8034 ***	0.8034 ***
	(0.0893)	(0.0898)	(0.0898)	(0.0911)	(0.0910)	(0.0900)
Observations	97	94	97	97	92	97

Note: * = $p < 0.10$, ** = $p < 0.05$, *** = $p < 0.01$. Clustered robust standard errors in parentheses.

We found that female CEOs have a negative impact on the operational efficiency of hospitals. This result remains unaltered for the two efficiency DEA models developed here. One of these two DEA models has a more economic-oriented output, while the other has a more healthcare-oriented output. These results, therefore, imply that women in CEO positions underperform in terms of economic and healthcare outcomes. The results remain stable in the three statistical models developed in the present study, reinforcing our findings' robustness and contribution. Our findings are in line with the results obtained by recent research conducted for general firms (e.g., [48]).

Theoretically, our findings can be explained from various points of view. Firstly, the literature sustains that female CEO appointments are often linked to organisations facing adverse conditions [81]. The practical implications of this are that hospitals with economic or healthcare problems ask to be managed by women. The limitation of women being promoted to leadership positions is reflected in the low proportion of female CEOs in the healthcare industry, where only 20% of CEOs are women, despite the fact that women make up 75% of the healthcare labour force [82].

Secondly, another potential explanation for the negative impact of female CEOs on hospital operational efficiency can be explained by the alternative leadership styles between women and men. In this sense, previous studies have found that women executives are more prone to adopt transformational leadership styles that emphasise team structures [83]. Under the transformational management style, the group coordinates between individuals because it is considered that the synergies bring advantages that result in an improved working atmosphere, which ultimately improves hospital performance. In other words, female CEOs use a management style that promotes the worker's welfare and, indirectly, the hospital's outcomes. In contrast, male leaders often adopt transactional leadership styles based on competition and hierarchy. Here, the achievement of the organisation's strategic objective is based on efficient structures of governance where the corporate guidelines are directly channelled from the apex to the bottom of the hospital.

Consequently, given that the hospitals are large and complex organisations where decision-making is decentralised, it is more difficult to apply the coordination mechanisms and the dynamism required by the transformational leadership styles proposed by female executives. Therefore, in the healthcare environments, women CEOs likely underperform compared to their male counterparts. Conversely, when workflow management follows the direct hierarchical structures designed by a transactional leadership style, it favours management's concretion and objectiveness, thus improving operational efficiency.

4. Discussion

Women are under-represented in management positions. As we have seen, in the healthcare sector women represent only 20% of management positions, while representing 75% of the workforce [82]. This study focuses on the existence of an association between the gender of the CEO and the institution's operational performance. While the results are clear and robust, confirming our hypothesis—i.e., higher operational efficiency levels when the CEO is male—the reasons behind these results can be analysed from different points of view. However, the robustness and consistency of the results obtained in an area where studies are scarce and with different results are relevant.

UET and PSM determined a series of personal characteristics or features that could define individuals' decision-making. The results obtained in institutions can be predicted according to their management teams' characteristics. Along the same lines, feminist social theory also finds a series of differential social factors or attributes that would justify different managers performance levels (not necessarily worse) depending on gender. In this sense, different management styles may lead to varying performance levels and would explain the lower operational efficiency resulting from our analysis. For instance, Ref. [84] found that women tend to take a more participatory and democratic style of decision-making, which could be beneficial in some sectors, but in complex and large organisations it may slow down decision-making, decreasing operational efficiency. In the same vein, women are more socially flexible than men [34]. This could make women more adaptable to political interference, shaping management decisions with political influences, which could harm the hospital's performance. Another feature typically associated with females is that women emphasise relationships over winning and have more excellent interpersonal skills [85]. These features could lead female directors to pay more attention to patient care and providing higher-quality services than to the performance, resulting in lower operational performance levels.

Another plausible reason for the lower levels of operational efficiency is related to social conditioning, which could be associated with overconfidence levels. Ref. [86] found that men are more predisposed to overconfidence than women. Overconfidence is related to individuals in positions of power [61]. These overconfidence levels, in turn, lead to more complex investments and organisational structures [61], which consequently result in higher levels of performance. In the same vein, Ref. [87] found that lower levels of overconfidence lead to lower indebtedness levels and lower levels of acquisitions that could, in turn, lead to a lower performance level. Additionally, Ref. [33] propose that females are more risk-averse than males, especially when financial decisions are concerned [34]. This could lead to an accumulation of sub-optimal choices that could explain a lower operational efficiency level.

Apart from these social features, some other external systematic factors could lead female CEOs to achieve lower operational performance levels. In line with the thesis of liberal feminists, we present that women could face resource constraints (both economic and in terms of access to information) that would justify possible differences in performance between men and women. We started this discussion by pointing out the substantial female under-representation, particularly in the healthcare sector. This underrepresentation is problematic in itself for various reasons. Firstly, the lower presence of women confers them an out-of-group status. In line with the concept above of homophily, the out-of-the-group status could hinder access to the necessary resources and support for the correct performance of managerial functions, which would justify the lower operational efficiency level.

Another possible reason for women's lower performance may be that, given the lesser presence of women in management positions, they are more likely to accept such positions in companies that are in difficult situations, an affect known as the "glass cliff". This fact is not exclusive to private companies. Ref. [88] found that government entities have a higher incidence of "glass cliff" in the US.

Another possible reason could be the one put forward by [89] that affirmed that gender stereotypes and male discrimination contributed significantly to gender disparities. Such a disparity affects the arrival of female CEOs. Ref. [90] present a negative effect on the performance of entities when a woman succeeds a man as CEO, as it is considered a deviation from the common practice of selecting a male CEO. In this sense, the presence of a woman in the CEO position is not necessarily related to a higher level of diversity, which would limit the benefits of her arrival in the position.

Indeed, the results of [91] show that institutions' gender diversity performance benefits are related to a balanced board of directors, not to "the mere token presence of women"—that is, the presence of a female CEO.

5. Limits and Future Research

Following the criteria of honesty and transparency that should guide scientific knowledge [92], we now develop this research's limitations and weaknesses. The present study's main limitation is related to the temporal constraint of the data analysed due to the absence of further information on CEOs' gender in other periods. This limitation is relevant when it comes to understanding the results obtained, since a longer time sequence could introduce variables that could be relevant in the explanation, such as experience in the position. For example, this temporal limitation is the basis of the research of [93]. These authors revised the results obtained by [94], who found that female CEOs were paid more than male CEOs. However, when [93] extended the sample and time frame, they found results that differed from the previous study.

Additionally, while the results are robust and undoubtedly measure an association of more efficient institutions when the CEO is male, it is necessary to recognise some additional caveats, such as potential reverse causality—that is, the possibility that underperforming institutions select female CEOs (glass cliff effect) [64]. Finally, this sample is specifically of trusts belonging to the English NHS. We should bear in mind that the results presented correspond to certain variables and regions with specific characteristics. The results obtained may vary when looking at countries with lower levels of development [48]. As indicated in [95], scientific research contributes to potential solutions to social problems, such as the under-representation of women in managerial positions. Such scientific contribution is essential in developing countries as a measure to reach the levels of developed countries.

In line with the above limitations, we call for the development of future research—i.e., research that goes beyond extending the object to other public systems within the European region is of interest; it might be useful to add a greater temporal dimension; it would be interesting to examine together the impact of the CEO's gender with their years of experience in the position, the financial situation of the entity before the arrival of the female CEO, and the diversity of the board of directors. It would also be relevant to extend the present research to other regions, beyond the countries of the European environment, contributing to the scientific evidence in developing countries. These additions would help us to better understand the causal connection of the results obtained.

6. Conclusions

Despite the limitations, this study contributes significantly to academic and political debate, generating evidence on female CEOs' roles in England NHS FT institutions' operational efficiency. It provides information that could support the establishment of policies to help overcome the present problems, providing background characteristics that could weigh down women's operational efficiency in management positions. The visibility of such features allows for more accurate plans to solve the gender imbalance in positions of responsibility. For instance, besides the quota system, some actions could better lead to overcoming some of the internal and external factors limiting female CEOs. For example, the lack of sponsorship of women within management teams in hospital systems hampers women's entry into such positions [28]. This situation limits the benefits of a more diverse management team, maintains female under-representation, and relegates women's role as tokens with limited institutional performance effects.

Author Contributions: Conceptualization, G.G.-R. and A.B.-O.; methodology, G.G.-R. and A.B.-O.; validation, A.B.-O., G.G.-R., M.T.M.-R., and M.C.-R.; formal analysis, G.G.-R. and A.B.-O.; investigation, G.G.-R. and A.B.-O.; resources, A.B.-O. and G.G.-R.; writing—original draft preparation, G.G.-R. and A.B.-O.; writing—review and editing, G.G.-R., A.B.-O., M.T.M.-R., and M.C.-R.; supervision, A.B.-O., M.C.-R., M.T.M.-R. All authors have read and agreed to the published version of the manuscript.

Funding: This research received no external funding.

Institutional Review Board Statement: Not applicable.

Informed Consent Statement: Not applicable.

Conflicts of Interest: The authors declare no conflict of interest.

References

1. Campbell, J.W. Efficiency, Incentives, and Transformational Leadership: Understanding Collaboration Preferences in the Public Sector. *Public Perform. Manag. Rev.* **2018**, *41*, 277–299. [CrossRef]
2. Narbón-Perpiñá, I.; De Witte, K. Local governments' efficiency: A systematic literature review—Part I. *Int. Trans. Oper. Res.* **2018**, *25*, 431–468. [CrossRef]
3. Wang, M.; Tao, C. Research on the Efficiency of Local Government Health Expenditure in China and Its Spatial Spillover Effect. *Sustainability* **2019**, *11*, 2469. [CrossRef]
4. Kandel, N.; Chungong, S.; Omaar, A.; Xing, J. Health security capacities in the context of COVID-19 outbreak: An analysis of International Health Regulations annual report data from 182 countries. *Lancet* **2020**, *395*, 1047–1053. [CrossRef]
5. Ferlie, E.; Pettigrew, A.; Ashburner, L.; Fitzgerald, L.; Ewan, S. *The New Public Management in Action*; Oxford University Press: Oxford, UK, 1996.
6. Eurostat. Healthcare Expenditure Statistics. 2017. Available online: https://ec.europa.eu/eurostat/statistics-explained/index.php/Healthcare_expenditure_statistics#Healthcare_expenditure (accessed on 31 December 2020).
7. Hood, C.; Dixon, R. What We Have to Show for 30 Years of New Public Management: Higher Costs, More Complaints. *Governance* **2015**, *28*, 265–267. [CrossRef]
8. Hughes, O.E. *Public Management and Administration*; Palgrave Macmillan: New York, NY, USA, 2012.
9. Nishii, L.; Gotte, A.; Raver, J.L. *Upper Echelon Theory Revisited: The Relationship Between Upper Echelon Diversity; The Adoption of Diversity Practices, and Organizational Performance*; CAHRS: Ithaca, NY, USA, 2007; pp. 1–14.

10. Hambrick, D.C.; Mason, P.A. Upper Echelons: The Organization as a Reflection of Its Top Managers. *Acad. Manag. Rev.* **1984**, *9*, 193–206. [CrossRef]
11. Carpenter, M.A.; Geletkanycz, M.A.; Sanders, W.G. Upper Echelons Research Revisited: Antecedents, Elements, and Consequences of Top Management Team Composition. *J. Manag.* **2004**, *30*, 749–778. [CrossRef]
12. Hambrick, D.C. Upper Echelons Theory: An Update. *Acad. Manag. Rev.* **2007**, *32*, 334–343. [CrossRef]
13. Dezsö, C.L.; Ross, D.G. Does female representation in top management improve firm performance? A panel data investigation. *Strat. Manag. J.* **2012**, *33*, 1072–1089. [CrossRef]
14. Peterson, R.S.; Smith, D.B.; Martorana, P.V.; Owens, P.D. The impact of chief executive officer personality on top management team dynamics: One mechanism by which leadership affects organisational performance. *J. Appl. Psychol.* **2003**, *88*, 795–808. [CrossRef] [PubMed]
15. Papadakis, V.M.; Barwise, P. How Much do CEOs and Top Managers Matter in Strategic Decision-Making? *Br. J. Manag.* **2002**, *13*, 83–95. [CrossRef]
16. Branch, G.; Hanushek, E.; Rivkin, S. *Estimating the Effect of Leaders on Public Sector Productivity: The Case of School Principals*; National Bureau of Economic Research: Cambridge, MA, USA, 2012.
17. Janke, K.; Propper, C.; Sadun, R. *The Impact of CEOs in the Public Sector: Evidence from the English NHS*; National Bureau of Economic Research: Cambridge, MA, USA, 2019.
18. Post, C.; Byron, K. Women on Boards and Firm Financial Performance: A Meta-Analysis. *Acad. Manag. J.* **2015**, *58*, 1546–1571. [CrossRef]
19. Abdullah, S.N.; Ismail, K.N.I.K.; Nachum, L. Does having women on boards create value? The impact of societal perceptions and corporate governance in emerging markets. *Strateg. Manag. J.* **2016**, *37*, 466–476. [CrossRef]
20. Shehata, N.; Salhin, A.; El-Helaly, M. Board diversity and firm performance: Evidence from the U.K. SMEs. *Appl. Econ.* **2017**, *49*, 4817–4832. [CrossRef]
21. Adams, R.B.; Ferreira, D. Women in the boardroom and their impact on governance and performance. *J. Financ. Econ.* **2009**, *94*, 291–309. [CrossRef]
22. Carter, D.A.; Dsouza, F.P.; Simkins, B.J.; Simpson, W.G. The Gender and Ethnic Diversity of US Boards and Board Committees and Firm Financial Performance. *Corp. Gov. Int. Rev.* **2010**, *18*, 396–414. [CrossRef]
23. Rhode, D.; Packel, A.K. Diversity on Corporate Boards: How Much Difference Does Difference Make? *SSRN Electron. J.* **2010**, *39*, 377–426. [CrossRef]
24. Simar, L.; Wilson, P.W. Estimation and inference in two-stage, semi-parametric models of production processes. *J. Econ.* **2007**, *136*, 31–64. [CrossRef]
25. Hoss, M.A.K.; Bobrowski, P.; McDonagh, K.J.; Paris, N.M. How gender disparities drive imbalances in health care leadership. *J. Heal. Leadersh.* **2011**, *3*, 59. [CrossRef]
26. Cheeseman-Day, A.; Christnacht, C. Women Hold 76% of all Health Care Jobs, Gaining in Higher Paying Occupations. Available online: https://www.census.gov/library/stories/2019/08/your-health-care-in-womens-hands.html (accessed on 14 August 2019).
27. Walsh, A.; Borkowski, S.C. Gender differences in factors affecting health care administration career development. *Hosp. Health Serv. Adm.* **1995**, *40*, 263.
28. Lapierre, T.A.; Zimmerman, M.K. Career advancement and gender equity in healthcare management. *Gend. Manag. Int. J.* **2012**, *27*, 100–118. [CrossRef]
29. Roemer, L. Women CEOs in Health Care: Did They Have Mentors? *Health Care Manag. Rev.* **2002**, *27*, 57–67. [CrossRef]
30. Ibarra, H.; Carter, N.M.; Silva, C. Why men still get more promotions than women. *Harv. Bus. Rev.* **2010**, *88*, 80–85.
31. Niederle, M.; Vesterlund, L. Do Women Shy Away from Competition? Do Men Compete Too Much? *Q. J. Econ.* **2007**, *122*, 1067–1101. [CrossRef]
32. Groysberg, B.; Bell, D. Dysfunction in the boardroom. *Harv. Bus. Rev.* **2013**, *91*, 89–97.
33. Apesteguia, J.; Azmat, G.; Iriberri, N. The Impact of Gender Composition on Team Performance and Decision Making: Evidence from the Field. *Manag. Sci.* **2012**, *58*, 78–93. [CrossRef]
34. Croson, R.; Gneezy, U. Gender Differences in Preferences. *J. Econ. Lit.* **2009**, *47*, 448–474. [CrossRef]
35. Huang, J.; Kisgen, D.J. Gender and corporate finance: Are male executives overconfident relative to female executives? *J. Financ. Econ.* **2013**, *108*, 822–839. [CrossRef]
36. Dezsö, C.L.; Ross, D.G. *'Girl Power': Female Participation in Top Management and Firm Performance*; University of Maryland Robert H Smith School of Business: College Park, MD, USA, 2008.
37. Khan, W.A.; Vieito, J.P. Ceo gender and firm performance. *J. Econ. Bus.* **2013**, *67*, 55–66. [CrossRef]
38. Fischer, E.M.; Reuber, A.; Dyke, L.S. A theoretical overview and extension of research on sex, gender, and entrepreneurship. *J. Bus. Ventur.* **1993**, *8*, 151–168. [CrossRef]
39. Zolin, R.; Watson, J. Gender and new venture outcomes: Not better or worse, just different. In Proceedings of the 2012 Australian Centre for Entrepreneurship Research and DIANA Conference (ACERE DIANA), Australian Centre for Entrepreneurship Research Exchange, Sydney, Australia, 3–5 February 2012; p. 118.
40. Galstian, C.; Hearld, L.; O'Connor, S.J.; Borkowski, N. The Relationship of Hospital CEO Characteristics to Patient Experience Scores. *J. Heal. Manag.* **2018**, *63*, 50–61. [CrossRef]

41. Silvera, G.A.; Clark, J.R. Women at the helm: Chief executive officer gender and patient experience in the hospital industry. *Health Care Manag. Rev.* **2019**. [CrossRef] [PubMed]
42. Gilligan, C. *In a Different Voice*; Harvard University Press: Cambridge, MA, USA, 1982.
43. Güth, W.; Levati, M.V.; Sutter, M.; Van Der Heijden, E. Leading by example with and without exclusion power in voluntary contribution experiments. *J. Public Econ.* **2007**, *91*, 1023–1042. [CrossRef]
44. Bolton, G.E.; Ockenfels, A. ERC: A Theory of Equity, Reciprocity, and Competition. *Am. Econ. Rev.* **2000**, *90*, 166–193. [CrossRef]
45. Eagly, A.H.; Carli, L.L. The female leadership advantage: An evaluation of the evidence. *Leadersh. Q.* **2003**, *14*, 807–834. [CrossRef]
46. Flett, G.L.; Hewitt, P.L.; De Rosa, T. Dimensions of perfectionism, psychosocial adjustment, and social skills. *Pers. Individ. Differ.* **1996**, *20*, 143–150. [CrossRef]
47. Manner, M.H. The Impact of CEO Characteristics on Corporate Social Performance. *J. Bus. Ethic* **2010**, *93*, 53–72. [CrossRef]
48. Jadiyappa, N.; Jyothi, P.; Sireesha, B.; Hickman, L.E. CEO gender, firm performance and agency costs: Evidence from India. *J. Econ. Stud.* **2019**, *46*, 482–495. [CrossRef]
49. Sheikh, S. The impact of market competition on the relation between CEO power and firm innovation. *J. Multinatl. Financ. Manag.* **2018**, *44*, 36–50. [CrossRef]
50. Acharya, A.G.; Pollock, T.G. Shoot for the Stars? Predicting the Recruitment of Prestigious Directors at Newly Public Firms. *Acad. Manag. J.* **2013**, *56*, 1396–1419. [CrossRef]
51. Ferris, G.R.; Perrewé, P.L.; Daniels, S.R.; Lawong, D.; Holmes, J.J. Social influence and politics in organisational research: What we know and what we need to know. *J. Leadersh. Organ. Stud.* **2017**, *24*, 5–19. [CrossRef]
52. Yetim, N. Social Capital in Female Entrepreneurship. *Int. Sociol.* **2008**, *23*, 864–885. [CrossRef]
53. McPherson, M.; Smith-Lovin, L.; Cook, J.M. Birds of a Feather: Homophily in Social Networks. *Annu. Rev. Sociol.* **2001**, *27*, 415–444. [CrossRef]
54. Lazarsfeld, P.F.; Merton, R.K. Friendship as a social process: A substantive and methodological analysis. *Freedom Control Mod. Soc.* **1954**, *18*, 18–66.
55. Terjesen, S.; Sealy, R.; Singh, V. Women Directors on Corporate Boards: A Review and Research Agenda. *Corp. Governance: Int. Rev.* **2009**, *17*, 320–337. [CrossRef]
56. Huang, J.; Diehl, M.R.; Paterlini, S. The influence of corporate elites on women on supervisory boards: Female di-rectors' inclusion in Germany. *J. Bus. Ethics* **2020**, *165*, 347–364. [CrossRef]
57. McDonald, M.L.; Westphal, J.D. Access Denied: Low Mentoring of Women and Minority First-Time Directors and Its Negative Effects on Appointments to Additional Boards. *Acad. Manag. J.* **2013**, *56*, 1169–1198. [CrossRef]
58. Ridgeway, C.L.; Correll, S.J. Limiting Inequality through Interaction: The End(s) of Gender. *Contemp. Sociol. A J. Rev.* **2000**, *29*, 110. [CrossRef]
59. Ding, W.W.; Murray, F.; Stuart, T.E. From Bench to Board: Gender Differences in University Scientists' Participation in Corporate Scientific Advisory Boards. *Acad. Manag. J.* **2013**, *56*, 1443–1464. [CrossRef]
60. Oakley, J.G. Gender-based Barriers to Senior Management Positions: Understanding the Scarcity of Female CEOs. *J. Bus. Ethics* **2000**, *27*, 321–334. [CrossRef]
61. Elsaid, E.; Ursel, N.D. Re-examining the Glass Cliff Hypothesis using Survival Analysis: The Case of Female CEO Tenure. *Br. J. Manag.* **2018**, *29*, 156–170. [CrossRef]
62. Boyd, D.; Crawford, K. Critical questions for big data: Provocations for a cultural, technological, and scholarly phenomenon. *Inf. Commun. Soc.* **2012**, *15*, 662–679. [CrossRef]
63. Mulcahy, M.; Linehan, C. Females and Precarious Board Positions: Further Evidence of the Glass Cliff. *Br. J. Manag.* **2014**, *25*, 425–438. [CrossRef]
64. Ryan, M.K.; Haslam, S.A. The Glass Cliff: Evidence that Women are Over-Represented in Precarious Leadership Positions. *Br. J. Manag.* **2005**, *16*, 81–90. [CrossRef]
65. Wagner, J.M.; Shimshak, D.G. Stepwise selection of variables in data envelopment analysis: Procedures and managerial perspectives. *Eur. J. Oper. Res.* **2007**, *180*, 57–67. [CrossRef]
66. Cooper, W.W.; Seiford, L.M.; Zhu, J. Data envelopment analysis: History, models, and interpretations. In *Handbook on Data Envelopment Analysis. International Series in Operations Research and Management Science*; Cooper, W., Seiford, L., Zhu, J., Eds.; Springer: Boston, MA, USA, 2011; Volume 164.
67. Gerdtham, U.G.; Löthgren, M.; Tambour, M.; Rehnberg, C. Internal markets and health care efficiency: A multiple output stochastic frontier analysis. *Health Econ.* **1999**, *8*, 151–164. [CrossRef]
68. Battilana, J.; Dorado, S. Building sustainable hybrid organisations: The case of commercial microfinance organisations. *Acad. Manag. J.* **2010**, *53*, 1419–1440. [CrossRef]
69. Magnussen, J. Efficiency measurement and the operationalisation of hospital production. *Health Serv. Res.* **1996**, *31*, 21–37.
70. Morey, R.; Fine, D.; Loree, S. Comparing the allocative efficiencies of hospitals. *Omega* **1990**, *18*, 71–83. [CrossRef]
71. McCallion, G.; McKillop, D.G.; Glass, J.C.; Kerr, C. Rationalising Northern Ireland hospital services towards larger providers: Best-practice efficiency studies and current policy. *Public Money Manag.* **1999**, *19*, 27–32. [CrossRef]
72. Tiemann, O.; Schreyögg, J. Effects of ownership on hospital efficiency in Germany. *Bus. Res.* **2009**, *2*, 115–145. [CrossRef]
73. Tiemann, O.; Schreyögg, J. Changes in hospital efficiency after privatisation. *Health Care Manag. Sci.* **2012**, *15*, 1–17. [CrossRef]

74. Linna, M.; Häkkinen, U.; Magnussen, J. Comparing hospital cost efficiency between Norway and Finland. *Health Policy* **2006**, *77*, 268–278. [CrossRef]
75. Banker, R.D.; Natarajan, R. Evaluating Contextual Variables Affecting Productivity Using Data Envelopment Analysis. *Oper. Res.* **2008**, *56*, 48–58. [CrossRef]
76. Farrell, M.J. The Measurement of Productive Efficiency. *J. R. Stat. Soc. Ser. A (General)* **1957**, *120*, 253–290. [CrossRef]
77. Drake, L.; Hall, M.J.; Simper, R. The impact of macroeconomic and regulatory factors on bank efficiency: A non-parametric analysis of Hong Kong's banking system. *J. Bank. Financ.* **2006**, *30*, 1443–1466. [CrossRef]
78. Charnes, A.; Cooper, W.W.; Rhodes, E. Measuring the efficiency of decision making units. *Eur. J. Oper. Res.* **1978**, *2*, 429–444. [CrossRef]
79. Banker, R.D.; Charnes, A.; Cooper, W.W. Some Models for Estimating Technical and Scale Inefficiencies in Data Envelopment Analysis. *Manag. Sci.* **1984**, *30*, 1078–1092. [CrossRef]
80. Greene, W. *Econometric Analysis*, 5th ed.; Prentice-Hall: Upper Saddle River, NJ, USA, 2003.
81. Dah, M.A.; Jizi, M.I.; Kebbe, R. CEO gender and managerial entrenchment. *Res. Int. Bus. Financ.* **2020**, *54*, 101237. [CrossRef]
82. Glass, C.; Cook, A. Do women leaders promote positive change? Analysing the effect of gender on business practices and diversity initiatives. *Hum. Resour. Manag.* **2017**, *57*, 823–837. [CrossRef]
83. Vecchio, R.P. Leadership and gender advantage. *Leadersh. Q.* **2002**, *13*, 643–671. [CrossRef]
84. Buttner, E.H. Examining Female Entrepreneurs' Management Style: An Application of a Relational Frame. *J. Bus. Ethics* **2001**, *29*, 253–269. [CrossRef]
85. Strebler, M. *Skills, Competencies and Gender: Issues for Pay and Training*; Grantham Book Services: Grantham, UK, 1997.
86. Lundeberg, M.A.; Fox, P.W.; Punćcohaŕ, J. Highly confident but wrong: Gender differences and similarities in confidence judgments. *J. Educ. Psychol.* **1994**, *86*, 114. [CrossRef]
87. Chen, G.; Crossland, C.; Huang, S. Female board representation and corporate acquisition intensity. *Strat. Manag. J.* **2014**, *37*, 303–313. [CrossRef]
88. Sabharwal, M. From Glass Ceiling to Glass Cliff: Women in Senior Executive Service. *J. Public Adm. Res. Theory* **2015**, *25*, 399–426. [CrossRef]
89. Weil, P.A.; Mattis, M.C. Narrowing the gender gap in healthcare management. *Healthc. Exec.* **2001**, *16*, 12–17. [PubMed]
90. Zhang, Y.A.; Qu, H. The Impact of CEO Succession with Gender Change on Firm Performance and Successor Early Departure: Evidence from China's Publicly Listed Companies in 1997–2010. *Acad. Manag. J.* **2016**, *59*, 1845–1868. [CrossRef]
91. Moreno-Gómez, J.; Lafuente, E.; Vaillant, Y. Gender diversity in the board, women's leadership and business performance. *Gend. Manag. Int. J.* **2018**, *33*, 104–122. [CrossRef]
92. Vuong, Q.H. Reform retractions to make them more transparent. *Nature* **2020**, *582*, 149. [CrossRef]
93. Gupta, V.K.; Mortal, S.C.; Guo, X. Revisiting the gender gap in CEO compensation: Replication and extension of Hill, Upadhyay, and Beekun's (2015) work on CEO gender pay gap. *Strat. Manag. J.* **2018**, *39*, 2036–2050. [CrossRef]
94. Hill, A.D.; Upadhyay, A.D.; Beekun, R.I. Do female and ethnically diverse executives endure inequity in the CEO position or do they benefit from their minority status? An empirical examination. *Strat. Manag. J.* **2015**, *36*, 1115–1134. [CrossRef]
95. Vuong, Q.-H. The (ir)rational consideration of the cost of science in transition economies. *Nat. Hum. Behav.* **2018**, *2*, 5. [CrossRef] [PubMed]

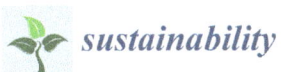

Article

Understanding the Spatial-Related Abstraction of Public Health Impact Goals and Measures: Illustrated by the Example of the Austrian Action Plan on Women's Health

Tatjana Fischer

Institute of Spatial Planning, Environmental Planning and Land Rearrangement,
University of Natural Resources and Life Sciences Vienna, Peter-Jordan-Straße 82, 1190 Vienna, Austria;
tatjana.fischer@boku.ac.at

Abstract: The influence of spatial aspects on people's health is internationally proven by a wealth of empirical findings. Nevertheless, questions concerning public health still tend to be negotiated among social and health scientists. This was different in the elaboration of the Austrian Action Plan on Women's Health (AAPWH). On the example of the target group of older women, it is shown whether and to what extent the inclusion of the spatial planning perspective in the discussion of impact goals and measures is reflected in the respective inter-ministerial policy paper. The retrospective analysis on the basis of a document analysis of the AAPWH and qualitative interviews with public health experts who were also invited to join, or rather were part of, the expert group, brings to light the following key reasons for the high degree of spatial-related abstraction of the content of this strategic health policy paper: the requirement for general formulations, the lack of public and political awareness for the different living situations in different spatial archetypes, and the lack of external perception of spatial planning as a key discipline with regard to the creation of equivalent living conditions. Nonetheless, this research has promoted the external perception of spatial planning as a relevant discipline in public health issues in Austria. Furthermore, first thematic starting points for an in-depth interdisciplinary dialogue were identified.

Keywords: space–health nexus; older women; spatial planning perspective; interdisciplinary expert dialogue; retrospective qualitative study; knowledge transfer; health policy analysis

Citation: Fischer, T. Understanding the Spatial-Related Abstraction of Public Health Impact Goals and Measures: Illustrated by the Example of the Austrian Action Plan on Women's Health. *Sustainability* **2021**, *13*, 773. https://doi.org/10.3390/su13020773

Received: 17 November 2020
Accepted: 12 January 2021
Published: 14 January 2021

Publisher's Note: MDPI stays neutral with regard to jurisdictional claims in published maps and institutional affiliations.

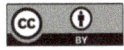

Copyright: © 2021 by the author. Licensee MDPI, Basel, Switzerland. This article is an open access article distributed under the terms and conditions of the Creative Commons Attribution (CC BY) license (https://creativecommons.org/licenses/by/4.0/).

1. Introduction

Women's health is in the focus of global interest [1,2] and therefore is a central concern of the WHO [3]. In line with the health-in-all-policies approach of the WHO, health should be implemented in all policies and become a focal subject of political action [4] in order to achieve the following UN Sustainability Goals [5]: SDG 3 "Good Health and Well-being" (in particular sub-target 3.8) [5] (p. 71), SDG 11 "Sustainable Cities and Communities" (in particular sub-targets 11.3, 11.7 and 11.a) [5] (p. 73) and SDG 17 "Partnerships for the Goals" (in particular sub-targets 17.14 and 17.17) [5] (p. 76).

In Austria (women's) health is already an important public responsibility [6,7]. This becomes evident when it comes to the international comparison of the availability and quality of the supply structures of health care facilities [8,9], the life expectancy of women (at old age) [10] and self-rated state of health [11]. Nevertheless, in Austria regional differences in the provision of ambulant social and care services and the spatial distribution of in-patient health and care facilities exist [12]. Other relevant issues are the increase in the absolute and relative proportion of older women in the population and a growing heterogeneity of women relating to educational level, fertility behavior and economic status related to life phases [13,14].

The Austrian Action Plan on Women's Health (AAPWH) [15] starts exactly here and defines general and target group-specific impact goals and measures in order to better satisfy the various needs and demands of women for the promotion of physical and mental health, taking into account the current position in the life cycle. Therefore, the AAPWH refers to the following three target groups: (1) "Girls and Young Women", referring to females going through puberty, or rather females aged 12 to 16 years [15] (p. 42), (2) "Women of Working Age", referring to women up to 60 years of age [15] (p. 53) and (3) "Older Women", referring to women aged 60 and older, or rather to women of retirement age [15] (p. 69).

1.1. AAPWH in Brief

The Austrian Action Plan on Women's Health (AAPWH) as an inter-ministerial strategic policy paper of the Federal Ministry of Social Affairs, Health and Consumer Protection and the Federal Ministry of Women, Families and Youth, Federal Chancellery of the Republic of Austria is unique in Europe [16].

It comprises ninety-eight pages and defines seventeen impact goals and forty measures and aims in order to achieve equity in the quality of life of women in Austria, which is fully in line with the European Health Goals [17] and in accordance with the principle of "leaving no one behind" [18].

Following the Health 2020 policy framework [19], the AAPWH was elaborated in an interdisciplinary and inter-ministerial development process consisting of sixty invited experts from different disciplines and an additional online-consultation process [15].

The AAPWH is published in German and is available online [20].

1.2. The Leading Role of Public Health and the Inclusion of the Author in the Circle of Public Health Experts

At the time the AAPWH was prepared, in Austria public health and women's health mainly were discussed among (public) health, nursing and social care experts, although health is a central subject of spatial planning due to the close interrelations between health and spatial aspects [21–23]. Moreover, spatial planning is perceived as a key scientific and policy sector-relevant discipline for public health [24]—particularly in the context of healthy cities [25].

The author of this article was therefore pleased to be invited to join the expert group on "Women in Old Age" on the recommendation of an expert who played a key role in the elaboration of the AAPHW.

With the participation in the expert group which dealt with public health impact goals and measures for older women, the author pursued two purposes: (1) raising the awareness of the working group members of the necessity of to taking into account the spatial dimension in the definition of impact goals and measures in the short run and (2) involving spatial planning as a cross-cutting, system- and action-oriented key professional discipline in the discussion on demand and supply planning in the long run by addressing:

1. The spatial-related reasons for health inequality (of women) and how they influence the future quality of ageing and being old in different spatial contexts or rather spatial archetypes, as well as to the negative consequences of an ongoing spatial polarization in structurally strong and structurally weak regions and
2. Presenting spatial planning approaches to create equivalent living conditions.

2. The Purpose of the Paper

This article discusses whether and to what extent the interdisciplinary discussion of health policy impact goals and measures, including the expertise of spatial planning, generates merit for evidence-informed health policy [26] with a focus on the target group of older women.

In the following paper this is illustrated by the example of the AAPWH. In this context, this Austrian pilot study addresses the following aspects:

1. The opportunities for and limitations of raising the awareness of public health experts about the relevance of the spatial dimension in defining impact goals and measures.
2. The factors that determine the degree of spatial abstraction of target group-specific impact goals and measures.
3. The frontiers of knowledge implementation in strategic policy papers.
4. Recommendations for spatial planning scholars who are interested in, or rather already engaged in, inter-sectoral collaboration and issues of public health.

Thus, this research not only fills a knowledge gap in Austria, but also complements the findings of (recent) thematically related studies from other European countries, namely the Netherlands [27] and the United Kingdom [28], which for their part discuss the need for and the merit of inter-sectoral collaboration between the public health and spatial planning sectors for the purpose of alleviating health inequalities on the basis of selected health-related (national) policy papers. In comparison to the study from Austria presented in this article, the above-mentioned studies neither focus on one specific target group, nor do they discuss the degree of spatial-relatedness of the formulated impact goals and measures in more detail.

3. The Space–Health Nexus and the Relevance of Spatial Planning

Space and health are interlinked in manifold ways. Amongst others, the availability and quality of affordable housing, the level of infrastructural provision for daily supply as well as for social, medical and nursing care, being embedded in a stable social surrounding and neighborhood, having access to a safe public space and the availability of accessible green and open spaces determine the well-being and quality of life, particularly of older people. This applies in particular to those who suffer from health restrictions, or rather dementia [22,29–32]. Against the background of demographic and climate change, particular importance must be attached to all of these aspects [33,34].

In this context, the particularities of different spatial archetypes (e.g., cities, small towns, remote rural areas) with regard to supply structures and the degree of supply with infrastructure, as well as public and open (green) spaces, but also with regard to the availability and structure of social networks, must not be disregarded. For example, the infrastructural supply in larger cities compared to rural, sparsely populated areas is more diverse and characterized by short trips, whereas rural areas tend to be better equipped with open or rather green spaces within walking distance [12,22]. With regard to infrastructure supply and accessibility, ageing in the rural periphery, or rather in dispersed (alpine) settlement structures, is particularly challenging [35].

Due to the continuing polarization in structurally strong and weak regions, the different supply structures with hospitals [36], the trend towards the retention of doctors in rural areas [37], changes of family and household structures as well as quality of ageing and being old differ not only between urban centers and rural peripheries, but also within a single municipality in alpine areas and dispersed settlement structures due to the lack of a comprehensive, adequate public transport system and the spatial locations of infrastructure and one's own place of residence [12].

Therefore, following the principle of health-in-all policies, the main task of spatial planning is to ensure an appropriate land use in order to provide people with green spaces, building land and traffic areas and to balance competing interests and needs, in order to provide livable settlement structures for people at all stages of life [22].

In German-speaking countries spatial planning as a cross-cutting subject and in its policy advisory function in connection with health issues in general and with regard to older people in particular takes on the following important tasks:

1. Ongoing spatial observation for the purpose of identifying changes in the infrastructural supply levels as well as for the derivation of fields of action, options and measures [12,38]
2. Identifying the right places for allocating (new) infrastructure as well as maintaining stable infrastructures [12]

3. The development of concepts and strategies that serve to create equal opportunities in access to infrastructure at the regional level [39].

Nonetheless, in Austria spatial planning is still is not involved in the strategic development of social care and health provision planning [12].

4. The Expert Group on "Women in Old Age"

The following initial situation formed the starting point for the expert group's discussions on impact goals and measures in the areas of health protection and health promotion of older women: their economic disadvantage compared to men of the same age; the special challenges in connection with role attributions and expectations with regard to the assumption of care for older people; and ageism [15].

In total, 35 national experts from various public health related professions and professional positions participated in this expert group in order to deal with the subject of women's health against the backdrop of various professional contexts. Four out of the 35 experts were men.

The participants held, or rather still hold, positions in administration (federal ministries, divisions for gender equality in the offices of federal governments), science and practice (amongst others, women's health care facilities, professional agencies, social insurance institutions, interest groups). An overview of the members of the expert group is provided in AAPHW [15], pages 85 and 86. Depending on their professional skills, some of the experts also joined the two working groups "Girls and Young Women" and "Women of Working Age".

Between April and November 2015, the expert group on "Women in Old Age" elaborated four target group-specific impact goals and ten measures and considered cross-target group-related impact goals and measures, taking into account already existing initiatives, projects and actors' landscapes in Austria. The number of impact goals and measures was predefined.

During this period the working group met three times for full-day workshops in Vienna (cf. Table 1).

Table 1. Overview of the agendas and working methods of the workshops of the expert group on "Women in Old Age".

Number of Workshop	Date, Location and Duration	Agenda [1]	Working Methods
Workshop No. 1	28 April 2015, Federal Ministry of Social Affairs, Health and Consumer Protection, 10.00 a.m. to 5 p.m.	Presentation of the project "Austrian Action Plan on Women's Health", Keynote speech given by the expert group leader Stocktaking of initiatives, and projects: focus on "Women in Old Age" and Development of 3 to 4 key topics Impact goals for the prioritized key topics	PowerPoint-presentation in plenary working in small groups/World Café (guided by key questions, result documentation using flipcharts) plenary discussion
Workshop No. 2	26 May 2015, Austrian National Public Health Institute, 10.00 a.m. to 5 p.m.	Retrospection on the project activities and results so far Feedback on the impact goals from the organizations involved in the making of AAPWH Completion of impact goals Compilation of good practices, agreements, Laws, regulations, concepts related to the impact goals Description of measures related to the impact goals and collection of ideas for cross-age topics Suggestions for the AAPWH's monitoring prioritization of measures	PowerPoint-presentation discussions in small groups and plenary discussion
Workshop No. 3	10 November 2015, Austrian National Public Health Institute, 10.00 a.m. to 5 p.m.	Discussion of the results of the online consultation and Project finalization [2]	PowerPoint-presentation and plenary discussion

[1] Sources: Minutes of Workshops No. 1 and No. 2 [40,41], [2] Source: Notes by the author of this paper. There are no minutes for Workshop No. 3.

The workshops were moderated and documented by the Austrian National Public Health Institute and the minutes were sent out to the expert group members by e-mail. Additionally, the experts were asked to seize the timespan between the workshops in order to prepare for the following session by completing defined work tasks.

5. Materials and Methods

5.1. Research Design

This is a qualitative, retrospective and descriptive research applying a mixed-methods approach which consists of (1) a theme-centered document analysis of the AAPWH focusing on the above-mentioned aspects and (2) semi-structured expert interviews with members of the expert group on "Women in Old Age" (cf. Figure 1) in order to avoid any misinterpretation from the author's reflection of the handwritten notes of the three workshops.

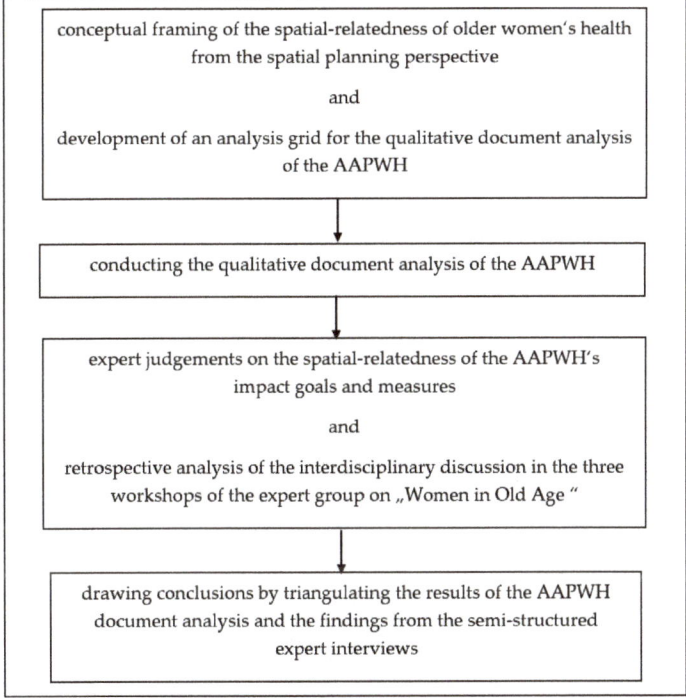

Figure 1. Research design and methodological steps.

As this research does not contain any experimental studies on human beings, no approval from an ethics committee was required. The research was carried out in compliance with the General Data Protection Regulation of the European Union.

5.2. Procedure

5.2.1. Development of an Analysis Grid for the Document Analysis of the AAPWH

As shown in Section 3, the interrelations between space and health (in old age) are complex and the (further) development of health protection and health promotion measures depends on the existing infrastructural level, the authorities and their legal competencies—in Austria the public health sector is characterized by federalism [42]—the financial margins of action in both the public and private sectors, and the heterogeneity of the (potential) demanders (among women in old age).

Basing on the author's research findings on the spatial-related challenges of the everyday life in old age as well as of caring for the elderly for various Austrian spatial contexts, the document analysis of the AAPWH addressed the following aspects:

1. The challenges of organizing and coping with everyday life, including the accessibility of infrastructure and the social inclusion of physically impaired, or rather mobility-reduced, older people, taking into account topography (alpine rural areas), settlement structures, population density, infrastructural supply structures, (limited) freedom of choice related to goods and services and changes in family and other social networks, as well as considering the differences between urban and rural places of residence [22,35,43]
2. The relevance of the region as the appropriate spatial reference of action with regard to the allocation of cost-intensive social infrastructures and the importance of regional centers or so-called central places as a result of the financially limited opportunities for action of low-income and/or ageing municipalities [12,44]
3. Taking into account the stakeholder group of long-distance caregivers. This group is considered to be of great importance in quantitative terms in Austria [45] due to the ongoing polarization into prosperous and unfavorable regions on the one hand and thus, regions with continuing population loss and growing urban centers on the other hand.

5.2.2. Document Analysis of the AAPWH

The analysis of the spatial-related aspects of the impact goals and measures addressing the target group "Women in Old Age" was carried out by means of a theme-centered document analysis according to Boyatzis [46] without the use of specific software. The procedure was as follows:

- In the first screening, the spatial references were checked. For this purpose, the text was searched for the following terms: "city/urban/urban space", "land/rural/rural space"; "local/communal"; "region/regional"; "municipality/district/province"; "public space/social space".
- In the second screening, the causalities between the state of health (or rather disadvantages and health inequalities) of women in old age and their housing and living environments were checked. To this end, all text paragraphs marked in the first screening as well as all impact goals and measures relevant to the target group on "Women in Old Age" were checked.
- In the third screening, interlinkages between the results of the first and the second screening were searched for. Moreover, the impact goals and measures were analyzed with a view to spatial-related differentiations of the theme-related recommendations for action.
- In the fourth screening, the AAPWH was checked for paragraphs which relate to a call for a more interdisciplinary (scientific) debate on the determinants of women's health. For this, the search terms "interdisciplinary" and "interdisciplinarity" were chosen.

5.2.3. Expert Judgements

The idea was to reflect on the spatial-related contents of the AAPWH and the discussion on the relevance of spatial-related aspects of well-being and health in older women in the context of the three workshops of the expert group on "Women in Old Age". For that purpose, semi-structured in-depth expert interviews were conducted with those members of the respective expert group who joined at least two out of the three workshops.

Aim of Expert Survey and Design of Questionnaire

The aim of the survey was to identify the key arguments of the experts: (1) regarding the reasons for the degree of spatial abstraction of the AAPHW's impact goals and measures for the target group of "Women in Old Age"; (2) to grasp the interviewed experts' perceptions of spatial planning experts (both, scientists and practitioners) as dialogue partners in the context of public health issues, and; (3) to explore the limitations of implementing profession-specific knowledge and spatial-related empirical evidence in strategic policy papers.

Based on the conceptual framework of the spatial relatedness of (women's) health in old age, the findings from the qualitative content analysis of the AAPWH, the workshop minutes as well as on the author's own handwritten notes, a catalogue of guiding questions consisting of 16 open questions was developed (cf. Table 2).

Table 2. Questionnaire for the expert interviews.

Theme	Questions (Verbatim)
General questions on the three workshops of the expert group on "Women in old age"	Q 1: How did you experience the interdisciplinary debate on the topic of "women in old age and health"? What challenges—in your opinion—were associated with the comprehensibility of the argumentation of experts from other disciplines?
Interrelations between health and space	Q 2: What do you associate with the terms "space" and "place"?" Q 3: What do you associate with the term "urban"? Q 4: What do you associate with the term "rural"? Q 5: If you interlink the three terms "rural", "older women" and "health", what will come to your mind? Q 6: How do you define quality of life? Q 7: What spatial aspects do you associate with "good" or "bad" quality of life in old age?
Perception of spatial planning as a professional discipline and retrospection on the discussions during the workshops	Q 8: What do you associate with the term "spatial planning"? Q 9: Did you deal with "spatial planning" as a discipline before the workshops? Q 10: What competences or fields of expertise do you ascribe to spatial planning? Q 11: What, in your opinion, constitutes "good spatial planning", and who do you think is responsible for that? Q 12: How did you experience the introduction of spatial planning arguments during the discussions in the workshops? Do you remember something special of it? If so, why and what? If not, why not? Q 13: Has "acquaintance with spatial planning" changed a) your perception of the discipline of spatial planning, b) your awareness of the relevance of spatial aspects to the quality of getting old (as a women), c) your way of thinking and reasoning? (Please explain.) Q 14: How do you deal with the fact that the target group-specific impact goals and measures are characterized by a high level of abstraction in spatial terms?
Outlook	Q 15: How, in your opinion, could it succeed in future to anchor spatial aspects more firmly in health and care-related policy papers as well as in public health recommendations for action? Q 16: May I ask you for your further thoughts.

Sampling and Data Collection

As mentioned above, this research intended to gather the opinion of those experts who joined in with the whole discussion process on impact goals and measures for women in old age. The selection criterion was defined as presence in at least two out of the three workshops. The experts were identified by comparing the attendance lists of the available workshop minutes. Twelve experts met the selection criteria. In January 2018 the experts were contacted by e-mail. Six out of twelve could be recruited for an interview.

The questionnaire was sent out to all experts by e-mail a few days prior to the interview in order to give them the opportunity to prepare for it.

The interviews took place between January and March 2018. In order to meet the preferences of the interviewees, the interviews took place either at their workplaces, by telephone or in external locations such as cafés. The interviews lasted at least 60 min and were recorded on tape.

Five out of the six interviewees gave their oral consent to use the findings for a poster presentation at the biannual conference of the Austrian Society for Geriatrics and

Gerontology in March 2018 in Austria [47] and for international publications on occasion. After the conference, the poster was sent out to the five interviewees as a PDF-file by e-mail.

Due to the fact that saturation had not yet been reached, the author decided to increase the sample size. Finally, two more national public health experts were interviewed in May 2018. One of them was invited to the expert group on "Women in Old Age", too, but did not attend the workshops; the other expert held and still holds a relevant position in the AAPHW development and implementation process. For these two interviews the same catalogue of guiding questions was applied as for the first wave of interviews—except for the questions Q 1, Q 12 and Q 13. That is why the interviews lasted about 30 min each.

The author of this paper pursued the strategy to recruit as many members of the expert group on "Women in Old Age" as possible for interviews. However, this was challenging due to the fact that some of the experts were on maternity leave or had since retired.

Finally, seven expert judgements were available for further analysis. Table 3 gives an overview of the profiles of all interviewed experts.

Table 3. Profile of the interviewed experts.

Identifier of the Interview Partners	Gender	Educational Background/Place of Work	Interview Method/Date of Interview
Interviewee 1	female	nursing and health care, humanities/ public health institution	live one-to-one interview, 19 January 2018
Interviewee 2	female	medical sciences/ health care facility	live one-to-one interview, 22 January 2018
Interviewee 3	female	nursing and health care/ professional association	live one-to-one interview, 23 January 2018
Interviewee 4	female	public health, nursing, social sciences/ interest group	live one-to-one interview, 30 January 2018
Interviewee 5	female	journalism and communication sciences/ interest group	phone interview, 27 February 2018
Interviewee 6	female	nursing and health care, humanities, public health/ blue-light organization	live one-to-one interview, 4 May 2018
Interviewee 7	female	natural sciences/ federal authority	live one-to-one interview, 4 May 2018
Interviewee 8 [1]	female	social work/ professional association	live one-to-one interview, 5 March 2018

Due to the small sample size, the respective function of the interviewees in the elaboration process of the Austrian Action Plan on Women's Health (AAPHW) as well as the exact designation of their place of work are not listed for data protection reasons. [1] This interviewee withdrew her consent to publish the results of the interview without giving any reasons.

Data Extraction

The tape recordings of the seven expert interviews were listened to several times and transcribed mutatis mutandis. Particularly pithy statements were transcribed verbatim in order to use them as direct quotations in this article.

The transcripts, which consist of four to six handwritten manuscript pages each, were analyzed according to the method of continuous comparison by Glaser and Strauss [48].

6. Results

6.1. Findings from the Document Analysis

It should be noted that the AAPWH argues that discrimination against women in terms of access to services regardless of age is associated with income, migration background and social disintegration, and not with where women live, work and care. Nationwide equal opportunities of access to infrastructure and other services is requested.

The content analysis shows that spatial aspects serve to describe the background of the challenges or disadvantages faced by older women. For example, with regard to the issue of violence prevention (Measure 5), the reference to public space is directly addressed. The term "violence in the public social space" is used here [15] (p. 33).

With regard to those impact goals and measures which specifically address the target group of older women, spatial-related aspects found their way in the text as follows:

- Spatial-related challenges in organizing and coping with everyday life
- The region as spatial reference of action as an appropriate spatial reference level for infrastructure measures

Impact Goal 17 *"Developing a differentiated, appreciative picture of the diverse realities of older women's lives and secure older women's opportunities for participation in society"* [15] (p. 79) identifies spatial-related challenges of organizing and coping with everyday life are referring to the need to *"design a public and safe space"* as a structural prerequisite for the *"social participation of older women"* [15] (p. 79). This is explained in more detail by *"Measure 38 Improving the living situation and ensuring the participation opportunities of older women in the long term"* [15] (p. 80f): *"Scientifically sound findings on the life situation of older women enable the targeted promotion of diverse, high-quality projects, initiatives and events close to home to ensure the participation opportunities of older women and to improve their life situation. The target group of this measure are in particular older women who are living alone, women with health restrictions, structurally caused mobility impairments and women with low income. Since there are differences between urban and rural areas with regard to older women's opportunities for participation, all activities must take into account spatially specific aspects"* [15] (p. 80f).

This measure expresses the awareness of spatial-related challenges experienced by older women with reduced mobility and limited participation opportunities and points out the importance of local daily supply structures and supportive initiatives.

The terms "urban", "rural" and "space-specific" are used in the text for the purpose of pointing out spatial differences.

Impact Goal 14 *"Ensuring gender-appropriate, individualized medical, psychosocial and nursing care up to old age, regardless of the [spatial] setting"* [15] (p. 71) addresses the need for nationwide and accessible infrastructures. This is specified by *"Measure 32 Establishing regional platforms for women's health"* [15] (p. 72), which is envisaged as a short-term measure and which refers to a specific spatial reference of action.

The regional level as an appropriate spatial reference of action is also addressed in Impact Goal 16 *"Women at old age and at risk of poverty are given conditions that enable them to maintain their capabilities for self-help and to live self-determined and autonomous lives"* [15] (p. 78). *"Measure 37 Establishing a one-stop shop"* for the application for and processing of *social benefits and for care counselling"* [15] (p. 79), which is assigned to this impact goal, may—among other measures—facilitate access to counselling and information services for women at risk of poverty in structurally weak rural areas—especially if the so-called "one-stop shops" are established regionally.

However, the term "region" is not further specified with regard to its catchment area or accessibility for older people who are not, or rather who are no longer capable of, driving a car.

On the other hand, the following objectives of the author of this paper are not directly addressed in the AAPHW:

- The subject of "long-distance caregiving". Nonetheless, this issue is addressed by Impact Goal 15 *"Creating framework conditions that enable the currently mainly female caregivers to maintain their own health, self-determination and dignity"* [15] (p. 74), specified by short-term *"Measure 36 Sensitizing companies to the situation of caregiving relatives and establishing counselling services"* [15] (p. 77).
- The mention of spatial planning as a crucial discipline in the discussion of (older) women's well-being and health. Nevertheless, the need for more interdisciplinarity was put in writing. This is shown by medium-term *"Measure 31 Strengthening interdisciplinary research on health issues specific to women in the third and fourth phases of life"* [15] (p. 72), which is related to Impact Goal 14 *"Ensuring gender-appropriate, individualized medical, psychosocial and nursing care up to old age, regardless of setting"* [15] (p. 71).

6.2. Findings from the Expert Interviews

According to the interviewed experts, the empirical findings presented in this section can be understood as the outcome of many years of professional experience, being up to date with the latest scientific knowledge (in some cases) as well as personal experiences and stories from the experts' private lives.

6.2.1. The Meaning of Space and Place for the Health of Older Women and the Urban–Rural Mindset

The interviewees conceptualized the terms "space" and "place" in different ways, addressing the material, or rather physical and social, characteristics of place, which in their view are relevant to the health of older women. Thus, they addressed selected features that are also assessed as important by geographical gerontologists [49]. From the point of view of the interviewed experts, "place" is a construct of natural surroundings, human intervention and political categorization. The significance for (older) women's health shows in several ways (cf. Figure 2):

1. The basic importance of unspoiled nature and appropriate sanitary conditions
2. Space as a basic prerequisite for personal development
3. The importance of opportunities for social participation. Therefore, space is *"a sphere where people are living together"* (I 6).

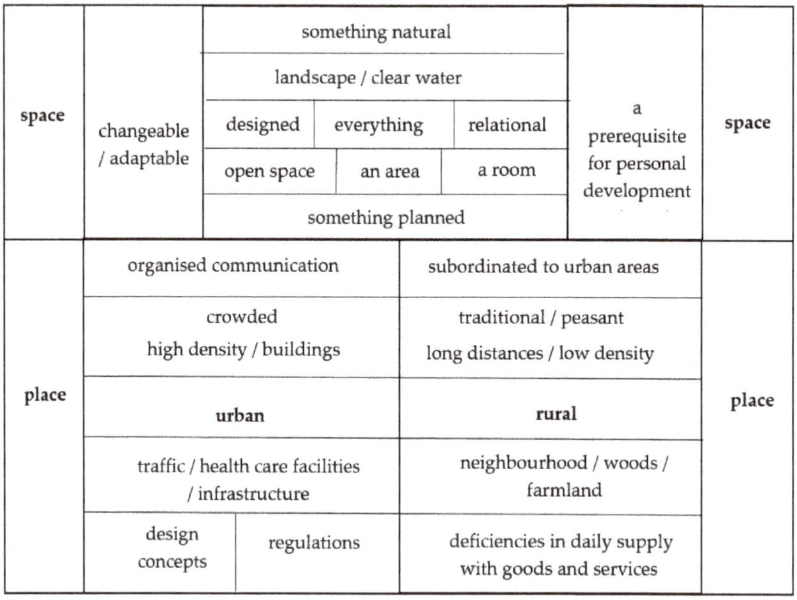

space	changeable / adaptable	something natural			a prerequisite for personal development	space
		landscape / clear water				
		designed	everything	relational		
		open space	an area	a room		
		something planned				
place	organised communication		subordinated to urban areas		place
	crowded high density / buildings		traditional / peasant long distances / low density		
	urban		**rural**		
	traffic / health care facilities / infrastructure		neighbourhood / woods / farmland		
	design concepts	regulations	deficiencies in daily supply with goods and services		

Figure 2. Public health experts' conceptualization of "space" and "place".

The interviewees thought in distinct spatial categories: "urban" and "rural" areas. Above all, they associated urban areas with high density and diversity of infrastructure, and rural areas with the exact opposite; low density and challenges with regard to the supply of goods and services in daily demand, and the provision of socio-medical services as well as the resulting restrictions in freedom of choice and accessibility of services and facilities.

6.2.2. Perceived Spatial-Related Challenges for Maintaining and Improving Quality of Life and Health of Women in Old Age in Urban and Rural Areas and the Tendency of Marginalization of Women Living in Rural Areas

From the interviewees' perspective, the quality of the built environment and of nature have a significant impact on health (see also [50]). In their opinion, it is essential to point out that the quality of housing and the living environment as well as the characteristics of the social networks of older women living in urban and rural areas differ fundamentally, which in turn results in differences in health care provision and quality of life for women in old age.

According to the interviewees, infrastructural deficiencies, long distances and a lack of public transport, eroding social networks and structural barriers in the built and residential environment coupled with health restrictions lead to challenges for living an independent life and participating in social life for women of all ages, regardless of the location of the place of residence. In the opinion of one interviewee, "*security in and of public spaces*" (I 3) is a key issue for older women living in cities.

The marginalization of especially very old women without a driving license in rural areas is the result of a thinned-out infrastructure supply, the lack of adequate cultural offerings, and poor public transport outside the main centers and villages. The changes of family structures and social environments imply a decline in informal support and increased loneliness. One interviewee commented as follows: "*In my opinion the interrelations of rurality, quality of life and women's health are more negative than positive—in the sense of a double devaluation. First, women care for men. The women are left behind. Second, women have no voice in society. Therefore, it is not so important to take care of them.*" (I 1)

Furthermore, related to the need of action, rural areas are perceived as subordinated to urban areas. According to one interviewee, the reasons for that are also rooted in misunderstandings, for example with regard to the quality of social cohesion: "*When they think of rural areas people are of the opinion that everything is still all right, and that is why many women are left behind*" (I 1).

One interviewee stated that the rhetoric of a healthier old age and growing old (as a woman) in the countryside compared to the city is also the result of a non-reflected use of clichés and therefore needs to be readjusted: "*You need to have to look at this in a more differentiated manner. In rural areas the availability of health care providers such as doctors, nurses, informal caregivers and various professional groups is more problematic*" (I 2).

At the same time, the same interviewee points out that the urban–rural dichotomy is insufficient in order to appropriately describe infrastructure-related differences in daily supply with goods and services. She points to the need for a spatially more differentiated discussion: "*Here [in rural areas] there are certain differences. The more peripheral the less available. It's as simple as that*" (I 2).

Moreover, it is difficult to derive valid spatial-related impacts on the entire collective of older women with regards to spatial health assessment and quality of life. The latter is why quality of life is something very individual and also depends on the respective demands and expectations. In this context some interviewees relate the questions concerning quality of life more to their own person than to the target group of women in old age.

6.2.3. The Significance of Spatial Planning for Public Health and the Merit of Integrating Spatial and Planning Sciences Scholars in the Debate on Older Women's Health

Only one out of the eight interviewees was already professionally in contact with spatial planning experts prior to the workshops of the expert group on "Women in Old Age". The working context referred to various projects of designing public spaces and accessibility, as well as of fall and accident prevention. The author of this article was already well known to two of the interviewees.

The significance of the professional discipline "spatial planning" is perceived as strategic and project-oriented as well as object-related and is often associated with the terms "housing" and "public space".

Some of the experts assign strategically important competencies to spatial planning by saying that spatial planning:

- ... is *"a political issue"* (I 2), which nevertheless *"is not yet on the radar."* (I 1, I 5)
- ... is *"a societal means of power"* (I 1), which organizes human coexistence.
- ... is addressed to all and *"being done by all"* (I 3).
- ... is about *"allocating spatial resources taking into account the needs of the population as well as of different target groups"* (I 4).
- ... *"must ensure that offers are maintained right down to the last corner"* (I 7).
- ... is an important task in which *"a great deal is about social responsibility"* (I 2).

Good spatial planning, in the eyes of the experts interviewed, is therefore: *"That one considers how an environment has to be designed so that people can cope with everyday life to a reasonable extent, regardless of their level of education and financial resources."* (I 2) This also includes providing opportunities *"in order to enable unplanned communication"* (ibid.).

Thus, those interviewees who took part in the workshops found the interdisciplinary dialogue with a spatial planning scholar enriching on the one hand and challenging, exciting and promising on the other hand.

Nonetheless, the following should always be borne in mind: *"Each expert speaks for him- or herself or rather for one's own profession"* (I 5).

The discussion of spatial references was also complicated by the fuzzy use of terms. Although the interdisciplinary discussion sharpened the subjective perception of space and place and helped to create (more) awareness of the importance of spatial planning as a focal subject, the experts do not remember any specific spatial planning-related arguments, or rather key messages.

6.2.4. Explanations for the Degree of Spatial-Related Abstraction of the Impact Goals and Measures and Its Determining Factors

The experts' judgements of the extent to which the integration of spatial planning expertise during the workshops influenced the way in which spatial references were taken into account in the impact goals and measures, and how the quality of their spatial relevance should ultimately be assessed, are controversial. Some of the interviewees were not surprised by the high level of spatial abstraction, as they know this from other contexts of work, and say: *"The spatial reference is not considered in the action plan, which is a pity."* (I 4)

According to another expert, spatial references serve at best as justification for the impact goals. Another expert believes that the author could be pleased that the terms *"space and region are addressed directly in the Action Plan"* (I 7).

Addressing the high level of provision and quality of both social and health care facilities in international comparison, an interviewee comments as follows: *"In Austria we discuss [health] at a relatively high level. Nevertheless, there is still so much to be done."* (I 2)

Moreover, there is an agreement on the need to pay more attention to spatial-related aspects in the context of the health of older women. However, in many cases, these aspects have been neglected in public affairs and politics:

- *"There is hardly any understanding of how individual life is related to spatial conditions."* (I 6)
- *"If it served the economy, this issue would carry more weight."* (I 1)

6.2.5. Recommendations for Spatial Planning Scholars

Established lobbies and power structures determine the implementation of inter- and transdisciplinary knowledge. Cross-cutting issues are nodded off, so they fall out of the prioritization phase. This could be alleviated by problem-centered evidence and ideas and strategies that address various spatial levels of action. An expert puts it as follows: *"You should approach from two directions: case study based from below; in the general view from above"* (I 6).

Furthermore, modifications are needed in the handling of knowledge production and knowledge transfer. There is disagreement among the interviewed public health experts on the merit of public consultation processes. The spectrum of opinions ranges from *"each consultation is useful"* (I 2) to thinking that consultation processes are a pure formality.

One expert recommends the following: a clear positioning and identification of content-related interfaces with other disciplines as well as investments in networking, which will help to increase the perception of spatial planning as a cross-cutting discipline. Furthermore, it must always be kept in mind that spatial conditions and critical events both determine the pressure for political action. Therefore, spatial planning can contribute to creating appropriate framework conditions for healthy ageing. That is why further in-depth discussions with spatial planning scholars are welcome.

7. Discussion

7.1. Methodological Strengths, Challenges and Limitations

This qualitative research is characterized by the application of mixed-methods and a retrospective multi-perspective reflection on the opportunities and limits of anchoring spatial aspects of women's health using the example of the making of a specific strategic policy paper. This research design can therefore be assigned to action research [51].

The crucial methodological challenge with regard to the realization of the research design was the development of a conceptual evidence-based framework [52] in order to be able to capture the spatial-relatedness of the health of older women with special regard to the Austrian situation, which was to serve as a basis for the analysis of the AAPWH as well as for the expert survey. At that time, in German-speaking countries the spatial planning scientific debate on its contributions to public health has just begun. In early summer 2017, in Potsdam (Germany) the first relevant congress entitled "Anchoring Health in Spatial Planning" was organized by the Academy for Spatial Development in the Leibniz Association.

That is why the author of this article decided to base the conceptual framework on her own empirical findings. The suitability of the conceptual framing was proven during the in-depth discussions with the experts.

After having completed the eight interviewees it became apparent that despite the small sample size, content saturation has occurred. This was due to the comprehensiveness of the described space–health nexus as well as to the explanations relating to the degree of spatial abstraction of the impact goals and measures. The latter is probably also related to the fact that the interviewed experts are outstanding professionals employed in the Austrian public health scene and have various (academic) educational backgrounds. Moreover, some of them also held and still hold leading positions in the making of the AAPWH and its implementation.

Related to the analysis of the material—namely, the qualitative content analysis of the AAPWH and the transcripts of the expert interviews—it can be critically noted that the content analysis was carried out exclusively by the author of this article. Thus, this article does not claim to speak for the whole spatial planning community in Austria, but intends to fuel the discussion among spatial planning theorists and practitioners on the reasons for the lack of involvement in defining gender-related health policy impact goals and measures.

7.2. Considerations on the Validity of the Questionnaire and Reliability of the Findings from the Expert Survey

Validity is a much-discussed topic in qualitative social research, especially with regard to the question 1. of whether the information obtained in this way is right or wrong, 2. what significance can be assigned to the findings and 3. how they can be put into the larger, or rather international, context [53].

Regarding the validity of the questionnaire applied for this research, it should be noted that it was suitable for capturing the complexity of the topic. This was proven by (1) the fluency of the interviews, (2) the ability of the interviewees to put themselves back to the year 2015 very quickly, (3) staying close to the topic during the entire interview and (4) the lack of critical comments on the methodological approach chosen to reflect the making of the AAPWH and its results, as well as on the guiding questions for the interviews.

With regard to the reliability of the results of the expert survey, it should be noted that (1) the statements are in line with the empirical evidence of spatial science research in Austria on the spatial-relatedness of health in old age and (2) the explanations of the degree of the spatial-related abstraction of the impact objectives and measures of the AAPWH are logical and conclusive. The experts' pragmatic attitude towards the predefined number of impact objectives and measures can be explained by their function in the AAPWH preparation process and is therefore perfectly understandable.

Looking at the applied research approach and the reliability of the expert judgements, it must be critically noted that more than two years passed between the third workshop of the expert group on "Women in Old Age" and the first expert interview. Whether and to what extent this time span had an effect on the quality of the content and the level of detail of the retrospective assessments cannot be assessed ex post. On the contrary, it should be emphasized that the willingness of the experts to reflect on the AAPHW in greater depth can be interpreted as a sincere interest in a cross-disciplinary discussion of health issues, including the spatial planning perspective.

7.3. The Merit of the Interdisciplinary Discussion within the Expert Group on "Women in Old Age" Including the Spatial Planning Perspective

The cross-disciplinary reflection on the impact goals and measures defined in the AAPWH has stimulated public health experts: (1) to take a different look at issues of (older) women's health; (2) to reflect on the principles of informed political decision making and the feasibility of taking into account the spatial-related complexity of challenges and problems, taking into account a predefined number of impact goals and measures; and (3) to become aware of the similarities and differences of the objectives and differences in the approaches of public health and spatial planning.

7.3.1. Identifying Health-Relevant Spatial Aspects and Dealing with Spatial-Relatedness of (Older) Women's Health: Similarities of and Differences between the Two Professions

Public health experts assign great importance to spatial aspects for the health protection and health promotion of women in different stages of life, or rather life situations—above all the accessibility as well as the availability and quality of health care and nursing facilities, as well as counselling services for those seeking information and advice.

It is interesting to note that the focus here is on the provision of social and health-related infrastructure facilities, and that the experts pay little attention to the importance of green spaces for maintaining health. With regard to the AAPWH this may be due to the fact that green space planning is not within the competence of the ministries responsible for the AAPWH. A follow-up of the cross-disciplinary dialogue on the importance of green infrastructure including the spatial planning perspective might perhaps lead to the involvement of other ministries in the AAPWH in the long run.

It was shown that public health experts ascribe a great importance to spatial planning with regards to health protection and health promotion (cf. Figure 2). Therefore, it is surprising that the interviewees have had little professional contact with other representatives of the discipline of spatial planning, or rather have not actively sought contact with them. Intensive cooperation between public health experts and spatial planning experts would be a good thing; both professions are dealing with cross-sectional issues [54,55], address important social and socio-political questions, put general interests at the center of their considerations, are used to working in a system- as well as target group-oriented manner and take the function of policy advisors. In addition, both professions, public health and spatial planning, call for a comprehensive discussion of health issues with particular attention to area-wide measures and equal access to infrastructure.

On the other hand, there are differences between public health and spatial planning experts with regard to dealing with spatial levels of action and the complexity of spatial-related inequalities of health in old age. When it comes to health and infrastructure disparities, spatial planning professionals think beyond urban–rural dichotomies and, within the framework of spatial research, draw attention to the importance of the functional interactions between different spatial archetypes in terms of the question of for what purposes people spend time in particular places and where health infrastructure should be located. The so-called multilocal lifestyle is becoming more and more important in this context [56].

7.3.2. Explanations for the Level of Spatial-Related Abstraction in the Impact Goals and Measures of the AAPWH

Despite the public health experts' basic understanding of the relevance of spatial-related aspects for the health and well-being of women of all ages, they do not think beyond distinct spatial categories, or rather the so-called urban–rural dichotomy. Moreover, they do not mind the absence of a clarification of the so-called "regional reference level of action" with regard to the defined impact goals and measures.

On the contrary, from the public health experts' perspective, the lack of a more precise spatial differentiation should be considered less a failure than a proof of the logic of dealing with cross-cutting and cross-sectional socio-political topics.

The experts' explanations of the standards and particularities of the preparation of inter-ministerial strategic policy—formal specifications such as the predefined number of impact objectives and measures as well as the length of the policy paper on the one hand, and the basic challenge of implementing the requirements of cross-cutting disciplines such as spatial planning on the other hand—can be interpreted as an important limitation of knowledge transfer in the context of evidence-based policy making [57]. A strategic argument for this may also be the political *"desire for a feasible plan"* (I 5) aiming at a win-win-situation for all involved stakeholders [27], which requires to include measures, which build on existing measures or rather be suitable to be integrated into existing actors' and supply landscapes as well as projects and initiatives. This also explains the political approval of the AAPHW and guarantees planning continuity. Despite all criticism, it should be noted that politically speaking *"it is not easy to get everything together"* (I 7).

Moreover, one expert recommends taking the AAPHW for what it is: a living inter-ministerial paper addressing the national level of and expressing the political commitment to the relevance of the subject of women's health in Austria without a defined expiry date and thus, serving as a strategic and operational anchor point for the implementation of changing focal topics in public administration units which are responsible for health provision (planning) at different spatial levels of action [58], encouraging the inter-sectoral and cross-disciplinary networking of experts within the framework of so-called focal points on selected, or rather emerging health topics.

7.4. Some Considerations on the Fit of Findings into an International Perspective

The results from this research are in line with the findings from other recent studies from the Netherlands [24,27,59] as well as from United Kingdom [28,60] on the general anchor and sticking points in inter-sectoral public health policy making, including the spatial planning perspective.

More generally formulated, the findings from Austria most likely may fit into the perspective of other high-income welfare states where (1) the creation of equivalent living conditions is a supreme political imperative, (2) the public sector takes a major role in the provision of services of general interest and (3) spatial planning is a public responsibility.

Furthermore, it is necessary to point out that the discussion on health-in-all-policies as well as the need for and the potential of inter-sectoral collaboration in order to protect and promote health—with particular regard to older women—in the Global North differs much from the Global South, since in the latter the basic (spatial-related) requirements for good health and well-being such as nutrition, sanitation, housing, security and medical care are still not met. Particularly, this situation limits the international transferability of the inferred conclusions of this research presented below and moreover, underlies the challenge of creating a geographically and socio-culturally overarching global mindset on public health in the foreseeable future [61].

8. Conclusions and Outlook

Conclusion 1: The degree of the spatial-related abstraction of the impact goals and measures can be explained by the fact that in Austria spatial planning as a cross-cutting discipline—as stated by Storm et al. [24]—has not yet been included in the strategic discourse on health protection and health promotion.

Conclusion 2: Both professions, public health and spatial planning, have similar ideas about the complexity of the space–health nexus and the importance of (governing) values in planning [58,62]. Thus, the joint dialogue in the expert group and the reflection on the impact goals and measures were experienced as fruitful on the part of both sides. The spatially differentiated approach and the way of reasoning in spatial planning can thus enrich the interdisciplinary discourse on women's health issues. For this reason, some of the interviewees also expressed their wish to keep in touch with the author of this article. This has already happened—for example in the context of network meetings or targeted information about current publications.

Conclusion 3: The need for a closer cooperation of public health and spatial planning—as claimed amongst others by Tomlinson et al. [63], by McKinnon et al. [60] as well as by Hendriks et al. [64] in general or Lowe et al. [65] for the urban context in particular—emerged during the expert discussions. A concrete thematic starting point for a further dialogue between the two disciplines could be the issue of long-distance caregiving, a topic still neglected in public health in Austria [45,66]. The main challenge of including "new" issues or target groups in the AAPWH is to integrate them into the right impact goal(s) and already existing measure(s).

Conclusion 4: It would be valuable to analyze the AAPWH in the context of an intertextual content analysis [67] with regard to the consideration of the spatial relatedness of the impact goals and measures for the two other target groups "Girls and Young Women" and "Women of Working Age" and subsequently—as shown here for the expert group of "Women in Old Age"—to reflect them in an interdisciplinary manner. An in-depth and continuous dialogue between public health and spatial planning experts may reveal cross-connections between target group-specific needs for action and thus perhaps bring to light the new cross-target group's priority themes, impact goals and measures including explicit and implicit spatial references.

Conclusion 5: Spatial and planning scholars must learn to understand that a change towards a comprehensive, or rather holistic, approach to health issues including the "spatial dimension" takes time. At the academic level, key representatives of other relevant disciplines (including, above all, public health) must be introduced to the mindset of spatial planning; at the political level, much effort is still needed to raise awareness and to sensitize all relevant stakeholders to the space–health nexus as a main reason for inequalities in (women's) health and to take ownership of the discovered interrelations [68,69]. Therefore, especially against the backdrop of demographic ageing, climate change and the impact of pandemics, as in line with the claim for more "evidence-informed public health policy" [26], spatial and planning scholars are encouraged to:

- Actively approach public health experts in science [29] and administration—the latter are focal points between scientists and political decision-makers [65]—and seize every opportunity for networking in order to bring expertise into the policy cycle in a timely manner [59].
- Describe complex and abstract issues in a low-threshold manner, depicting them visually and, for this purpose, explain the space–health nexus for example by means of storytelling, in order to convey the key messages appropriately [26].
- Discuss the impact goals and measures of the AAPWH in the light of the sound empirical evidence of spatial planning research together with public health experts, in order to bring these findings closer to policy makers [28].

Funding: This research received no external funding.

Institutional Review Board Statement: Ethical review and approval were waived for this study, due to the character of this research. It does not count as investigative medical research.

Informed Consent Statement: Informed consent was obtained from seven out of eight involved experts in this research. Therefore, this article only relates to findings from experts who gave consent.

Data Availability Statement: No new data were created or analyzed in this study. Data sharing is not applicable to this article.

Acknowledgments: The author would like to thank all interviewees for their support and openness. The open access publishing was supported by the BOKU Vienna Open Access Publishing Fund.

Conflicts of Interest: The author declares no conflict of interest.

References

1. Nour, N.M. Global women's health—A global perspective. *Scand. J. Clin. Lab. Investig. Suppl.* **2014**, *244*, 8–12; discussion 11–12. [CrossRef] [PubMed]
2. Peters, S.A.E.; Woodward, M.; Jha, V.; Kennedy, S.; Norton, R. Women's health: A new global agenda. *BMJ Glob. Health* **2016**, *1*, e000080. [CrossRef] [PubMed]
3. Manandhar, M.; Hawkes, S.; Buse, K.; Nosrati, E.; Magar, V. Gender, health and the 2030 agenda for sustainable development. *Bull. World Health Organ.* **2018**, *96*, 644–653. [CrossRef]
4. Rudolph, L.; Caplan, J.; Ben-Moshe, K.; Dillon, L. *Health in All Policies: A Guide for State and Local Governments*; American Public Health Association and Public Health Institute: Washington, DC, USA; Oakland, CA, USA, 2013.
5. World Bank, W. *Atlas of Sustainable Development Goals 2018. From World Development Indicators*; World Bank Publications: Washington, DC, USA, 2018; ISBN 978-1-4648-1250-7.
6. Rásky, É. Women's Health Network: State of Affairs, Concepts, Approaches, Organizations in the Women's Health Movement. Country Report Austria. Available online: https://www.gesundheit-nds.de/ewhnet/Country%20Reports/AustriaE.PDF (accessed on 1 October 2020).
7. Habimana, K.; Bachner, F.; Bobek, J.; Ladurner, J.; Ostermann, H. Das Österreichische Gesundheitswesen im Internationalen Vergleich. Wissenschaftlicher Ergebnisbericht.: Im Auftrag des Bundesministeriums für Gesundheit. Available online: https://www.sozialministerium.at/dam/jcr:32d88746-dd2b-4e38-bd6b-a7622200da71/das_oesterreichische_gesundheitswesen_im_internationalen_vergleich.pdf (accessed on 1 October 2020).
8. Barber, R.M.; Fullman, N.; Sorensen, R.J.D.; Bollyky, T.; McKee, M.; Nolte, E.; Abajobir, A.A.; Abate, K.H.; Abbafati, C.; Abbas, K.M.; et al. Healthcare Access and Quality Index based on mortality from causes amenable to personal health care in 195 countries and territories, 1990–2015: A novel analysis from the Global Burden of Disease Study 2015. *Lancet* **2017**, *390*, 231–266. [CrossRef]
9. OECD. Health at a Glance 2017: OECD Indicators. Available online: https://www.oecd-ilibrary.org/social-issues-migration-health/health-at-a-glance-2017_health_glance-2017-en (accessed on 1 October 2020).
10. World Health Organization. World Health Statistics 2020: Monitoring Health for the SDGs, Sustainable Development Goals. Available online: https://www.who.int/data/gho/publications/world-health-statistics (accessed on 1 October 2020).
11. Simon, G.; Benischke, C. FRAUEN (60+) IN ÖSTERREICH. FAKTEN, FRAGEN, FORSCHUNGSLÜCKEN: GRUNDLAGEN ZUM EMPOWERMENT. Available online: https://www.sozialministerium.at/dam/jcr:a37b8996-5183-4e8e-af82-9712926ccef2/Frauen%2060+.%202019.pdf (accessed on 1 October 2020).
12. Fischer, T. Versorgung mit sozialer Infrastruktur. In *Stöglehner, Gernot (Hrsg.): Grundlagen der Raumplanung 2. Strategien, Themen, Konzepte.*; Facultas: Wien, Austria, 2020; pp. 235–267, ISBN 978-3-7089-1755-9.
13. Bundesministerium für Arbeit, Soziales, Gesundheit und Konsumentenschutz. Demographischer Wandel—Geänderte Rahmenbedingungen für den Sozialstaat? Available online: https://www.sozialministerium.at/dam/jcr:6375bc0a-d6a7-4c93-879e-b2e7acb13668/dokument_demographischer_wandel_22_11_2019_barrierefrei.pdf (accessed on 1 October 2020).
14. Mayrhuber, C. Erwerbsunterbrechungen, Teilzeitarbeit und ihre Bedeutung für das FrauenLebenseinkommen. Available online: http://www.forschungsnetzwerk.at/downloadpub/Studie_Lebenseinkommen%202017_end.pdf (accessed on 1 October 2020).
15. Bundesministerium für Bundesministerium für Arbeit, Soziales, Gesundheit und Konsumentenschutz. In *Aktionsplan Frauengesundheit. 40 Maßnahmen für Die Gesundheit von Frauen in Österreich*; Sozialministerium: Wien, Auatria, 2018.
16. Austrian Presidency of the Council of the European Union, Federal Chancellery of Austria, Federal Minister for Women, Families and Youth, Division III—Women and Equality. Gender Equality in Austria. Milestones, Successes and Challenges. Available online: https://www.frauen-familien-jugend.bka.gv.at/dam/jcr:67b5975f-358e-474e-9b3c-5c81b3167fca/Gleichstellung_Broschuere_Ratsvorsitz_EN_RZ16.pdf (accessed on 5 January 2021).
17. World Health Organization (WHO). Regional Office for Europe. Health 2020. A European Policy Framework and Strategy for the 21st Century. Available online: https://www.euro.who.int/en/publications/abstracts/health-2020.-a-european-policy-framework-and-strategy-for-the-21st-century-2013 (accessed on 1 October 2020).

18. Buzeti, T.; Madureira Lima, J.; Yang, L.; Brown, C. Leaving no one behind: Health equity as a catalyst for the sustainable development goals. *Eur. J. Public Health* **2020**, *30*, i24–i27. [CrossRef]
19. World Health Organization (WHO). Regional Office for Europe. Intersectoral Action between Health, Social Protection and Labour Market Policy. Available online: https://www.euro.who.int/__data/assets/pdf_file/0017/413018/Intersectoral-action-between-health,-social-protection-and-labour-market-policy.pdf (accessed on 1 October 2020).
20. Federal Ministry of Social Affairs, Health, Care and Consumer Protection. Available online: https://broschuerenservice.sozialministerium.at/Home/Download?publicationId=480 (accessed on 13 January 2021).
21. Baumgart, S. Räumliche Planung und öffentliche Gesundheit—eine historische Verknüpfung. In *Planung für Gesundheitsfördernde Städte. Forschungsberichte der ARL 08*; Baumgart, S., Köckler, H., Ritzinger, A., Rüdiger, A., Eds.; ARL: Hannover, Germany, 2018; pp. 20–36, ISBN 978-3-88838-085-3. Available online: https://webcache.googleusercontent.com/search?q=cache:BjWo1P517gIJ:https://shop.arl-net.de/planung-fuer-gesundheitsfoerdernde-staedte.html+&cd=2&hl=de&ct=clnk&gl=at&client=firefox-b-d (accessed on 13 January 2021).
22. Fischer, T.; Stöglehner, G. Gesundheitsbezogene Lebensqualität im Alter als Thema der Raumplanung. Zusammenhänge und Handlungsoptionen. In *Gesundheitliche Lebensqualität im Alter. Ein Interdisziplinäres Handbuch für Health Professionals*; Kolland, F., Dorner, T.E., Eds.; MANZ Verlag: Wien, Austria, 2020; pp. 27–41, ISBN 978-3-214-13158-6.
23. UN-HABITAT & World Health Organization. Integrating Health in Urban and Territorial Planning: A Sourcebook. Available online: https://apps.who.int/iris/handle/10665/331678 (accessed on 4 January 2021).
24. Storm, I.; den Hertog, F.; van Oers, H.; Schuit, A.J. How to improve collaboration between the public health sector and other policy sectors to reduce health inequalities?—A study in sixteen municipalities in the Netherlands. *Int. J. Equity Health* **2016**, *15*, 97. [CrossRef]
25. Barton, H.; Tsourou, C. *Healthy Urban Planning. A WHO Guide to Planning for People*; Published on Behalf of the World Health Organization Regional Office for Europe by Spon: London, UK, 2000; ISBN 0-415-24327-0.
26. Sisnowski, J.; Street, J.M. Evidence-Informed Public Health Policy. In *International Encyclopedia of Public Health*; Elsevier: Amsterdam, The Netherlands, 2017; pp. 57–65, ISBN 9780128037089.
27. Storm, I.; Aarts, M.-J.; Harting, J.; Schuit, A.J. Opportunities to reduce health inequalities by 'Health in All Policies' in the Netherlands: An explorative study on the national level. *Health Policy* **2011**, *103*, 130–140. [CrossRef]
28. Ige-Elegbede, J.; Pilkington, P.; Bird, E.L.; Gray, S.; Mindell, J.S.; Chang, M.; Stimpson, A.; Gallagher, D.; Petrokofsky, C. Exploring the views of planners and public health practitioners on integrating health evidence into spatial planning in England: A mixed-methods study. *J. Public Health* **2020**. [CrossRef]
29. Baumgart, S.; Köckler, H.; Ritzinger, A.; Rüdiger, A. (Eds.) *Planung für Gesundheitsfördernde Städte. Forschungsberichte der ARL 08*; Hannover, Germany, 2018; ISBN 978-3-88838-085-3. Available online: https://webcache.googleusercontent.com/search?q=cache:BjWo1P517gIJ:https://shop.arl-net.de/planung-fuer-gesundheitsfoerdernde-staedte.html+&cd=2&hl=de&ct=clnk&gl=at&client=firefox-b-d (accessed on 13 January 2021).
30. Phillips, J.; Walford, N.; Hockey, A.; Foreman, N.; Lewis, M. Older people and outdoor environments: Pedestrian anxieties and barriers in the use of familiar and unfamiliar spaces. *Geoforum* **2013**, *47*, 113–124. [CrossRef]
31. Mehrabi, F.; Béland, F. Effects of social isolation, loneliness and frailty on health outcomes and their possible mediators and moderators in community-dwelling older adults: A scoping review. *Arch. Gerontol. Geriatr.* **2020**, *90*, 104119. [CrossRef]
32. Morrisby, C.; Joosten, A.; Ciccarelli, M. Do services meet the needs of people with dementia and carers living in the community? A scoping review of the international literature. *Int. Psychogeriatr.* **2018**, *30*, 5–14. [CrossRef] [PubMed]
33. Harper, S. The Convergence of Population Ageing with Climate Change. *Popul. Ageing* **2019**, *12*, 401–403. [CrossRef]
34. Haq, G.; Whitelegg, J.; Kohler, M. *Growing Old in a Changing Climate: Meeting the Challenges of an Ageing Population and Climate Change*; Stockholm Environment Institute: Stockholm, Sweden, 2008. [CrossRef]
35. Fischer, T. Aging in rural areas in Austria—On the interrelations of spatial aspects and the quality of life of today's older generation. *Eur. Countrys.* **2009**, *1*. [CrossRef]
36. Rechel, B.; Džakula, A.; Duran, A.; Fattore, G.; Edwards, N.; Grignon, M.; Haas, M.; Habicht, T.; Marchildon, G.P.; Moreno, A.; et al. Hospitals in rural or remote areas: An exploratory review of policies in 8 high-income countries. *Health Policy* **2016**, *120*, 758–769. [CrossRef] [PubMed]
37. Allen, P.; May, J.; Pegram, R.; Shires, L. 'It's mostly about the job'—Putting the lens on specialist rural retention. *Rural Remote Health* **2020**, *20*, 5299. [CrossRef] [PubMed]
38. ARL—Akademie für Raumentwicklung in der Leibniz-Gemeinschaft. Raumordnung: Anwalt für Gleichwertige Lebensverhältnisse und Regionale Entwicklung—Eine Positionsbestimmung. = Positionspapier aus der ARL 115. Available online: https://www.arl-net.de/de/blog/raumordnung-anwalt-f%C3%BCr-gleichwertige-lebensverh%C3%A4ltnisse-und-regionale-entwicklung-eine (accessed on 5 October 2020).
39. Akademie für Raumforschung und Landesplanung. Daseinsvorsorge und Gleichwertige Lebensverhältnisse neu Denken—Perspektiven und Handlungsfelder. Hannover. = Positionspapier aus der ARL 108. Available online: https://shop.arl-net.de/daseinsvorsorg-und-gleichwertige-lebensverhaeltnisse-neu-denken.html (accessed on 5 October 2020).
40. Austrian National Public Health Institute. *Minute of Workshop No. 1 of the expert group "Women in Old Age" Title of document: Minute_28_04_2015.pdf*, Document not available to the public.

41. Austrian National Public Health Institute. *Minute of Workshop No. 2 of the expert group "Women in Old Age". Title of document: Minute_26_05_2015.pdf*, Document not available to the public.
42. Hofmarcher, M.M.; Rack Herta, M. *Gesundheitssysteme im Wandel: Österreich*; WHO Regionalbüro für Europa im Auftrag des Europäischen Observatoriums für Gesundheitssysteme und Gesundheitspolitik: Kopenhagen, Denmark, 2006.
43. Fischer, T. Raumrelevante Aspekte des Altseins und Älterwerdens im ländlichen Raum Österreichs und in der Metropolregion Wien. In *Europäische Raumentwicklung: Metropolen und Periphere Regionen*; Güldenberg, E., Ed.; Lang: Frankfurt am Main, Germany, 2009; pp. 93–108, ISBN 3631588771.
44. Fischer, T. Räumliche Disparitäten und gleichwertige Lebensverhältnisse. In *Stöglehner, Gernot (Hrsg.): Grundlagen der Raumplanung 2. Strategien, Themen, Konzepte.*; Facultas: Wien, Austria, 2020; pp. 303–324, ISBN 978-3-7089-1755-9.
45. Fischer, T.; Jobst, M. Capturing the Spatial Relatedness of Long-Distance Caregiving: A Mixed-Methods Approach. *Int. J. Environ. Res. Public Health* **2020**, *17*, 6406. [CrossRef] [PubMed]
46. Boyatzis, R.E. *Transforming Qualitative Information: Thematic Analysis and Code Development*, 1st ed.; Sage Publications: Thousand Oaks, CA, USA, 1998.
47. Fischer, T. Zur Verankerung raum-und planungswissenschaftlicher Anliegen im Aktionsplan Frauengesundheit—Ein Erfahrungsbericht [Poster]. In *Forum Geriatrie und Gerontologie Bad Hofgastein. Altern Multiprofessionell: Praxis und Forschung, 8.–10.*; Kongresszentrum Bad Hofgastein: Bad Hofgastein, Österreich, 2018.
48. Glaser, B.G.; Strauss, A.L. *Grounded Theory. Strategien Qualitativer Forschung*, 1st ed.; Huber: Bern, Switzerland, 1998.
49. Wiles, J. Conceptualizing place in the care of older people: The contributions of geographical gerontology. *J. Clin. Nurs.* **2005**, *14*, 100–108. [CrossRef]
50. Harris, P.; Kent, J.; Sainsbury, P.; Thow, A.M. Framing health for land-use planning legislation: A qualitative descriptive content analysis. *Soc. Sci. Med.* **2016**, *148*, 42–51. [CrossRef]
51. Hult, M.; Lennung, S.-Å. Towards a definition of action research: A note and bibliography. *J. Manag. Stud.* **1980**, *17*, 241–250. [CrossRef]
52. Walt, G.; Shiffman, J.; Schneider, H.; Murray, S.F.; Brugha, R.; Gilson, L. 'Doing' health policy analysis: Methodological and conceptual reflections and challenges. *Health Policy Plan.* **2008**, *23*, 308–317. [CrossRef]
53. Huber, A. Die Angst des Wissenschaftlers vor der Ästhetik. *Forum Qual. Soz.* **2001**. [CrossRef]
54. Schmitt, P.; Wiechmann, T. Unpacking Spatial Planning as the Governance of Place. *Disp. Plan. Rev.* **2018**, *54*, 21–33. [CrossRef]
55. Freedman, D.A.; Bess, K.D.; Tucker, H.A.; Boyd, D.L.; Tuchman, A.M.; Wallston, K.A. Public health literacy defined. *Am. J. Prev. Med.* **2009**, *36*, 446–451. [CrossRef]
56. Danielzyk, R.; Dittrich-Wesbuer, A.; Hilti, N.; Tippel, C. (Eds.) *Multilokale Lebensführungen und Räumliche Entwicklungen—Ein Kompendium*; Print-on-Demand; ARL—Akademie für Raumentwicklung in der Leibniz-Gemeinschaft: Hannover, Austria, 2020; ISBN 978-3-88838-098-3.
57. Levy, C. Gender and the environment: The challenge of cross-cutting issues in development policy and planning. *Environ. Urban.* **1992**, *4*, 134–149. [CrossRef]
58. Mirzoev, T.N.; Green, A.T. Planning, for Public Health Policy. In *International Encyclopedia of Public Health*; Elsevier: Amsterdam, The Netherlands, 2017; pp. 489–499, ISBN 9780128037089.
59. Peters, D.T.J.M.; Raab, J.; Grêaux, K.M.; Stronks, K.; Harting, J. Structural integration and performance of inter-sectoral public health-related policy networks: An analysis across policy phases. *Health Policy* **2017**, *121*, 1296–1302. [CrossRef]
60. McKinnon, G.; Pineo, H.; Chang, M.; Taylor-Green, L.; Strategy, A.J.; Toms, R. Strengthening the links between planning and health in England. *BMJ* **2020**, *369*, m795. [CrossRef] [PubMed]
61. Vuong, Q.H.; Napier, N.K. Acculturation and global mindsponge: An emerging market perspective. *Int. J. Intercult. Relat.* **2015**, *49*, 354–367. [CrossRef]
62. Albrechts, L. Strategic (Spatial) Planning Reexamined. *Environ. Plan B Plan Des.* **2004**, *31*, 743–758. [CrossRef]
63. Tomlinson, P.; Hewitt, S.; Blackshaw, N. Joining up health and planning: How Joint Strategic Needs Assessment (JSNA) can inform health and wellbeing strategies and spatial planning. *Perspect. Public Health* **2013**, *133*, 254–262. [CrossRef] [PubMed]
64. Hendriks, A.-M.; Habraken, J.; Jansen, M.W.J.; Gubbels, J.S.; de Vries, N.K.; van Oers, H.; Michie, S.; Atkins, L.; Kremers, S.P.J. 'Are we there yet?'—Operationalizing the concept of Integrated Public Health Policies. *Health Policy* **2014**, *114*, 174–182. [CrossRef]
65. Lowe, M.; Whitzman, C.; Giles-Corti, B. Health-Promoting Spatial Planning: Approaches for Strengthening Urban Policy Integration. *Plan. Theory Pract.* **2018**, *19*, 180–197. [CrossRef]
66. Fischer, T.; Jobst, M. On the Suitability and Potential of Nursing Care Discussion Forums as a Health Promotion Measure for Long-Distance Caregiving Relatives: Evidence from Upper Austria. *Healthcare* **2019**, *7*, 139. [CrossRef] [PubMed]
67. Allen, G. *Intertextuality*, 2nd ed.; Routledge: London, UK, 2011; ISBN 9780203829455.
68. Clark, H.; Taplin, D. Theory of Change Basics: A Primer on Theory of Change. Available online: https://www.theoryofchange.org/wp-content/uploads/toco_library/pdf/ToCBasics.pdf (accessed on 15 October 2020).
69. Smith, M.K.; Argyris, C. Chris Argyris: Theories of Action, Double-Loop Learning and Organizational Learning. The Encyclopedia of Informal Education. Available online: www.infed.org/thinkers/argyris.htm (accessed on 15 October 2020).

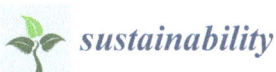

Article

Economic and Social Factors That Predict Readmission for Mental Health and Drug Abuse Patients

Quang "Neo" Bui * and Emi Moriuchi

Rochester Institute of Technology, 105 Lomb Memorial Drive, Rochester, NY 14623, USA; emoriuchi@saunders.rit.edu
* Correspondence: qnbbbu@rit.edu; Tel.: +1-585-475-4411

Abstract: According to the United Nations, curtailing the rise of mental illness and drug abuse has been an important goal for sustainable development of member states. In the United States, reducing readmission rates for mental health and drug abuse patients is critical, given the rising health care costs and a strained health care system. This study aims to examine economic and social factors that predict readmission likelihood for mental health and drug abuse patients in the state of New York. Patient admission data of 25,846 mental health patients and 32,702 drug abuse patients with multiple visits in New York hospitals in 2015 were examined. Findings show that economic factors like income level and payment type impact readmission rates differently: The poorest patients were less likely to get readmitted while patients with higher incomes were likely to experience drug relapse. Regarding social factors, mental health patients who lived in neighborhoods with high social capital were less likely to be readmitted, but drug abuse patients in similar areas were more likely to be readmitted. The findings show that policy-makers and hospital administrators need to approach readmission rates differently for each group of patients.

Keywords: readmission; social capital; economics; mental health; drug abuse

---

Citation: Bui, Q.N.; Moriuchi, E. Economic and Social Factors That Predict Readmission for Mental Health and Drug Abuse Patients. *Sustainability* **2021**, *13*, 531. https://doi.org/10.3390/su13020531

Received: 17 November 2020
Accepted: 6 January 2021
Published: 8 January 2021

Publisher's Note: MDPI stays neutral with regard to jurisdictional claims in published maps and institutional affiliations.

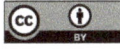

Copyright: © 2021 by the authors. Licensee MDPI, Basel, Switzerland. This article is an open access article distributed under the terms and conditions of the Creative Commons Attribution (CC BY) license (https://creativecommons.org/licenses/by/4.0/).

"The inclusion of noncommunicable diseases under the health goal is a historical turning point. Finally, these diseases are getting the attention they deserve. Through their 169 interactive and synergistic targets, the Sustainable Development Goals (SDGs) seek to move the world towards greater fairness that leaves no one behind."

Dr Chan, 2013 WHO Director-General

1. Introduction

In 2013, the 66th World Health Assembly adopted a comprehensive plan to curtail the rise of mental illness and drug abuse worldwide [1]. The then World Health Organization (WHO) director, Dr. Chan, called this a "historical turning point" that moved the world toward a more sustainable future. Since then, treating mental health and drug abuse has always been integrated into the United Nations (UN) platform to promote sustainable development among member states [2]. Responding to this, various studies have focused on factors that can predict and curtail mental illness and drug abuse in various contexts [3–7].

In the United States (US), mental health and drug abuse patients have steadily increased in recent years. According to the 2017 National Survey on Drug Use and Health, nearly one in five US adults suffered from a mental health condition, and one in eight US adults struggled with both alcohol and drug use disorders [8]. The Mental Health America institute estimated that youth mental health is worsening with an increase of 4.3% over five years for youth age 12–17 [9]. The opioid crisis, which has killed 128 people every day due to overdose [10], is an example of severe drug abuse issues in the US. In addition, with the Covid-19 pandemic in 2020, it is estimated that there will be even more people suffering from the psychological impacts of lock-downs due to emotional stress and financial distress [3].

In addition, there is a sustainability crisis in the US public health care system [11]. It has a declining tax base and diminishing social values that are encouraging more private sector choices, and there are two views on addressing the sustainability of the US public health care system [12,13]. First, while there may be economies in more efficient administration of the public health care system that will address sustainability concerns, more scrutiny is needed of how funding is provided. Those who maintain that the system is unsustainable would argue that public funding and administration is part of the problem. The solution may be that Americans have to accept less-comprehensive public health insurance, with more services being paid for out-of-pocket or by private insurance. In this situation, supporters of this view would believe that the private-for-profit insurance companies are the source of the health expenditure increase. A second view is based on the rising cost of health care, which is threatening to overwhelm the public health care system. Thus, a major structural reform of the system is required to encourage better public management as it has the opportunity to provide greater efficiency in the form of faster service and greater choice for Americans [14]. Furthermore, the use of public funds to provide health care suggests that when the expenditure for health care increases, either taxes must be increased or public services reduced. Thus, to avoid such negative effects, public health care needs to maintain quality while addressing the individual's health needs accurately (e.g., differentiating illness accurately).

Against this backdrop, this study seeks to identify economic and social factors that predict readmission rates of mental health and drug abuse patients in the state of New York. Understanding these factors will help policy-makers and health administrators pursue high-quality health care and improve public health in a sustainable manner without exhausting limited resources.

This study's focus on the state of New York is motivated by the state's high readmission rates, with 93% of hospitals estimated to be penalized for such high rates [15]. In 2008, it is estimated that 15% of all hospital stays in NY result in readmission, costing $3.7 billion per year [16]. Reducing readmission rates has become a priority for state public health officials. In addition, the state has a high growth of mental health and drug abuse patients, ranking fifth in the nation [17]. This makes it more critical to understand the factors that impact readmission rates for mental health and drug abuse patients in the state of New York.

2. Conceptual Foundation
2.1. Readmission Rates in the US Health System

Compared to other developed countries, hospitals in the United States have higher readmission rates [18]. Given the rapid rise of health care costs and rampant inefficiencies in the health care system, reducing readmission rates has been a crucial goal for quality health care and sustainable development in the US [19]. To combat this issue, in the US, since 2013, Medicare reimbursement has been linked to hospital 30-day readmission rates for acute myocardial infarction (AMI), heart failure (HF), and pneumonia (PN). Subsequently, reducing readmission rates has become an important indicator of hospital performance in the US, and a growing number of studies have examined factors that contribute to reduced readmissions. To date, prior studies have suggested a plethora of factors, ranging from hospital and treatment characteristics [20–22] to patient-level social and economic factors [23–25]. These studies make it clear that readmission is a complex issue dependent not only on hospital-related factors but also on out-of-hospital factors such as social support [25], economic means [20,26], community factors [24], or even county-level characteristics [23].

Because readmission rates historically grow out of the concern from the Centers for Medicare and Medicaid Services (CMS) for AMI, HF, and PN patients, most readmission rate research has focused on patients with chronic conditions [20,22,25]. Recent studies have investigated readmission rates for all medical care services [23,24], for insured patients [21,26], or for patients with recent surgery or with pneumonia [27]. However, hospital readmissions for other different types of patients, including mental health and drug abuse patients, are still understudied. Studies have found that mental health and drug abuse patients indeed have a higher risk of readmission compared to other groups [28,29]. Thus, the objective of this study is to examine factors that contribute to readmission rates among mental health and drug abuse patients in the state of New York.

In addition, while some studies have looked at readmission rates for mental health and drug abuse patients [5,27,30,31], they often aggregate findings for both types of patients as one category. This study argues that such analyses can be incomplete as mental health patients possibly differ from drug abuse patients in terms of demographic factors, service utilization patterns, and diagnostic services [4]. Thus, this study aims to compare results for each type of patient to understand specific influential factors for their readmission rates.

2.2. Conceptual Model

Building on prior research, it is hypothesized that the likelihood of readmission for a patient will be explained by three groups of factors: Hospital treatments, economic factors, and social factors. First, the nature of treatments that patients receive can determine how likely they are to relapse and be readmitted. This is especially important for mental health and drug abuse patients [32], and prior studies have pointed out that those two types of patients utilize treatments and service hours differently [4]. Specifically, drug abuse patients had more treatments and longer stays than mental health patients [4], while prior diagnostic history was a strong predictor for readmission rates among mental health patients [30,33]. Thus, this study hypothesizes that these differences in hospital treatments will explain the readmission rate for mental health versus drug abuse patients.

Second, various studies have attributed readmission rates to economic factors, especially whether patients have access to economic means to afford hospital visits [20,21,25,26]. For mental health and drug abuse patients, economic factors can also reflect their neighborhood living conditions as low-income patients often cluster in poor areas and are more prone to mental health problems or entrenched drug usage. For instance, several studies have associated homelessness with a higher risk of readmission for mental health patients [30,34,35]. Thus, it is hypothesized that economic factors can help explain the readmission rates for mental health and drug abuse patients.

Finally, recent studies have posited that social factors also predict patient readmission rates [23,24]. Instead of relying on economic factors as a proxy for social impacts, these studies explored the supporting characteristics of patient living environment or community health system factors. For example, several researchers have suggested that follow-up in community hospitals can reduce readmission rates for mental health patients [30,31]. Others have identified stronger community support can reduce readmission rates in general [24,33,36]. Compared to hospital treatment factors (hospital-controllable) and economic factors (patient-controllable), these community factors are uncontrollable for hospitals and patients. Thus, they can provide a complete understanding of readmission rates. In this paper, it is hypothesized that social factors play a critical role in readmission rates of mental health and drug abuse patients because those patients need a wide range of social support to overcome their issues.

In sum, this study's conceptual model (Figure 1) uses hospital treatments, economic factors, and community factors to explain readmission rates for mental health and drug abuse patients. One model is built for each type of patient, and the findings are compared and contrasted to unveil insights that can inform policy-makers on how to reduce readmission rates for those patients. Next, data sources and variables used in the analysis are discussed.

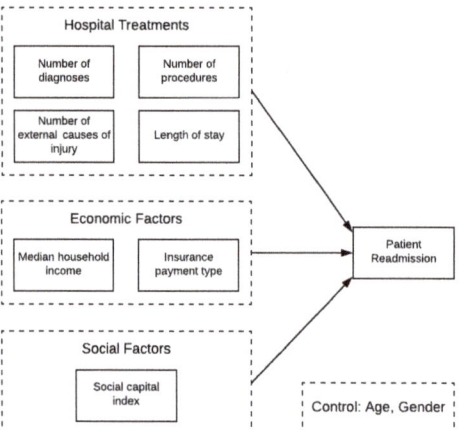

Figure 1. Conceptual model.

3. Materials and Methods

3.1. Data Sources and Variables

The study used 2015 discharge data from the New York State Inpatient Databases (SID) by the Healthcare Cost and Utilization Project (HCUP), and Agency for Healthcare Research and Quality [37]. The original dataset contained 2.29 million records. The unique patient identifier was used in the dataset to filter out patients with multiple hospital visits in 2015, and patients who received services classified as mental health and drug abuse services. This left 120,140 patients.

To distinguish mental health versus drug abuse patients, the ICD-10 Procedure Coding System (ICD-10-PCS) was used to identify specific services received by patients during their hospital visits. Specifically, mental health patients were those who received service coded 218 (psychological and psychiatric evaluation and theory) while drug abuse patients were those who received service coded 219 (alcohol and drug rehabilitation/detoxification). Excluding patients with missing data, the final datasets contained 25,846 mental health patients and 32,702 drug abuse patients.

From the patient's visit date and length of stay, a calculation was made as to whether the visit was readmission within 30 days of last visit discharge. This gave a primary outcome variable for hospital readmission (1/0 indicator). The independent variables come from three groups: Hospital treatments, economic factors, and social factors, with demographics as control variables.

Hospital treatments included the number of diagnoses received during a visit, the number of procedures received during a visit, the number of external causes of injury, and length of stay [5,30,31,38]. Following prior studies [5,21], economic factors, such as the median household income for a patient's zip code, and insurance type of primary payer were used. Insurance payment method includes private (self-pay, group insurance) and public (Medicare, Medicaid). Income was determined based on New York State's income categories (e.g., 1 = under poverty <$12,760 for an individual, <$24,600 for a family of four). Demographics included sex and age [30].

Social factors came from the social capital index for a patient's county [39]. The social capital index is developed by the Northeast Regional Center for Rural Development (http://aese.psu.edu/nercrd), and it is calculated using an array of individual and community factors to measure the socio-economic growth of a community. Prior studies have suggested that social capital within a community will impact patient readmission rates [23,24,40]. For this study, the social capital index is particularly relevant as supporting communities are likely to help reduce readmission rates for mental health and drug abuse patients [24,36].

3.2. Statistical Analysis

To estimate the likelihood of readmission for patients, a multinomial logistic regression was used. This type of regression uses maximum likelihood estimation to predict the probability of category membership on a dependent variable based on multiple independent variables. Goodness of fit analyses were conducted to accurately specify the model, in which a gamma distribution and log link were selected.

The sample size was split into two groups: Mental health patients with a total of 25,846 cases, and drug abuse patients with a total of 32,702 cases. The assumption of multinomial logistic regression in this study was that readmission due to a diagnosed illness is not related to the readmission for another diagnosed illness. In our mental health patient sample, a majority of the patients were hospitalized based on the occurrence of an emergency (82.1%), and 61.1% identified as male. The average age was 42 years old, and the average length of stay was 14 days. On the other hand, 52.4% of drug abuse patients were hospitalized due to an emergency, and 75.4% identified as male. The mean age was 43 years old. The average length of stay was 6.5 days.

Our model is as follows. The dependent variable Y = 0 if not readmitted, Y = 1 if readmitted.

$$y_i = (y_{i1}, y_{i2}, \ldots, y_{ir})^T$$

Readmission = length of stay + number of diagnoses + number of procedures + number of external causes + median household income + payment type + social capital + sex + age.

4. Results

4.1. Mental Health Patients

A multinomial logistic regression was performed to model the relationship between the predictors and type of illness in the two groups (mental health issues and drug abuse). The traditional 0.05 criterion of statistical significance was employed for all tests. For mental health patients, the final model showed a good fit between model and data, $\chi^2(14, N = 25,846) = 199.70$, Nagelkerke $R^2 = 0.01$, $p < 0.001$. Goodness-of-fit results showed that Pearson Chi-square was insignificant ($p = 0.41$), which indicated that the model fit the data well. Table 1 shows that for mental health patients, their readmission rates are significantly predicted by length of stay, number of diagnoses, number of procedures, median income, payment type, social capital, gender, and age.

Consistent with prior studies [22], our results showed that for mental health patients, their readmission likelihood was predicted by hospital treatments: Specifically, by the number of diagnoses and the number of procedures, but not the number of external causes. While the more diagnoses a patient had, the lower the readmission odds (negative coefficient), the more procedures a patient had, the higher the readmission odds (positive coefficient). A one-unit increase in the number of diagnoses will lead to a 0.02 decrease in the relative log odds of being readmitted as a mental patient, while a one-unit increase in the number of procedures will result in a 0.025 increase in the readmission odds. Length of stay appears as a significant predictor, but its beta was small, indicating its low impact.

Economic factors showed positive impacts on readmission likelihood, but the effects varied. Specifically, median income level as a whole showed a negative significant impact ($p < 0.05$) on readmission, and for every unit increase in the income level, there was a 0.08 unit decrease in readmission odds. However, among different income categories, patients who fell under the poverty line tended not to be readmitted ($\beta = -0.79$, $p < 0.05$), while the effects of income were negated for other income levels. On the other hand, the payment method (i.e., insurance coverage) also had an impact on readmission odds, but only among patients who used Medicare or Medicaid ($\beta = -0.30$, $p < 0.05$; $\beta = -0.39$, $p < 0.01$, respectively).

Table 1. Findings from Multinomial Logistic Regression for Mental Health vs. Drug Abuse Patients.

Independent Variables (IV)	Descriptive	Mental Health (SE)	Descriptive	Drug Abuse (SE)
Hospital Treatments				
Length of Stay		−0.00 ** (0.00)		0.04 ** (0.00)
Number of Diagnoses		−0.02 ** (0.00)		−0.017 ** (0.00)
Number of Procedures		0.025 * (0.01)		0.005 n.s. (0.02)
Number of External Causes		0.035 n.s. (0.03)		−0.046 n.s. (0.03)
Economic Factors				
Median Income		−0.05 ** (0.01)		−0.06 ** (0.01)
$0–$25,000	39.0%	−0.079 * (0.04)	35.9%	−0.073 * (0.03)
$25,001–$30,000	18.4%	−0.045 n.s. (0.04)	17.5%	0.103 ** (0.04)
$30,001–$35,000	16.6%	0.030 n.s. (0.05)	18.2%	0.087 * (0.04)
$35,001+	25.9%	0 (0)	28.4%	0 (0)
Payment Type		−0.08 ** (0.02)		−0.13 ** (0.01)
Medicare	30.0%	−0.297 * (0.13)	12.4%	−0.240 ** (0.08)
Medicaid	54.3%	−0.391 ** (0.13)	66.3%	−0.093 n.s. (0.07)
Private Insurance	12.4%	−0.089 n.s. (0.13)	15.9%	0.280 ** (0.08)
Self-pay	2.0%	−0.084 n.s. (0.16)	2.6%	0.360 ** (0.11)
No Charge	1.3%		0.1%	−0.689 n.s. (0.40)
Other			2.8%	
Social Factor				
Social Capital		−0.04 * (0.01)		0.04 ** (0.01)
Demographic				
Proportion of Male	58.6%	−0.27 ** (0.02)	75.6%	−0.36 ** (0.03)
Age		0.00 * (0.00)		−0.01 ** (0.00)

* $p < 0.05$, ** $p < 0.01$.

Additionally, the results showed that a one-unit increase in the social capital status is associated with a 0.04 decrease in the relative log odds of being readmitted to the hospital as a mental health patient. The beta shows a negative result, which suggests that patients who have higher social capital (which reflects the social environment of their neighborhood) will have lower readmission odds. This finding is aligned with prior studies that have suggested the positive impacts of social influences on readmission rates [24,25].

Age was also found to have a significant positive impact on readmission odds ($p < 0.05$). Income level showed a negative significant impact ($p < 0.05$) on readmission. For every unit increase in the income level, there is a 0.08 unit decrease in readmission odds.

4.2. Drug Abuse Patients

Table 1 shows that for drug abuse patients, significant predictors for their readmission were length of stay, number of diagnoses, income level, payment method, social capital, gender, and age. The model has a good fit, $\chi^2(15, N = 32,702) = 791.54$, Nagelkerke $R^2 = 0.04$, $p < 0.001$. Goodness-of-fit results also show that Pearson Chi-square was insignificant ($p = 0.28$), which indicates that the model fits the data well.

Among hospital treatment factors, only length of stay and number of diagnoses were significant predictors for readmission odds among drug abuse patients. Interestingly, every day remaining hospitalized was associated with a 0.04 increase in the readmission odds ($\beta = 0.04$). On the other hand, a one-unit increase in the number of diagnoses was associated with a 0.017 decrease in relative log odds of being readmitted ($\beta = -0.017$, $p < 0.01$).

As with mental health patients, economic factors also had a significant impact on readmission odds for drug abuse patients. At the aggregate level, income level had a significant negative impact on readmission odds. A one-level increase in the variable income level is associated with a decrease in the relative odds of being readmitted. While only income below the poverty line impacted readmission odds for mental health patients, higher income brackets also impacted drug abuse patients (below the poverty line, between $24,000–$35,000, and above $35,000). More interestingly, patients below the poverty line saw reduced readmission odds while patients with higher income levels saw a higher chance of being readmitted as a drug abuse patient.

Payment through Medicare, self-pay, and private insurance, but not through Medicaid, had a positive impact on readmissions. Specifically, every one-unit increase in the use of Medicare is associated with a decrease of 0.24 units in readmissions odds ($\text{Exp}(\beta) = 0.79$).

On the other hand, every one-unit increase in self-pay is associated with a 0.28-unit increase in readmission and a 0.36-unit increase for private insurance payer.

Social capital had an opposite effect on drug abuse patients compared to mental health patients. The results showed that a one-unit increase in social capital is associated with a 0.05 increase in being readmitted as an opioid patient ($\beta = 0.05$, $p < 0.01$). Combined with the findings related to the income level above, this further confirms that drug abuse patients who have more disposable income and live in good neighborhoods are more likely to relapse.

For demographics, every year increase in age is associated with a 0.01 decrease in the relative log odds ($Exp(\beta) = 1.01$) of being readmitted. Moreover, males were more likely to be readmitted than females.

4.3. Patients with Both Mental Health and Drug Abuse Issues

The number of patients who have been diagnosed to have two types of illness (drug abuse and mental health) is 4226. Similar to the two models above, a multinomial logistic regression was performed to model the relationship between the predictors and their readmission likelihood. The traditional 0.05 criterion of statistical significance was employed. The final model showed a good fit between model and data, $\chi^2(15, N = 4226) = 1021.23$, Nagelkerke $R^2 = 0.01$, $p < 0.001$. Goodness-of-fit results showed that Pearson Chi-square was insignificant ($p = 0.54$), which indicated that the model fit the data well. Table 2 shows that significant unique contributions were made by all the factors except the number of external causes and age.

Table 2. Findings from Multinomial Logistic Regression for Patients with both Mental Health and Drug Abuse.

Independent Variables (IV)	Descriptive	Mental Health and Drug Abuse (SE)
Hospital Treatments		
Length of Stay		0.00 ** (0.01)
Number of Diagnoses		−0.02 ** (0.01)
Number of Procedures		0.14 ** (0.04)
Number of External Causes		−0.01 n.s. (0.10)
Economic Factors		
Median Income		−0.04 ** (0.01)
$0–$25,000	33.0%	−0.04 ** (0.02)
$25,001–$30,000	20.1%	0.07 ** (0.02)
$30,001–$35,000	18.6%	0.07 ** (0.02)
$35,001+	28.2%	0
Payment Type		−0.08 ** (0.01)
Medicare	25.0%	−0.08 n.s. (0.05)
Medicaid	55.6%	−0.12 ** (0.05)
Private Insurance	14.9%	0.23 ** (0.05)
Self-pay	2.3%	0.27 ** (0.07)
No Charge	0.0%	−0.53 n.s. (0.30)
Other	2.2%	0
Social Factor		
Social Capital		0.05 ** (0.01)
Demographic		
Proportion of Male	63.1%	−0.26 ** (0.01)
Age		−0.00 n.s. (0.00)

* $p < 0.05$, ** $p < 0.01$.

When the data were analyzed based on a patient who has been diagnosed with two types of illness, length of stay had a positive significant impact on readmission odds. For every day in the hospital, there is an increase of 0.01 units in relative log odds of being readmitted as a patient. The number of procedures had a positive significant impact on readmission odds. For every increase in the number of procedures done on the patient, there is an increase of 0.12 units in the odds of being readmitted as a patient. Being a patient who fell under the poverty line had a significant negative impact on being readmitted. For every increase in income bracket, there is a decrease of 0.22 units of being readmitted as a patient. The odds ratio is Exp (β) = 0.81. For dual illness patients, the results showed that payment method did have an impact on their readmission odds. Additionally, social capital did not have an impact on patients' readmission odds. The results showed that males were more likely to be readmitted than females.

5. Discussion

This study examines contributing factors that predict readmission likelihood for mental health and drug abuse patients. Readmission rates in the United States have been high for many years [8,18], and many institutions have been faced with financial penalties for high readmission rates [27]. To address these concerns, hospitals are seeking a new path forward to reduce readmissions. Several studies have reported different ways of reducing the readmissions rate. These include improving patient safety at hospital discharge [41], enhancing medication reconciliation [42], and improving the transition from inpatient to outpatient setting [43]. However, these prior studies often focus on chronic diseases [20,22,25] or combine mental health and drug abuse patients into one group [5,27,32]. This study separates these two groups of patients to discern differences in factors that impact their respective readmission odds. The findings showed some similarities and differences. For both groups, hospital treatments, economic factors, and social factors played significant roles in predicting readmissions. However, their effects varied across the two groups. Specifically, the number of procedures was a significant predictor for mental health patients' readmissions, but not for drug abuse patients, while length of stay was a significant predictor for drug abuse patients' readmissions but not for mental health patients. This is a contrasting finding with prior studies as researchers have associated lower length of stay with lower readmission rates for mental health patients [31,32]. Interestingly, for mental health patients, the number of procedures had a positive impact, and the number of diagnoses had a negative impact. Prior research has often associated the number of procedures with lower readmission rates [22,38], but has not scrutinized the number of diagnoses. Future study is needed to explain the underlying reason.

In terms of economic factors, the findings confirm prior studies that economic factors matter [5,34], however, prominent differences between the two types of patients were found. Patients in higher income levels were likely readmitted for drug abuse issues but not mental health issues, and private insurance and self-pay significantly predicted readmissions of drug abuse patients but not mental health patients. Relating back to the Affordable Care Act, mental health is covered by Medicare and Medicaid, so this finding that only Medicare and Medicaid patients are frequently readmitted makes sense. This finding also suggests that healthcare accessibility through economic means has different effects on different types of patients. This seems to indicate that patients with more disposable income are likely to relapse to drug abuse. This finding is also related to social capital impact when an opposite effect is observed: High social capital locations were associated with a higher chance of readmission for drug abuse, but lower readmission odds for mental health patients. This is a surprising finding given prior studies have often associated well-off communities with lower admission rates overall [23,24,31,36,43]. Thus, the findings indicate that community-based support should be strategically allocated for each type of disease, as found in this current study.

The findings have several implications for societal sustainability. First, this study illustrates the importance of healthcare accessibility to the reduction of readmission rates for mental health and drug abuse patients. It echoes prior studies and suggests policy-makers pay greater attention to economic inequality as a direct influencer on community well-being [23,24]. For instance, given patients with high income levels who live in neighborhoods with high social capital actually have higher readmission odds for drug abuse issues, community leaders in well-off areas can consider incorporating rehabilitation facilities to address the issue. Second, the findings inform hospital administrators of various factors that can be used as an indicator of potential readmission among mental health and drug abuse patients. By identifying potential relapse, hospitals can reduce inefficiencies and get closer to a more sustainable healthcare system [19]. Finally, the findings show differences between mental health and drug abuse patients, which suggests the need for different policies to reduce readmission rates for each group of patients. For instance, patients with lower socio-economic means are likely to suffer from mental illness, thus governmental-level support is needed to help this population (e.g., extending coverage for mental illness).

The study is not without limitations. The data focused solely on New York State, thus, the findings are generalizable only to states that have similar demographics and populations. However, nation-wide data would be more comprehensive in addressing the shortfall for this study. A second limitation is that this data set is focused only on one year of readmission data. A longitudinal data set would benefit the study of these readmission rates in a time series manner. In other words, other determinants, such as a change in public policy due to a change in political parties, could be used to compare the difference in insurance cost and how that will impact readmission rates.

6. Conclusions

Hospitals in the United States are financially penalized for having a higher than expected thirty-day readmission rate among patients who have comorbid mental health diagnoses or other symptoms. Traditionally, hospitals have been categorizing readmission rates between drug abuse patients with mental health patients [5,27,31,32]. It is also unknown what the effect of distinguishing the readmission data into its respective disease could have on readmission rates. While many patients are comorbid patients, this study found that although the effects vary in each group, it is important to have different and separate policies to reduce readmission rates for patients with different types of diseases. Prior studies argued that providing support to mental health patients after their discharge helps with reducing physical health readmissions [36]. In addition, prior studies found that alcohol dependence and other mental disorders are associated with inpatient admission or emergency department (ED) visits [5]. In that same study, the authors found that insurance types were predictors of readmission. This study contributes to the existing literature by utilizing hospital discharge data from the state of New York to understand predictors for readmission rates of mental health and drug abuse patients. This study investigated not only the hospital-controllable and patient-controllable factors (i.e., hospital treatments and economic factors) but also uncontrollable factors, such as social determinants, to predict the readmission odds of mental health and drug abuse patients. Considering the high rate of readmissions and ED use in the United States [18], and the concomitant spending by patients, such efforts to address these knowledge gaps could improve patient outcomes and reduce readmission rates, which leads to a reduction of health care costs in a sustainable manner.

Author Contributions: All authors have contributed equally to the conceptualization, analysis, writing, and preparation of this study. All authors have read and agreed to the published version of the manuscript.

Funding: This research received no external funding.

Informed Consent Statement: Not applicable.

Data Availability Statement: This study uses 2015 discharge data from New York, State Inpatient Databases (SID), Healthcare Cost and Utilization Project (HCUP), Agency for Healthcare Research and Quality (https://www.hcup-us.ahrq.gov/).

Conflicts of Interest: The authors declare no conflict of interest.

References

1. WHA. *Comprehensive Mental Health Action Plan 2013–2020*; WHO: Geneva, Switzerland, 2013.
2. UN. *Transforming Our World: The 2030 Agenda for Sustainable Development*; UN: New York, NY, USA, 2015.
3. Rajkumar, R.P. Covid-19 And Mental Health: A Review Of The Existing Literature. *Asian J. Psychiatry* **2020**, *52*, 1–5. [CrossRef] [PubMed]
4. Havassy, B.E.; Alvidrez, J.; Mericle, A.A. Disparities in Use of Mental Health and Substance Abuse Services by Persons with Co-occurring Disorders. *Psychiatr. Serv.* **2009**, *60*, 217–223. [CrossRef] [PubMed]
5. Smith, M.W.; Stocks, C.; Santora, P.B. Hospital Readmission Rates and Emergency Department Visits for Mental Health and Substance Abuse Conditions. *Community Mental Health J.* **2015**, *51*, 190–197. [CrossRef] [PubMed]
6. Nguyen, M.H.; Le, T.T.; Meirmanov, S. Depression, Acculturative Stress, and Social Connectedness among International University Students in Japan: A Statistical Investigation. *Sustainability* **2019**, *11*, 878. [CrossRef]
7. Castiblanque, R.P.; Calatayud, P.J.B. Inequalities and the Impact of Job Insecurity on Health Indicators in the Spanish Workforce. *Sustainability* **2020**, *12*, 6425. [CrossRef]
8. NSDUH. *Key Substance Use and Mental Health Indicators in the United States: Results from the 2017 National Survey on Drug Use and Health*; Center for Behavioral Health Statistics and Quality, Substance Abuse and Mental Health Services Administration: Rockville, MD, USA, 2018.
9. Mental Health America. The State of Mental Health in America. Available online: https://mhanational.org/issues/state-mental-health-america (accessed on 30 June 2020).
10. National Institute on Drug Abuse. Opioid Overdose Crisis. Available online: https://www.drugabuse.gov/drug-topics/opioids/opioid-overdose-crisis (accessed on 30 June 2020).
11. Scheirer, M.A.; Dearing, J.W. An Agenda for Research on the Sustainability of Public Health Programs. *Am. J. Public Health* **2011**, *101*, 2059–2067. [CrossRef]
12. Shelton, R.C.; Cooper, B.R.; Stirman, S.W. The Sustainability of Evidence-Based Interventions and Practices in Public Health and Health Care. *Annu. Rev. Public Health* **2018**, *39*, 55–76. [CrossRef]
13. Bircher, J.; Kuruvilla, S. Defining Health By Addressing Individual, Social, And Environmental Determinants: New Opportunities For Health Care And Public Health. *J. Public Health Policy* **2014**, *35*, 363–386. [CrossRef]
14. Shi, L.; Singh, D.A. *Delivering Health Care in America: A System Approach*; Jones & Bartlett Learning: New York, NY, USA, 2014.
15. Rau, J. Under Trump, Hospitals Face Same Penalties Embraced By Obama. *Kaiser Health News*, 3 August 2017.
16. Chollet, D.; Barrett, A.; Lake, T. *Reducing Hospital Readmissions in New York State: A Simulation Analysis of Alternative Payment Incentives*; NYS Health Foundation: New York, NY, USA, 2011.
17. World Population Review. Mental Health Statistics By State 2020. Available online: https://worldpopulationreview.com/state-rankings/mental-health-statistics-by-state#dataTable (accessed on 30 June 2020).
18. Gusmano, M.; Rodwin, V.; Weisz, D.; Cottenet, J.; Quantin, C. Comparison of Rehospitalization Rates in France and the United States. *J. Health Serv. Res. Policy* **2015**, *20*, 18–25. [CrossRef]
19. Fineberg, H.V. A Successful and Sustainable Health System—How to Get There from Here. *N. Engl. J. Med.* **2012**, *366*, 1020–1027. [CrossRef]
20. Basu, J.; Avila, R.; Ricciardi, R. Hospital Readmission Rates in U.S. States: Are Readmissions Higher Where More Patients with Multiple Chronic Conditions Cluster? *Health Serv. Res.* **2016**, *51*, 1135–1151. [CrossRef] [PubMed]
21. Chakraborty, H.; Axon, R.N.; Brittingham, J.; Lyons, G.R.; Cole, L.; Turley, C.B. Differences in Hospital Readmission Risk across All Payer Groups in South Carolina. *Health Serv. Res.* **2017**, *52*, 1040–1060. [CrossRef] [PubMed]
22. Clark, D.E.; Ostrander, K.R.; Cushing, B.M. A Multistate Model Predicting Mortality, Length of Stay, and Readmission for Surgical Patients. *Health Serv. Res.* **2016**, *51*, 1074–1094. [CrossRef] [PubMed]
23. Aswani, M.S.; Kilgore, M.L.; Becker, D.J.; Redden, D.T.; Sen, B.; Blackburn, J. Differential Impact of Hospital and Community Factors on Medicare Readmission Penalties. *Health Serv. Res.* **2018**, *53*, 4416–4436. [CrossRef] [PubMed]
24. Herrin, J.; St. Andre, J.; Kenward, K.; Joshi, M.S.; Audet, A.M.J.; Hines, S.C. Community Factors and Hospital Readmission Rates. *Health Serv. Res.* **2015**, *50*, 20–39. [CrossRef] [PubMed]
25. Navathe, A.S.; Zhong, F.; Lei, V.J.; Chang, F.Y.; Sordo, M.; Topaz, M.; Navathe, S.B.; Rocha, R.A.; Zhou, L. Hospital Readmission and Social Risk Factors Identified from Physician Notes. *Health Serv. Res.* **2018**, *53*, 1110–1136. [CrossRef]
26. Zingmond, D.S.; Liang, L.J.; Parikh, P.; Escarce, J.J. The Impact of the Hospital Readmissions Reduction Program across Insurance Types in California. *Health Serv. Res.* **2018**, *53*, 4403–4415. [CrossRef]
27. Kripalani, S.; Theobald, C.N.; Anctil, B.; Vasilevskis, E.E. Reducing hospital readmission rates: Current strategies and future directions. *Annu. Rev. Med.* **2014**, *65*, 471–485. [CrossRef]
28. Becker, M.; Boaz, T.; Andel, R.; Hafner, S.; Becker, M.A.; Boaz, T.L. Risk of Early Rehospitalization for Non-Behavioral Health Conditions Among Adult Medicaid Beneficiaries with Severe Mental Illness or Substance Use Disorders. *J. Behav. Health Serv. Res.* **2017**, *44*, 113–121. [CrossRef]
29. Singh, G.; Wei, Z.; Yong-Fang, K.; Sharma, G.; Zhang, W.; Kuo, Y.-F. Association of Psychological Disorders With 30-Day Readmission Rates in Patients With COPD. *CHEST* **2016**, *149*, 905–915. [CrossRef]
30. Rylander, M.; Colon-Sanchez, D.; Keniston, A.; Hamalian, G.; Lozano, A.; Nussbaum, A.M. Risk Factors for Readmission on an Adult Inpatient Psychiatric Unit. *Qual. Manag. Health Care* **2016**, *25*, 22–31. [CrossRef] [PubMed]

31. Mark, T.; Tomic, K.; Kowlessar, N.; Chu, B.; Vandivort-Warren, R.; Smith, S. Hospital Readmission Among Medicaid Patients with an Index Hospitalization for Mental and/or Substance Use Disorder. *J. Behav. Health Serv. Res.* **2013**, *40*, 207–221. [CrossRef] [PubMed]
32. Swindle, R.W.; Phibbs, C.S.; Paradise, M.J.; Recine, B.P.; Moos, R.H. Inpatient Treatment For Substance Abuse Patients With Psychiatric Disorders: A National Study of Determinants of Readmission. *J. Subst. Abuse* **1995**, *7*, 79–97. [CrossRef]
33. Huynh, C.; Ferland, F.; Blanchette-Martin, N.; Ménard, J.-M.; Fleury, M.-J. Factors Influencing the Frequency of Emergency Department Utilization by Individuals with Substance Use Disorders. *Psychiatr. Q.* **2016**, *87*, 713–728. [CrossRef] [PubMed]
34. Lam, C.N.; Arora, S.; Menchine, M. Increased 30-Day Emergency Department Revisits Among Homeless Patients with Mental Health Conditions. *Westwen J. Emerg. Med.* **2016**, *17*, 607–612. [CrossRef]
35. Khatana, S.A.M.; Wadhera, R.K.; Choi, E.; Groeneveld, P.W.; Culhane, D.P.; Kushel, M.; Kazi, D.S.; Yeh, R.W.; Shen, C. Association of Homelessness with Hospital Readmissions—An Analysis of Three Large States. *J. Gen. Intern. Med.* **2020**, *35*, 2576–2583. [CrossRef]
36. Benjenk, I.; Chen, J. Effective Mental Health Interventions To Reduce Hospital Readmission Rates: A Systematic Review. *J. Hosp. Manag. Health Policy* **2018**, *2*, 45. [CrossRef]
37. AHRQ. *HCUP State Inpatient Databases*; Healthcare Cost and Utilization Project/Agency for Healthcare Research and Quality: Rockville, MD, USA, 2015.
38. Bardhan, I.; Oh, J.H.; Zheng, Z.Q.; Kirksey, K. Predictive Analytics for Readmission of Patients with Congestive Heart Failure. *Inf. Syst. Res.* **2015**, *26*, 19–39. [CrossRef]
39. Rupasingha, A.; Goetz, S.J.; Freshwater, D. The Production of Social Capital in US Counties. *J. Socio-Econ.* **2006**, *35*, 83–101. [CrossRef]
40. Bui, Q.N.; Hansen, S.; Liu, M.; Tu, Q. From Meaningful Use to Meaningful Results: Revisiting the Productivity Paradox in the Case of Health Information Technology. *Commun. ACM* **2018**, *61*, 78–85. [CrossRef]
41. Hansen, L.O.; Young, R.S.; Hinami, K.; Leung, A.; Williams, M.V. Interventions To Reduce 30-Day Rehospitalization: A Systematic Review. *Ann. Intern. Med.* **2011**, *155*, 520–528. [CrossRef] [PubMed]
42. Rennke, S.; Nguyen, O.K.; Shoeb, M.H.; Magan, Y.; Wachter, R.M.; Ranji, S.R. Hospital-Initiated Transitional Care Interventions As A Patient Safety Strategy: A Systematic Review. *Ann. Intern. Med.* **2013**, *158*, 433–440. [CrossRef] [PubMed]
43. Hesselink, G.; Zegers, M.; Vernooij-Dassen, M.; Barach, P.; Kalkman, C.; Flink, M.; Ön, G.; Olsson, M.; Bergenbrant, S.; Orrego, C.; et al. Improving Patient Discharge And Reducing Hospital Readmissions By Using Intervention Mapping. *BMC Health Serv. Res.* **2014**, *14*, 389. [CrossRef] [PubMed]

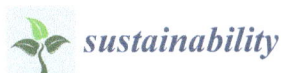

Article

Inequalities and the Impact of Job Insecurity on Health Indicators in the Spanish Workforce

Raúl Payá Castiblanque * and Pere J. Beneyto Calatayud

Department of Sociology and Social Anthropology, University of Valencia, Av. dels Tarongers 4b, 46022 Valencia, Spain; Pere.J.Beneyto@uv.es
* Correspondence: raul.paya@uv.es; Tel.: +34-650-157-401

Received: 15 June 2020; Accepted: 7 August 2020; Published: 10 August 2020

Abstract: In a context of high job insecurity resulting from social deregulation policies, this research aims to study health and substance abuse inequalities in the workplace from a gender perspective. To this end, a transversal study was carried out based on microdata from the National Health Survey in Spain—2017, selecting the active population and calculating the prevalence of the state of health and consumption, according to socio-occupational factors (work relationship, social occupational class, time and type of working day). Odds ratios adjusted by socio-demographic variables and their 90% confidence intervals were estimated by means of binary logistic regressions stratified by sex. The results obtained showed two differentiated patterns of health and consumption. On the one hand, unemployed people and those from more vulnerable social classes showed a higher prevalence of both chronic depression and anxiety and of hypnosedative and tobacco use. On the other hand, the better positioned social classes reported greater work stress and alcohol consumption. In addition, while unemployment affected men's health more intensely, women were more affected by the type of working day. The study can be used to design sustainable preventive occupational health policies, which should at least aim at improving the quantity and quality of employment.

Keywords: job insecurity; health and consumption indicators; gender inequalities; sustainable preventive policies

1. Introduction

More than a decade has passed since the financial crisis and the stagnation of the global economy in 2008 (the great recession) began and austerity policies (the great aggression) imposed by the Troika (formed by the European Commission, the European Central Bank and the International Monetary Fund) based on a political exchange of "neoliberal intergovernmentalism" that forced the member states of the European Union with economic difficulties, especially the countries of the South (Spain, Greece and Portugal), to deregulate the labor market and labor relations [1,2] with the "conditionality" of obtaining financial aid and bank bailouts [3]. These policies have led to a radical transformation of industrial relations models and the breakdown of the fragile balances achieved during decades of social dialogue by deregulating the three historical collective mechanisms that have acted in the defense and protection of workers: protection of legality, trade union intervention and business coverage [4]. This aggression has meant a great regression that, on the one hand, has led the most disadvantaged social classes to even worse living conditions, and, on the other hand, has slipped the middle classes into economic fragility, extending economic and social vulnerability to large social strata [5].

In this regard, with regard to the extent of social and economic vulnerability in the field of health, a study by Stuckler et al. [6,7] in post-communist countries found that massive privatization programs in the health system increased short-term adult male mortality rates by 12.8% among the most disadvantaged social classes. On a national level, the impact of austerity policies on the health of the Spanish population has been the subject of numerous investigations from the public health field, concluding that the effects on the population are heterogeneous and controversial, endangering the sustainability of the national health system [8–12]. In particular, important differences have been identified between the Autonomous Communities in terms of the management of the economic crisis and austerity policies. While the government of the Basque Country did not implement austerity policies during the crisis, in La Rioja, Madrid and the Balearic Islands, privatization policies were implemented in the health system [8]. In addition, the study conducted by Del Pozo-Rubio et al. [10] showed how the co-payment of dependency introduced in Spain through the Resolution of 13 July 2012 meant, on the one hand, an unequal application of co-payments between the Autonomous Communities, with Andalusia, Valencia and Catalonia having the highest levels of co-payment, and, on the other hand, how the co-payment went from 20% in the national average before the reform to 53.54% after the reform. Thus, these studies would confirm both the inequalities between social classes and between the different regions of Spain. In addition, there is empirical evidence on problems of technical quality (misdiagnosis or inappropriate diagnosis) and interpersonal quality (poorer treatment and communication) in the public health system related to cuts in the health workforce, which affects the whole population, but especially people with fewer resources and immigrants [12]. These cuts and privatizations could explain how since the beginning of the economic crisis in Spain, there has been a significant slowdown in the reduction of the cancer mortality rate [11], which would be related in some way to the studies by Stuckler and others [6,7]. This context of economic crisis jeopardizes the sustainability of the welfare state, as the protection system (healthcare and social benefits) is financed in most European countries through employers' and workers' contributions to work performance. As a result, austerity measures reduce state revenues, which are largely dependent on full employment and decent wage policies, leading to severe cuts in public health and other social expenditures [13]. High unemployment rates in turn erode the bargaining power of workers and their class organizations, feeding back into the spiral of deregulation and deterioration of working conditions and occupational health [14].

In this context and for the purposes of this research, there has been an increase in job insecurity both in the European Union (EU) in general and in Spain in particular [15]. Job insecurity can be defined as a perceived threat to the continuity and stability of employment as currently experienced [16] or the loss of well-being resulting from job uncertainty [17]. Different domains or facets of job insecurity can be drawn from these definitions. The first would be uncertainty in a threefold dimension: (a) uncertainty about whether or not employment will eventually be lost; (b) uncertainty about when it will occur, i.e., when the job will be lost; and (c) uncertainty about the consequences of the loss of employment [18]. The second domain would be the threat, since the uncertainty of loss of employment is comparable to the severity of the threat [19]. That is, depending on the possibilities of finding new employment and the degree of dependence on wages for survival, the degree of threat will be greater or lesser, and therefore, is related to some theories of human needs (for example, Maslow's pyramid) [20]. Finally, there is a third dimension that refers to the powerlessness or absence of strategies available to workers to resist the threat of dismissal [21–23]. Thus, the lack of protection (trade unions, working without a contract, unemployment benefit systems, and so on) makes it more or less likely that they will resist the threat of unemployment [22]. In the scientific literature, various ways can be found to study and make job insecurity operational in order to measure it. On the one hand, there are studies that focus on the analysis of perceived or subjective insecurity [24], understood as an interpretation or evaluation by the worker of a series of external signs that have to do with job continuity [25]. On the other hand, there are studies that focus on the analysis of attributed insecurity [26], that is, on the objective signs of insecurity (contractual situation, position of the worker in the company, working conditions, etc.) that do not depend on the worker's perception [24]. Although there are various ways of studying job insecurity, the fact is that perceived or subjective insecurity and attributed or objective insecurity are related, insofar as, although perceived insecurity depends on personal and contextual factors, which may lead some workers to overestimate the probability of losing their jobs, the fact is that there is empirical evidence that correlates the subjective dimension with the objective one [27]. In fact, it has been shown that temporary contracts are associated with greater self-perceived insecurity [28–30] and the transformation of temporary contracts into permanent contracts with a greater perception of security [31]. The focus of this research is on attributed insecurity and therefore requires further analysis. In this regard, the previous literature has identified four types of studies related to objective insecurity: (a) research that focuses on studying insecurity dynamically through unstable employment trajectories [32,33]; (b) insecurity produced by closures, restructuring or downsizing, including those workers not affected by layoffs [34,35]; (c) job insecurity from the point of view of the type of contract or contractual relationship (temporary or permanent) [36,37]; and (d) research that studies job insecurity from a multidimensional point of view not only based on the contractual relationship but also including other elements such as occupational social class or working time, approaching the concept of job insecurity [38–41]. From the classification given, this study is part of the proposals for measuring insecurity attributed from a multidimensional perspective. It should be noted that this holistic perspective is related to labor precariousness, since this construct is broader and contemplates insecurity but not in an isolated manner [25].

Focusing on the health effects of perceived job insecurity, previous studies have identified how a subjective perception of insecurity leads to an erosion of job satisfaction [42], increased feelings of anxiety [15], or high levels of stress comparable to those who are unemployed [16]. However, the psychological health effects of job insecurity can be modulated by subjective employability [43]. In other words, subjective employability differs from objective employability (observable contextual conditions such as contractual conditions [44]) because it focuses on people's belief that they can easily find a new job based on their genuine skills, such as work experience or educational level [45], and that previous studies have shown that it is associated with lower levels of psychological risk when unemployment is addressed proactively [45–47].

With regard to the health effects of attributed or objective job insecurity, it has been shown that unemployment exposes individuals to greater psychological risk [48,49]. Specifically, unemployment has been associated with a worse self-perceived general health status [50], increased mental illness such as anxiety and depression [51,52], psychosomatic and sleep disorders [43,49], the use of hypnosedatives [50,53], addictive behaviors such as the consumption of alcohol, tobacco or drugs [50,53,54], and even family conflicts and suicides [48]. If we focus on the multidimensional perspective of this study, previous research has observed elements of job insecurity attributed to the increase in psychosomatic disorders and unhealthy habits, such as the use of hypnosedatives and addictive substances that erode people's health [55–60]. Specifically, with regard to contractual status, working conditions and occupational social class, it has been identified that (a) people on temporary contracts use health services less frequently for fear of being absent from work and dismissed [55]; (b) working long hours has been associated with higher levels of alcohol consumption [55]; (c) night work has been associated with regular smoking [56]; (d) high levels of occupational stress have been associated with a higher prevalence of alcohol consumption [57,58] and the use of hypnosedatives [59]; and (e) the more vulnerable manual social classes have been associated with poor mental health [60] and regular tobacco use [55].

From the findings of the previous literature, it is possible to observe multiple and complex bilateral and multilateral relationships between socio-professional factors, on the one hand, and the spiral of constant health deterioration on the other. For example, work-related stress has been associated with depression or anxiety [60,61]. These mental disorders are in turn linked to the use of hypnosedatives [59] and addictive behavior [57,58]. Even among the most disadvantaged manual workers, alcohol consumption has been found to be associated with an increased likelihood of losing their job [62], which deepens the feedback between social vulnerability and health impairment.

Given the complexity and current occupational vulnerability in Spain and the scarce specific and partial studies that study the associations between mental health, the use of hypnosedatives and the consumption of addictive substances in the workplace, it is necessary to carry out more extensive analyses to explore possible patterns of relationships between all the aforementioned variables of health and consumption of the active population in the labor market, in order to establish sustainable health and employment policies that reverse the health emergency situation caused, to a certain extent, by the economic crisis management policies themselves. Therefore, the main objective of this research is to explore, holistically and jointly, the possible patterns between the main occupational factors of attributed or objective job insecurity (type of contract or employment relationship, occupational social class, working time and type of working day) and the various health factors (general and mental state, consumption of hypnosedatives, tobacco and alcohol) in the Spanish active population. In addition, several studies indicate that the different gender roles in the area of reproductive tasks [63,64] and the precarious working conditions that affect working women most intensely [65,66] make them more likely to refer to psychosomatic disorders and to consume more hypnosedatives [67–69]. In light of these findings, it is considered relevant to address the objective of this research to explore health and consumption patterns by stratifying the working population sample by sex.

2. Materials and Methods

2.1. Sample and Study Population

In order to achieve the proposed objectives, the use of the microdata from the questionnaire for adults from the National Health Survey (ENSE, 2017) [70], carried out by the Ministry of Health, Consumption and Social Welfare of Spain, was considered the most suitable source for carrying out the study, since for each Autonomous Community, an independent sample was designed, which allowed for having a large and representative sample of the entire country [71]. The sample carried out was a polytopic one. In the first stage the census sections were selected and in the second stage the main family dwellings were selected. In each dwelling, an adult person aged 16 years old or over was selected to carry out the adult questionnaire. The fieldwork was extended between the months of October 2016 and October 2017, for the purpose of collecting data that might be affected by seasonality. The total size of the ENSE survey for adults in 2017 was 23,089 persons, with a high response rate of 95%. Information was collected through personal interviews. The same was complemented, in exceptional cases, by means of a telephone interview. For the present study, only the active population was selected. The active population was considered to be those persons who were of working age (16 years old or over in Spanish legislation) and who carried out a professional activity, as well as those persons of working age who were unemployed and who were actively seeking employment [72]. Thus, the sample for this research was 12,260 persons between the ages of 16 and 64 years old. Specifically, the study included a sample of 6299 men (5163 (82%) employed and 1136 (18%) unemployed) and 5931 women (4610 (77.3%) employed and 1351 (22.7%) unemployed) (Table 1).

Table 1. Sociodemographic characteristics of the active population in Spain, health status, consumption of hypnosedatives, tobacco and alcohol, according to sex.

Variables	Men (n = 6299; 51.4%)	Women (n = 5961; 48.6%)	p-Value [b]
	n (%) [a]	n (%) [a]	
Self-perceived health status			<0.001
Bad	1168 (18.5)	1486 (24.9)	
Good	5131 (81.5)	4475 (75.1)	
Visits to the family doctor			<0.001
No	1902 (30.2)	1069 (17.9)	
Yes	4397 (69.8)	4892 (82.1)	
Depression			<0.001
No	6012 (95.5)	5391 (90.4)	
Yes	285 (4.5)	566 (9.5)	
DK/DA	2 (0.0)	4 (0.1)	

Table 1. *Cont.*

Variables	Men (n = 6299; 51.4%) n (%) [a]	Women (n = 5961; 48.6%) n (%) [a]	p-Value [b]
Chronic anxiety			<0.001
No	5960 (94.6)	5302 (89.0)	
Yes	334 (5.3)	651 (10.9)	
DK/DA	5 (0.1)	8 (0.1)	
Stress			<0.001
No	2670 (51.7)	2209 (48.1)	
Yes	2484 (48.1)	2388 (51.8)	
DK/DA	9 (0.2)	3 (0.1)	
Tranquilizers, relaxants, sleeping pills			<0.001
No	2840 (45.0)	3137 (52.6)	
Yes	369 (5.9)	601 (10.1)	
DK/DA	3090 (49.1)	2223 (37.3)	
Antidepressants, stimulants			<0.001
No	3072 (48.7)	3431 (57.6)	
Yes	137 (2.2)	307 (5.1)	
DK/DA	3090 (49.1)	2223 (37.3)	
Smoke			<0.001
No	4148 (65.9)	4205 (70.6)	
Yes	2144 (34.1)	1753 (29.4)	
DK/DA	7 (0.1)	3 (0.0)	
Alcohol			<0.001
No	2102 (33.4)	3384 (56.8)	
Yes	4192 (66.6)	2573 (43.2)	
DK/DA	5 (0.1)	4 (0.1)	
Type of contract or employment situation			<0.001
Entrepreneur	370 (5.9)	182 (3.1)	
Official	505 (8.0)	607 (10.2)	
Indefinite salaried	2754 (43.7)	2517 (42.2)	
Temporary employee	769 (12.2)	788 (13.2)	
Autonomous	742 (11.8)	460 (7.7)	
Without contract	23 (0.4)	56 (0.9)	
Unemployed	1136 (18%)	1351 (22.7)	
Occupational Category			<0.001
Managers with more than 10 workers	732 (11.6)	759 (12.8)	
Managers with fewer than 10 workers	525 (8.3)	584 (9.8)	
Intermediate technicians	1190 (18.9)	1270 (21.4)	
Qualified supervisors	957 (15.2)	582 (9.8)	
Qualified manual technicians	2045 (32.5)	1808 (30.3)	
Unqualified manual technicians	809 (12.8)	924 (15.5)	
DK/DA	41 (0.7)	34 (0.6)	
Working time			<0.001
Full time	4894 (94.8)	3616 (78.5)	
Part time	268 (5.2)	987 (21.4)	
DK/DA	1 (0.0)	7 (0.1)	

Table 1. *Cont.*

Variables	Men (n = 6299; 51.4%) n (%) [a]	Women (n = 5961; 48.6%) n (%) [a]	p-Value [b]
Type of working day			<0.001
Split shift	2105 (40.8)	1379 (29.9)	
Continue in the morning	1383 (26.8)	1638 (35.9)	
Continue in the afternoon	117 (2.3)	201 (4.4)	
Continue through the night	68 (1.3)	37 (0.8)	
Shifts	39 (0.8)	183 (4)	
Irregular or variable day according to the days	757 (14.8)	616 (13.4)	
Other types	637 (12.5)	506 (10.9)	
DK/DA	57 (1.1)	50 (1.0)	
Age			0.006
16–24	230 (3.7)	200 (3.4)	
25–34	946 (15.0)	1022 (17.1)	
35–44	1924 (30.5)	1844 (30.9)	
45–54	1851 (29.4)	1851 (29.0)	
≥55	1348 (21.4)	1168 (19.6)	
Nationality			0.014
Spanish	5516 (87.6)	5131 (86.1)	
Foreigner	783 (12.4)	830 (13.9)	
Marital status			<0.001
Single	1937 (30.7)	1667 (28.0)	
Married	3840 (61)	3310 (55.7)	
Widower	54 (0.9)	181 (3.0)	
Divorced	463 (7.4)	789 (13.3)	
DK/DA	5 (0.1)	14 (0.2)	
Education level			<0.001
Primary	860 (13.7)	604 (10.1)	
Secondary	4077 (64.7)	3501 (58.7)	
Tertiary	1362 (21.6)	1856 (31.1)	
Type of family life			<0.001
Married	3597 (57.1)	2813 (47.2)	
Domestic partner	189 (3.0)	137 (2.3)	
Do not live together	2513 (39.9)	3010 (50.5)	
Family care work			<0.001
No	5706 (90.6)	5216 (87.5)	
Yes	592 (9.4)	745 (12.5)	
Monthly household income			0.781
Less than 1050 euros per month	1983 (31.5)	5216 (87.5)	
From 1050 to less than 2200 euros	2739 (43.5)	745 (12.5)	
From 2200 to less than 4500 euros	1540 (24.4)	1465 (24.6)	
More than 4500 euros per month	37 (0.6)	26 (0.5)	

[a] n = number; % = percentage of total sample; [b] p value = sex differences calculated using Chi-square test, with 95% confidence level. DK/DA= Does not know/does not answer.

2.2. Dependent, Independent and Covariant Adjustment Variables

Nine dichotomised dependent variables were used. The general health status was evaluated on the basis of two questions: (a) "In the last twelve months, would you say your health status has been very good, good, fair, bad, very bad?" This question was dichotomized into 0 = Bad health (fair/bad/very bad) and 1 = Good health (very good/good); and (b) "When was the last time you consulted your general practitioner or family doctor for yourself?" The variable was dichotomized into 0 = No (12 months ago or more/Never) and 1 = Yes (Within the last 4 weeks/Between 4 weeks and 12 months). It is worth mentioning that the self-perceived health variable was dichotomized following common practices in public health studies [73–75]. In addition, we studied the relationship between the self-perceived health variable constructed with twenty-five indicators of pathologies diagnosed by health professionals, finding in all cases a statistically significant relationship that shows how people with good self-perceived health present a lower frequency of being diagnosed with pathologies (Table A1, Appendix A) and, therefore, demonstrate the validity of the constructed variable.

With regard to the state of mental health, three variables were used. Two of them refer to whether the person interviewed suffered from depression in the last 12 months (0 = No; 1 = Yes) or chronic anxiety (0 = No; 1 = Yes). The third variable, corresponding to work stress, was measured through the following question: "Globally and taking into account the conditions in which you carry out your work, indicate how you consider the level of stress of your work according to a scale from 1 (not at all stressful) to 7 (very stressful)". The question was dichotomized by the median which was 4, with 0 = No (from 1 to 4) and 1 = Yes (from 5 to 7). The consumption of hypnosedatives was measured through two questions referring to whether in the last 12 months the person interviewed had consumed tranquilizers, relaxants and/or sleeping pills (0 = No; 1 = Yes), or whether he/she took antidepressants and/or stimulants (0 = No; 1 = Yes). Finally, addictive behaviors were measured through two questions: (a) "Could you tell me if you smoke?"—the question was dichotomized into 0 = No (I don't currently smoke, but have smoked before/I don't smoke or have never smoked regularly) and 1 = Yes (Yes, I smoke daily/I do smoke, but not daily); and (b): "During the past 12 months, how often have you had alcoholic beverages of any kind?"—it was dichotomized by the median; this resulted in 0 = No (Never/No in last 12 months/3 days per month to less than 1 day in a month) and 1 = Yes (Daily or almost daily/6 to 1 days per week).

The independent variables correspond to the main socio-labor characteristics present in the ENSE survey itself. These are: the type of contract or employment situation, the socio-labor category, the working time and the type of working day. It is worth noting that it was not necessary to transform any of the four independent variables, since the ENSE already provided them in an adequate manner to carry out the study. The socio-demographic adjustment variables were age, nationality, marital status, level of education, the income of the family household, type of family life and family care work, following the guidelines of previous studies with similar characteristics [54,56,76]. These variables were selected because they interact predictably with gender roles and can affect men and women differently and act as confounding variables [59–62]. In fact, to avoid selection problems in the female labor force, these studies incorporate family status and care work as adjustment variables, since the reproductive and productive spheres are interconnected [60]. However, in order to verify the presence or absence of selection bias in the female labor force derived from their lower level of participation in the labor market, the Heckman two-stage model was used. The results obtained (Table A2) show that there is no selection bias in any of the nine dependent variables derived from the fact that the correlation coefficients of the error terms of the two equations (Rho) are close to zero and are not significant. Therefore, the likelihood test carried out to verify the null hypothesis of independence between the equations is not rejected. In addition, it can be seen how the coefficients of each variable show how women who are married or live with a partner and in households where there are care jobs have less participation in the labor market. These findings would reinforce the robustness of the results of the present study. Finally, it should be mentioned that the answers "don't know" and "don't respond" were eliminated from the statistical analyses.

2.3. Statistical Analysis

First, a descriptive analysis of the absolute and relative (%) frequencies of all the variables used was performed, and the differences between men and women were recorded using the chi-square test ($p < 0.05$) (Table 1). Secondly, before stratifying the sample by sex, in order to compare differences between health and consumption indicators between men and women, adjusted odds ratios (aOR) were calculated for all socio-labor and demographic variables and their 90% confidence intervals, using logistic regression models, establishing men as the reference category (Figure 1 and Table 2). Third, once the comparison between both sexes was made, the sample was stratified between the male and female labor force to find associations between socio-labor factors and health and consumption indicators. To this end, as in the previous case, logistical regressions adjusted for all socio-labor and demographic variables were carried out for both the male (Table 3) and female labor forces (Table 4). The regression models were based on the most favorable socio-labor categories (Employment status = Entrepreneur; Socio-labor category = Manager with more than 10 workers; Working time = Full time; Type of workday = Start), following the criteria of favorability used in previous studies with similar characteristics [54]. The goodness of fit of the models was evaluated using the Hosmer–Lemeshow test. The calculations were performed with the SPSS program (version 24) which allows the analysis of complex samples.

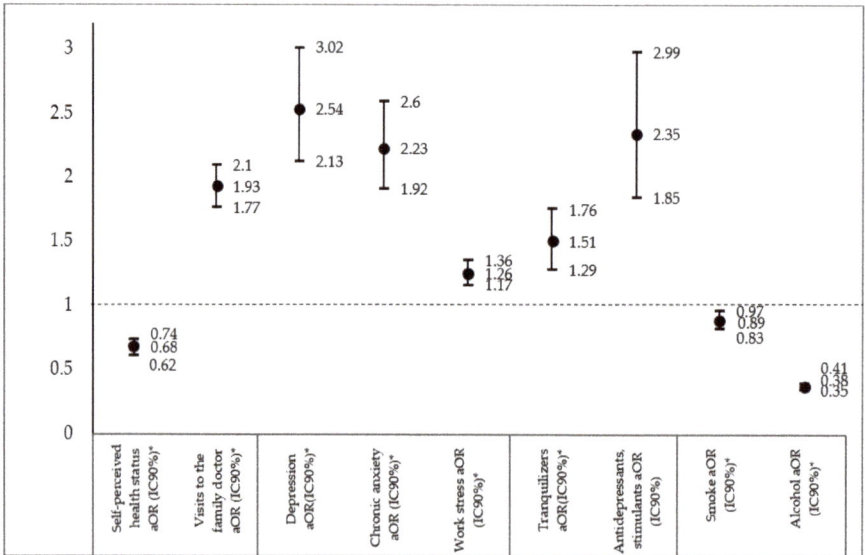

Figure 1. Logistic regressions between health and consumption indicators by sex. OR: adjusted odds ratio for the four socio-labor variables included in the table (type of contract or employment situation, occupational category, household income, working time and type of working day) and the demographic variables (age, nationality, marital status, level of education, type of family life, family care work, monthly household income) with men as the reference category; IC90%: confidence interval; * significance level of the p-value < 0.10.

Table 2. Regressions of health and consumption indicators with the interactions between gender with the type of work relationship and occupational social class.

	Health Status Last 12 Months		You Have Suffered from Mental Disorders in the Last 12 Months			Consumption of Sedative Hypnotics in the Last 12 Months		Use of Addictive Substances in the Last 12 Months	
	Self-Perceived Health Status aOR (IC90%) [a]	Visits to the Family Doctor aOR (IC90%) [a]	Depression aOR (IC90%) [a]	Chronic Anxiety aOR (IC90%) [a]	Work Stress aOR (IC90%) [a]	Tranquilizers aOR (IC90%) [a]	Antidepressants, Stimulants aOR (IC90%) [a]	Smoking aOR (IC90%) [a]	Alcohol aOR (IC90%) [a]
Entrepreneurs	1 [b]	1 [b]	1 [b]	1 [b]	1 [b]	1 [b]	1 [b]	1 [b]	1 [b]
Officials	1.57 (1.27–1.90) [g]	0.58 (0.4–0.69) [g]	1.44 (1.06–1.9) [f]	1.68 (1.28–2.2) [g]	1.04 (0.90–1.21)	1.52 (1.17–1.9) [g]	1.67 (1.14–2.44) [f]	0.70 (0.59–0.83) [g]	0.41 (0.3–0.47) [g]
Indefinite wage earners	1.72 (1.55–1.90) [g]	0.53 (0.4–0.58) [g]	1.78 (1.52–2.0) [g]	1.85 (1.59–2.1) [g]	1.30 (1.19–1.4) [g]	1.36 (1.17–1.58) [g]	1.46 (1.16–1.84) [g]	0.84 (0.77–0.92) [g]	0.40 (0.3–0.44) [g]
Temporary employees	1.54 (1.30–1.83) [g]	0.54 (0.4–0.63) [g]	2.33 (1.84–2.9) [g]	1.94 (1.65–2.4) [g]	0.80 (0.7–0.91) [f]	1.06 (0.81–1.39)	2.06 (1.48–2.89) [g]	0.86 (0.75–0.98) [e]	0.39 (0.3–0.45) [g]
Freelancers	1.65 (1.40–1.96) [g]	0.39 (0.3–0.45) [g]	1.70 (1.27–2.33) [g]	1.57 (1.17–2.1) [g]	0.96 (0.81–1.12)	1.42 (1.06–1.89) [f]	1.58 (1.05–2.3) [f]	0.67 (0.55–0.81) [g]	0.39 (0.3–0.46) [g]
Without contract	1.85 (0.73–4.66)	0.49 (0.24–1.06)	4.03 (2.22–7.3) [g]	3.96 (2.2–7.0) [g]	0.58 (0.3–0.95) [e]	1.71 (0.87–3.41)	4.01 (1.92–8.3) [g]	0.35 (0.20–0.64) [g]	0.26 (0.1–0.44) [g]
Unemployed	1.03 (0.91–1.17)	0.56 (0.49–0.64) [g]	3.19 (2.71–3.2) [g]	3.15 (2.69–3.6) [g]	– [d]	1.96 (1.65–2.31) [g]	2.95 (2.36–3.69) [g]	0.89 (0.79–0.99) [e]	0.27 (0.2–0.30) [g]
Managers with more than 10 employees	1 [b]	1 [b]	1 [b]	1 [b]	1 [b]	1 [b]	1 [b]	1 [b]	1 [b]
Managers with fewer than 10 employees	0.97 (0.84–1.12)	1.34 (1.16–1.5) [g]	1.48 (1.2–1.82) [g]	1.42 (1.15–1.7) [g]	0.90 (0.76–1.05)	1.38 (1.14–1.67) [f]	1.72 (1.33–2.22) [g]	0.70 (0.61–0.81) [g]	0.50 (0.4–0.56) [g]
Intermediate technicians	0.81 (0.74–0.88) [g]	1.69 (1.51–1.8) [g]	1.74 (1.5–1.97) [g]	1.97 (1.74–2.2) [g]	1.14 (1.02–1.2) [e]	1.68 (1.50–1.88) [g]	1.72 (1.47–2.02) [g]	0.75 (0.69–0.82) [g]	0.44 (0.4–0.48) [g]
Qualified supervisors	0.68 (0.62–0.75) [g]	2.32 (2.0–2.69) [g]	2.03 (1.7–2.32) [g]	2.23 (1.94–2.5) [g]	0.86 (0.74–1.02)	2.01 (1.78–2.27) [g]	2.02 (1.71–2.39) [g]	0.70 (0.63–0.79) [g]	0.29 (0.2–0.32) [g]
Qualified manual technicians	0.64 (0.60–0.69) [g]	1.99 (1.81–2.1) [g]	2.45 (2.23–2.6) [g]	2.27 (2.05–2.5) [g]	1.14 (1.03–1.2) [e]	1.95 (1.78–2.13) [g]	2.29 (2.03–2.59) [g]	0.75 (0.69–0.80) [g]	0.28 (0.2–0.30) [g]
Unqualified manual technicians	0.59 (0.54–0.65) [g]	2.18 (1.91–2.5) [g]	2.43 (2.1–2.73) [g]	2.45 (2.16–2.7) [g]	0.91 (0.79–1.06)	1.95 (1.74–2.18) [g]	2.22 (1.90–2.59) [g]	0.72 (0.65–0.80) [g]	0.24 (0.2–0.26) [g]

[a] OR: odds ratio adjusted for the four socio-labor variables included in the table (type of contract or employment situation, occupational category, working time and type of working day) and the demographic variables (age, nationality, marital status, level of education, type of family life, family care work, monthly household income); IC 90%: confidence interval; [b] Reference category. In interactions the reference category is men; [c] Insufficient sample size for analysis; [d] Indicators measured only in employed persons; [e] Significance level of value of $p < 0.1$; [f] Significance level value of $p < 0.05$; [g] Significance level value of $p < 0.01$.

Table 3. Adjusted logistic regression between socio-labor determinants and health and consumption indicators in the male labor force.

	Health Status Last 12 Months		You Have Suffered from Mental Disorders in the Last 12 Months			Consumption of Sedative-Hypnotics in the Last 12 Months		Use of Addictive Substances in the last 12 Months	
	Self-Perceived Health Status aOR (IC90%) [a]	Visits to the Family Doctor aOR (IC90%) [a]	Depression aOR (IC90%) [a]	Chronic Anxiety aOR (IC90%) [a]	Work Stress aOR (IC90%) [a]	Tranquilizers aOR (IC90%) [a]	Antidepressants, Stimulants aOR (IC90%) [a]	Smoke aOR (IC90%) [a]	Alcohol aOR (IC90%) [a]
Entrepreneurs	1 [b]	1 [b]	1 [b]	1 [b]	1 [b]	1 [b]	1 [b]	1 [b]	1 [b]
Officials	1.04 (0.77–1.41)	1.04 (0.81–1.34)	1.67 (0.87–3.21)	1.84 (0.97–3.47)	0.60 (0.47–0.7) [g]	1.60 (0.96–2.66)	3.33 (1.11–9.91)	0.71 (0.55–0.92) [f]	0.85 (0.66–1.11)
Indefinite wage earners	1.07 (0.84–1.36)	1.01 (0.84–1.26)	1.01 (0.57–1.77)	1.57 (0.90–2.73)	0.78 (0.6–0.94) [f]	1.13 (0.73–1.74)	1.85 (0.68–5.03)	0.94 (0.77–1.16)	0.86 (0.69–1.05)
Temporary employees	0.91 (0.69–1.21)	1.13 (0.89–1.44)	1.52 (0.81–2.87)	1.63 (0.88–3.03)	0.55 (0.4–0.68) [g]	0.89 (0.53–1.52)	3.43 (1.19–9.93) [f]	1.27 (1.01–1.60) [f]	0.81 (0.64–1.03)
Freelancers	1.04 (0.79–1.36)	0.75 (0.59–0.9) [e]	1.18 (0.63–2.22)	1.83 (1.01–3.3) [e]	0.47 (0.2–1.03)	0.92 (0.55–1.53)	2.67 (0.93–7.67)	0.91 (0.77–1.14)	0.92 (0.73–1.17)
Without contract	1.07 (0.41–2.79)	1.07 (0.49–2.33)	3.44 (0.87–13.5)	- [c]	0.64 (0.5–0.79) [f]	- [c]	5.53 (0.75–40.74)	1.59 (0.77–3.31)	0.56 (0.27–1.16)
Unemployed	0.57 (0.38–0.89) [g]	1.15 (0.83–1.60)	5.53 (2.4–12.2) [g]	5.92 (2.8–12,4) [g]	- [d]	3.09 (1.60–5.95) [g]	6.75 (1.91–23.83) [g]	1.75 (1.28–2.41) [g]	0.51 (0.3–0.71) [g]
Managers with more than 10 employees	1 [b]	1 [b]	1 [b]	1 [b]	1 [b]	1 [b]	1 [b]	1 [b]	1 [b]
Managers with fewer than 10 employees	0.89 (0.73–1.10)	1.27 (1.06–1.5) [e]	1.54 (0.98–2.31)	1.44 (0.98–2.11)	0.89 (0.73–1.09)	1.63 (1.21–2.20) [f]	1.43 (0.83–2.48)	1.36 (1.12–1.64) [g]	0.93 (0.78–1.10)
Intermediate technicians	0.80 (0.67–1.00)	1.24 (1.06–1.4) [e]	2.10 (1.5–2.95) [g]	1.60 (1.16–2.2) [f]	0.87 (0.74–1.04)	1.34 (1.0–1.79)	1.75 (1.11–2.75) [e]	1.41 (1.20–1.66) [g]	0.87 (0.75–1.05)
Qualified supervisors	0.76 (0.67–1.00)	1.39 (1.18–1.6) [e]	1.78 (1.25–2.5) [f]	1.59 (1.13–2.2) [f]	0.84 (0.69–1.02)	1.48 (1.13–1.94) [f]	1.89 (1.19–3.01) [f]	1.81 (1.53–2.14) [g]	1.01 (0.86–1.17)
Qualified manual technicians	0.69 (0.64–0.91) [f]	1.24 (0.99–1.65)	2.22 (1.58–3.1) [g]	1.76 (1.27–2.4) [g]	0.63 (0.69–1.02)	1.36 (1.00–1.77)	1.77 (1.13–2.77) [f]	2.07 (1.76–2.42) [g]	0.88 (0.76–1.01)
Unqualified manual technicians	0.57 (0.48–0.69) [g]	1.20 (0.96–1.44)	2.39 (1.67–3.4) [g]	2.40 (1.71–3.4) [g]	0.51 (0.5–0.76) [g]	1.92 (1.44–2.56) [g]	2.30 (1.42–3.71) [g]	2.62 (2.19–3.13) [g]	0.68 (0.58–0.8) [g]
Full-time	1 [b]	1 [b]	1 [b]	1 [b]	1 [b]	1 [b]	1 [b]	1 [b]	1 [b]
Part-time	0.87 (0.67–1.17)	1.09 (0.87–1.37)	1.64 (0.98–2.74)	1.48 (0.94–2.35)	0.60 (0.49–0.7) [g]	1.54 (1.01–2.34) [e]	1.64 (0.83–3.24)	1.23 (0.99–1.53)	0.85 (0.68–1.05)
Split shift	1 [b]	1 [b]	1 [b]	1 [b]	1 [b]	1 [b]	1 [b]	1 [b]	1 [b]
Continues in the morning	0.95 (0.81–1.11)	1.11 (0.98–1.26)	1.38 (1.00–1.91)	1.18 (0.88–1.58)	0.70 (0.6–0.79) [g]	1.18 (0.90–1.56)	0.92 (0.58–1.48)	1.15 (1.02–1.31)	0.87 (0.77–1.00)
Continues in the afternoon	0.77 (0.51–1.15)	1.23 (0.87–1.74)	1.59 (0.72–3.52)	2.04 (1.08–3.8) [e]	0.79 (0.58–1.10)	1.71 (0.92–3.18)	0.93 (0.27–3.17)	0.97 (0.69–1.37)	0.75 (0.54–1.05)
Continues in the evening	0.73 (0.45–1.19)	1.09 (0.70–1.70)	1.02 (0.31–3.40)	0.40 (0.07–2.10)	0.72 (0.47–1.09)	1.05 (0.35–2.88)	2.98 (1.04–8.53) [e]	1.11 (0.72–1.71)	0.80 (0.52–1.22)
Shifts	0.82 (0.52–0.99) [e]	1.25 (1.07–1.4) [f]	1.37 (0.93–2.02)	1.67 (1.21–2.3) [g]	1.01 (0.87–1.16)	1.36 (0.99–1.87)	1.27 (0.76–2.13)	1.01 (0.86–1.17)	0.81 (0.7–0.94) [f]
Irregular	1.16 (0.94–1.43)	0.90 (0.77–1.05)	0.54 (0.3–0.96) [e]	1.06 (0.72–1.57)	1.05 (0.90–1.22)	0.88 (0.60–1.30)	0.37 (0.16–0.90) [e]	1.09 (0.92–1.28)	0.89 (0.76–1.04)

[a] OR: odds ratio adjusted for the four socio-labor variables included in the table (type of contract or employment situation, occupational category, working time and type of working day) and the demographic variables (age, nationality, marital status, level of education, type of family life, family care work, monthly household income); IC90%: confidence interval; [b] Reference category; [c] Insufficient sample size for analysis; [d] Indicators measured only in employed persons; [e] Significance level value of $p < 0.1$; [f] Significance level value of $p < 0.05$; [g] Significance level value of $p < 0.01$.

Table 4. Adjusted logistic regression between socio-labour determinants and health and consumption indicators in the female labour force.

	Health Status Last 12 Months		You Have Suffered from Mental Disorders in the Last 12 Months			Consumption of Sedative Hypnotics in the Last 12 Months		Use of Addictive Substances in the Last 12 Months	
	Self-Perceived Health Status aOR (IC90%) [a]	Visits to the Family Doctor aOR (IC90%) [a]	Depression aOR (IC90%) [a]	Chronic Anxiety aOR (IC90%) [a]	Work Stress aOR (IC90%) [a]	Tranquilizers aOR (IC90%) [a]	Antidepressants, Stimulants aOR (IC90%) [a]	Smoke aOR (IC90%) [a]	Alcohol aOR (IC90%) [a]
Businesswomen	1 [b]	1 [b]	1 [b]	1 [b]	1 [b]	1 [b]	1 [b]	1 [b]	1 [b]
Officials	1.04 (0.74–1.46)	1.08 (0.75–1.54)	0.84 (0.49–1.43)	0.91 (0.56–1.47)	0.88 (0.66–1.17)	1.52 (0.89–2.59)	1.00 (0.50–2.02)	0.69 (0.50–1.05)	0.86 (0.65–1.15)
Indefinite salaried	1.08 (0.79–1.45)	1.09 (0.79–1.51)	0.95 (0.60–1.53)	0.97 (0.63–1.49)	1.18 (0.91–1.53)	1.27 (0.78–2.08)	0.91 (0.48–1.73)	0.91 (0.69–1.21)	0.85 (0.66–1.11)
Temporary salaried	1.04 (0.74–1.44)	1.06 (0.75–1.51)	1.20 (0.72–1.99)	1.00 (0.62–1.59)	0.76 (0.57–1.01)	1.00 (0.58–1.73)	1.33 (0.67–2.65)	1.00 (0.74–1.35)	0.80 (0.60–1.06)
Autonomous	1.05 (0.75–1.48)	0.92 (0.64–1.33)	0.96 (0.56–1.63)	0.84 (0.51–1.38)	0.81 (0.60–1.08)	1.32 (0.76–2.29)	0.97 (0.47–1.99)	0.72 (0.52–1.00)	0.85 (0.63–1.14)
Without contract	0.97 (0.54–1.74)	1.20 (0.59–2.45)	1.92 (0.56–1.63)	1.96 (0.96–4.00)	0.62 (0.60–1.08)	1.42 (0.61–3.29)	2.58 (0.99–6.76)	2.60 (1.01–6.7) [e]	0.56 (0.3–0.98) [f]
Unemployed	0.56 (0.39–0.79) [f]	1.34 (0.91–1.96)	2.70 (1.59–4.5) [f]	2.00 (1.23–3.26) [e]	—[d]	2.29 (1.30–4.00) [f]	1.87 (0.89–3.82)	1.92 (1.03–3.61) [e]	0.52 (0.38–0.7) [g]
Directives with more than 10 employees	1 [b]	1 [b]	1 [b]	1 [b]	1 [b]	1 [b]	1 [b]	1 [b]	1 [b]
Directives with fewer than 10 employees	1.03 (0.86–1.24)	0.88 (0.73–1.07)	1.07 (0.82–1.40)	1.00 (0.76–1.30)	0.69 (0.5–0.84) [g]	1.09 (0.85–1.39)	1.20 (0.86–1.70)	1.34 (1.11–1.61) [g]	0.96 (0.83–1.12)
Intermediate technicians	0.86 (0.74–1.01)	1.08 (0.88–1.20)	1.27 (1.02–1.5) [e]	1.40 (1.13–1.7) [f]	0.85 (0.91–1.53)	1.31 (1.08–1.60) [f]	1.25 (0.95–1.64)	1.68 (1.43–1.96) [g]	0.93 (0.82–1.05)
Qualified supervisors	0.74 (0.63–0.87) [g]	1.44 (1.18–1.7) [f]	1.43 (1.14–1.8) [f]	1.53 (1.22–1.9) [g]	0.67 (0.7–0.99) [e]	1.48 (1.20–1.82) [g]	1.43 (1.07–1.90) [f]	1.76 (1.47–2.10) [g]	0.67 (0.5–0.78) [g]
Qualified manual technicians	0.69 (0.60–0.79) [g]	1.22 (1.04–1.4) [e]	1.78 (1.45–2.1) [g]	1.59 (1.29–1.9) [g]	0.86 (0.5–0.83) [g]	1.48 (1.22–1.79) [g]	1.68 (1.30–2.19) [g]	1.92 (1.64–2.25) [g]	0.61 (0.5–0.69) [g]
Unqualified manual technicians	0.62 (0.53–0.72) [g]	1.34 (1.10–1.6) [f]	1.82 (1.46–2.2) [f]	1.76 (1.49–2.2) [g]	0.72 (0.7–0.98) [f]	1.52 (1.24–1.87) [g]	1.69 (1.28–2.23) [g]	1.96 (1.64–2.33) [g]	0.50 (0.4–0.57) [g]
Full-time	1 [b]	1 [b]	1 [b]	1 [b]	1 [b]	1 [b]	1 [b]	1 [b]	1 [b]
Part-time	0.87 (0.76–1.00)	1.03 (0.88–1.20)	1.50 (1.22–1.8) [g]	1.21 (1.00–1.47)	0.59 (0.4–0.61) [g]	1.16 (0.93–1.43)	0.96 (0.71–1.30)	0.99 (0.87–1.36)	0.91 (0.81–1.03)
Split shift	1 [b]	1 [b]	1 [b]	1 [b]	1 [b]	1 [b]	1 [b]	1 [b]	1 [b]
Continues in the morning	0.83 (0.7–0.96) [f]	0.96 (0.82–2.12)	1.32 (1.03–1.6) [f]	1.18 (0.94–1.46)	0.88 (0.78–1.00)	1.41 (1.11–1.7) [f]	1.14 (0.82–1.58)	1.05 (0.92–1.21)	0.93 (0.82–1.06)
Continues in the afternoon	0.64 (0.48–0.84) [g]	0.91 (0.66–1.25)	2.38 (1.63–3.4) [g]	1.95 (1.35–2.8) [e]	0.67 (0.5–0.86) [g]	1.32 (0.86–2.03)	1.12 (0.63–2.00)	0.93 (0.70–1.24)	0.79 (0.61–1.02)
Continues in the evening	1.14 (0.57–2.26)	1.03 (0.49–2.18)	1.59 (0.63–3.97)	0.93 (0.33–2.56)	1.54 (0.87–2.74)	0.82 (0.29–2.34)	1.08 (0.31–3.75)	1.32 (0.72–2.41)	0.65 (0.35–1.18)
Shifts	1.07 (0.86–1.31)	0.91 (0.74–1.13)	1.13 (0.82–1.56)	0.93 (0.69–1.26)	1.34 (1.13–1.5) [g]	1.54 (1.13–2.0) [f]	1.19 (0.80–1.81)	1.31 (1.09–1.5) [f]	0.92 (0.78–1.09)
Irregular	0.87 (0.70–1.07)	1.14 (0.91–1.45)	1.56 (1.14–2.1) [g]	1.35 (1.01–1.8) [e]	1.02 (0.86–1.22)	1.59 (1.16–2.1) [g]	1.27 (0.82–1.95)	1.15 (0.96–1.37)	1.15 (0.96–1.37)

[a] OR: odds ratio adjusted for the four socio-labor variables included in the table (type of contract or employment situation, occupational category, working time and type of working day) and the demographic variables (age, nationality, marital status, level of education, type of family life, family care work, monthly household income); IC90%: confidence interval; [b] Reference category; [c] Insufficient sample size for analysis; [d] Indicators measured only in employed persons; [e] Significance level value of $p < 0.1$; [f] Significance level value of $p < 0.05$; [g] Significance level value of $p < 0.01$.

3. Results

The descriptive analysis showed, on the one hand, that working women presented a worse state of self-perceived health in the last 12 months (24.9%), visited their family doctor more frequently (82.1%), suffered from a higher prevalence of depression (9.5%), chronic anxiety (10.9%), occupational stress (51.8%), and consumed tranquilizers (10.1%) and antidepressants (5.1%) more frequently. On the other hand, the consumption of tobacco and alcohol was higher in men (34.1% and 66.6%, respectively) (Table 1).

The regression models (Figure 1), would confirm the associations found in the descriptive analyses, to the extent that women were 1.47 times more likely to report poor health perceived by themselves than men (aOR = 0.68; IC90%:0.62–0.74) and 1.93 times more likely to visit the family doctor (aOR = 1.93; IC90%:1.77–2.1). In addition, women had a worse mental health status as they were 2.54 times more likely to suffer from depression (aOR = 2.54; IC90%:2.13–3.02), 2.23 and 1.26 times more likely to remit chronic anxiety and stress, respectively, compared to men. A similar situation occurred in the consumption of hypnosedatives, since women were more likely to consume tranquilizers (aOR = 1.51; IC90%:1.29–1.76) and antidepressants (aOR = 2.35; IC90%:1.85–2.99). However, men were 2.63 times more likely to consume alcohol (aOR = 0.38; IC90%: 0.35–0.41).

In order to deepen the analysis of the differences between the male and female labor force, regressions of the nine health and consumption indicators were carried out with the interactions between gender and the type of labor relationship and the occupational social class. The results obtained (Table 2) show that the gender differences found in Figure 1 increase both in work situations and in more vulnerable social classes. Specifically, women working without a contract were found to be 4.03 times more likely to suffer from depression (aOR = 4.03; IC90% = 2.22–7.3), 3.96 times more likely to report chronic anxiety (aOR = 3.96; IC90% = 2.2–7), or 4.01 times more likely to take antidepressants (aOR = 4.01; IC90% = 1.92–8.3) than men working without a contract. Similar situations were identified in unemployed women who were more likely to suffer from depression (aOR = 3.19; IC90% = 2.71–3.2), chronic anxiety (aOR = 3.15; IC90% = 2.69–3.6) and antidepressant use (aOR = 2.95; IC90% = 2.36–3.69) compared to unemployed men. With regard to the social occupational class, the most relevant gender differences were also found in psychosomatic pathologies and the consumption of hypnosedatives among both qualified and unqualified manual technicians, although these associations were less intense.

3.1. Relationships between Socio-Labour Characteristics and Consumption Indicators in the Male Labour Force

Regression analyses on the male labor force (Table 3) found how unemployment correlated with poorer health and consumption standards, as unemployed workers were 1.75 times more likely to report poorer self-perceived health (aOR = 0.57; IC90%: 0.38–0.89), 5.53 and 5.92 times more likely to suffer from depression and chronic anxiety, respectively (aOR = 5.53; IC90%:2.49–12.26; aOR = 5.92; IC90%: 2.83–12.42, respectively), compared to employers. In addition, unemployed workers were also more likely to use tranquilizers (aOR = 3.09; IC90%: 1.60–5.95), antidepressants (aOR = 6.75; IC90%: 1.91–23.83), and tobacco (aOR = 1.75; IC90%: 1.28–2.41). However, the employers presented greater probability of suffering labor stress with respect to the rest of labor situations, arriving to present 1.56 times larger probabilities of referring to stress than the workers without a contract (aOR = 0.64; IC90%: 0.51–0.79). In addition, employers were more likely to consume alcohol than unemployed workers (aOR = 0.51; IC90%: 0.37–0.71).

In reference to occupational social class, both skilled and unskilled manual technicians were associated with worse health standards (general and mint) and consumption of hypnosedatives compared to managers with more than 10 employees. Nevertheless, the highest differences were found in unskilled manual workers who were 1.75 times more likely to have worse self-perceived health status (aOR = 0.57; CI90%: 0.48–0.69), as well as being more likely to suffer from depression (aOR = 2.39; IC90%: 1.67–3.44), chronic anxiety (aOR = 2.40; IC90%: 1.71–3.42) and to take tranquilizers (aOR = 1.92; IC90%: 1.44–2.56), antidepressants (aOR = 2.30; IC90%: 1.42–3.71) or tobacco (aOR = 2.62; IC90%: 2.19–3.13). However, managers with more than 10 employees were 1.96 times more likely to report job stress (aOR = 0.51; IC90%: 0.40–0.63) and 1.47 more likely to consume alcohol (aOR = 0.68; IC90%: 0.58–0.80) compared to unskilled manual technicians.

Finally, the most noteworthy results regarding working time were that, on the one hand, part-time workers reported a smaller likelihood of suffering work stress (aOR = 0.60; IC90%: 0.49–0.7) and, on the other hand, that those who worked shifts appeared more likely to report a worse state of self-perceived health (aOR = 0.82; IC90%: 0.52–0.99), visiting their family doctor more (aOR = 1.25; IC90%: 1.07–1.40) and reporting chronic anxiety (aOR = 01.67; IC90%: 1.21–2.3) compared to those who worked split shifts.

3.2. Relationships between Socio-Labour Characteristics and Consumption Indicators in the Female Labour Force

In reference to the female labor force, the results obtained (Table 4) showed similar findings to those identified in men regarding the labor situation, insofar as unemployed women presented a lower probability of referring to a good state of self-perceived health (aOR = 0.56; IC90%: 0.39–0.79) and a higher probability of suffering from depression (aOR = 2.70; IC90%: 1.59–4.58), chronic anxiety (aOR = 2.00; IC90%: 1.23–3.26) or taking tranquilizers (aOR = 2.29; IC90%: 1.30–4.00) and tobacco (aOR = 1.92; IC90%: 1.03–3.61) with respect to female entrepreneurs. However, the highest probabilities were found in women working without a contract, who were 1.92 times more likely to suffer from depression (aOR = 1.92; IC90%: 1.12–4.1) and 2.60 times more likely to smoke tobacco (aOR = 2.60; IC90%: 1.01–6.70) than female entrepreneurs. Furthermore, coinciding again with the results for the male workforce, associations were observed between female managers and work stress or alcohol consumption, insofar as women working without a contract were less likely to suffer work stress (aOR = 0.62; IC90%: 0.36–0.8) or consume alcohol (aOR = 0.56; IC90%: 0.3–0.98) than female entrepreneurs.

In reference to occupational social class, again, coinciding with men, both qualified and unqualified manual techniques were associated with worse health and consumption of hypnosedatives compared to managers with more than 10 employees. The largest differences were found in unskilled manual workers who were 1.61 more likely to have worse self-perceived health (aOR = 0.62; CI90%: 0.53–0.72), as well as a higher probability of suffering from depression (aOR = 1.82; IC90%: 1.46–2.27) or chronic anxiety (aOR = 1.76; IC90%: 1.41–2.20) and of taking tranquilizers (aOR = 1.52; IC90%: 1.24–1.87), antidepressants (aOR = 1.69; IC90%: 1.28–2.23) or tobacco (aOR = 1.96; IC90%: 1.64–2.33). However, managers with more than 10 employees were 1.39 times more likely to report job stress (aOR = 0.72; IC90%: 0.58–0.89) and 2.00 times more likely to consume alcohol (aOR = 0.50; IC90%: 0.43–0.57) compared to unskilled manual technicians.

Finally, with reference to the working day, unlike the male working population, women working the afternoon shift or irregular days were those who presented the most significant associations with general and mental health indicators. Women working continuous afternoon shifts were 1.56 times more likely to report self-perceived ill health (aOR = 0.64; IC90%: 0.48–0.84), 2.38 times more likely to suffer from depression (aOR = 2.38; IC90%:1.63–3.4) and 1.95 times more likely to suffer from chronic anxiety (aOR = 1.95; IC90%: 1.35–2.8) than women working split shifts. On the other hand, workers with irregular working hours also presented a higher likelihood of reporting depression (aOR = 1.56; IC90%: 1.14–2.1), chronic anxiety (aOR = 1.35; IC90%: 1.01–1.8) and consumption of tranquilizers (aOR = 1.59; IC90%: 1.16–2.1). In terms of working time, part-time workers were more likely to suffer from depression (aOR = 1.50; IC90%: 1.22–1.8) and less likely to report job-related stress (aOR = 0.59; IC90%: 0.40–0.61).

4. Discussion

The results obtained (Table 1 and Figure 1) confirm some results of previous studies, as the prevalence of poor self-perceived health, mental disorders and hypnosedative use is higher in women [77,78], while alcohol consumption is higher in men [77–79]. Furthermore, as shown in Table 2, the differences between men and women increase in the most unstable employment situations (working without a contract or unemployed) and in the most vulnerable occupational social classes (skilled and unskilled manual workers) to the extent that the odds ratios identified in these categories are higher both in psychosomatic pathologies and in the consumption of hypnosedatives.

Likewise, it is confirmed for both sexes that unemployment is related to worse self-perceived health, the fact of suffering from depression and the consumption of hypnosedatives [51,54,77]. However, as noted in the introduction, subjective employability could influence as a possible moderator the relationship between job insecurity and negative mental health outcomes. It would be interesting in future studies to have measurement variables of subjective employability to observe their interaction with attributed job insecurity and health and consumption outcomes.

Continuing with the analysis, it is worth mentioning that the impact of unemployment is greater among the male labor force for several reasons. First, because unemployed workers are more than twice as likely to suffer from depression as employed women. Second, while the unemployed have had a high prevalence of chronic anxiety and antidepressant use compared to actively working men, no differences in antidepressant use have been found between currently working and unemployed women, and the relationships identified for chronic anxiety are much smaller than those of men. This situation could be explained by the division of family roles and responsibilities between men and women, as previous studies have shown [60,80]. However, these hypotheses merit specific analysis in future studies, rather than the multidimensional analysis sought in this research, since, while there are important differences between the probabilities of the female and male workforces, when the sample is stratified by sex, they are no longer comparable.

Previous research has found that temporary workers and those with job instability make less frequent visits to the family doctor [55] and have a higher prevalence of mental disorders [53]. However, in our study we found that self-employed workers are the least likely to make medical visits and the most likely to suffer from depression and chronic anxiety. Despite the divergences between the results and the complexity of the relationships, there may be a pattern derived from the stronger perception of distress among precarious workers when they perceive high job insecurity [53], which may lead them not to absent themselves from work for fear of being fired and, consequently, not attending the doctor and opting to self-medicate. In fact, the Sixth European Survey on Working Conditions 2015 [81], identified that 44% of workers with permanent contracts declared that they had worked while sick during the last year, while among self-employed workers the rate was 50%, which could confirm that the productive need makes the self-employed worker not absent from work, even if he is sick. On the other hand, a study conducted in public hospitals identified that professionals with temporary employment contracts were more likely to self-medicate [82], which would explain why people who feel a high degree of job insecurity, whether as self-employed or temporary workers, tend not to be absent from work when they have health problems, and opt for self-medication. However, these hypotheses should be evaluated in future research. We could also consider that the precarious working conditions to which temporary workers are subjected may mean that they do not have sufficient financial resources to take out private health insurance and therefore go to the doctor less often. However, Spain has a universal health system, so this hypothesis for the Spanish case would be ruled out.

Since the aim of this research is to explore and describe, as a whole, the associations between factors of job insecurity and the different health and consumption indicators, we can observe different relationship patterns, depending on the work situation and the occupational social class. On the one hand, it has been identified that unemployed people, who belong to the most vulnerable social classes, suffer more frequently depression and chronic anxiety. These mental disorders, in turn, are associated, as shown by previous studies, with the increased consumption of hypnosedatives [58] and tobacco [83]. This would explain, to a certain extent, the patterns and associations of social vulnerability with mental disorders, consumption of hypnosedatives and tobacco obtained in our study.

The occupational classes with the highest status in Tables 3 and 4, on the other hand, have reported greater stress than manual occupational classes, and both male and female managers with more than 10 employed people have also reported greater job stress, which would refute the findings identified in previous studies [84]. The greater occupational stress of these groups could be derived from the intensification of work in the most qualified "knowledge" jobs as they are more intensely exposed than manual workers to psychosocial risk factors such as emergencies to perform tasks, time pressure, speed or short term in the execution of work, role dysfunction, self-management, etc. [85–90]. The fact that the occupational classes with the highest status are also associated with the highest alcohol consumption would in turn confirm other previous findings [54]. There are two hypotheses that could explain the higher alcohol consumption in the better-positioned occupational social classes. The first is that differences in consumption across classes are explained by cultural patterns and by reduced access to such substances by blue-collar workers [54]. The second hypothesis is that higher consumption of alcohol by these groups is associated with a greater need to combat stress [57]. Both hypotheses could explain the relationships found in this study between occupational social classes with higher status, work stress and alcohol consumption.

We can also see the influence of the relationship between professional situation and social class on working time. On the one hand, if we consider (albeit with certain nuances) that part-time work is part of precarious employment [74], the results obtained show that this partiality is associated with a higher prevalence of depression in women. On the other hand, the results show that full-time work is associated with greater job stress in both sexes. Previous studies record similar results, insofar as this research has associated a higher number of working hours with higher occupational stress [55].

Finally, with regard to the type of working day, the results obtained show significant differences between the sexes. Although few associations have been identified in men, with shift work being the most damaging to general and mental health, multiple associations have been identified in women. In particular, it should be noted that the continuous afternoon shift is the one with the highest prevalence of depression and chronic anxiety, while the irregular shift is also associated with the highest probability of suffering from depression, chronic anxiety and the use of tranquilizers. These results differ from those of previous studies associating mental disorders with shift work [56,91], and further research is needed to improve the understanding of this relationship. However, it was observed that while the work situation or occupational social class affected men more, the type of working day affected women more. This could again be explained by the division of gender roles, which implies a greater workload for women in the family setting [60,80].

Limitations

The study presents some common limitations of the use of this type of survey. Firstly, the most important limitation is that there may be a risk of reverse causality, and therefore the findings identified should be considered as associations rather than causal relationships. This is a common limitation in this type of study [56–61]. Secondly, except for Figure 1 and Table 2, in which differences between men and women can be compared, the results obtained from the separate regressions for the male and female labor force (Tables 3 and 4), as explained in the discussion, do not have comparable parameters, since the variance-covariance matrix is calculated separately. This situation would also occur in work of a similar nature [56–61]. However, it should be remembered that the objective of the research is to look for patterns that will allow more concrete comparative analyses to be carried out in future studies. Thirdly, there could be information and response biases of complacency on the part of participants, or of responding to what is considered socially acceptable. In this sense, more favored social classes and men, associated with stronger and more powerful roles, may be unwilling to acknowledge certain health problems because of social stigma. This attitude may result in an underrecording of mental pathologies or substance use. In fact, this situation could explain the low number of affirmative responses about mental disorders (depression or chronic anxiety) or the high number of unanswered cases about the use of hypnosedatives. On the other hand, there could be selection bias, for example, in the most vulnerable occupational classes due to the possibility of dropouts, or the increase in the number of unanswered questions. All this may favor the underregistration of pathologies and consumption. In addition, the underrepresentation of some categories (e.g., non-contract work, shift work, night work) prevents some more comprehensive stratified analyses. In the future it might be interesting to stratify the analysis by sex and age simultaneously or by a more disaggregated occupational social class, but the sample size would only allow a subset of analysis in those cases, leading to a reduction of possible analyses. The impossibility of having socio-occupational variables (e.g., number of working hours, production rates, social support) can also act as a confounder. It would therefore be useful to include them in future editions of the ENSE survey. Finally, it is worth mentioning that the associations found cannot be evaluated as "causal", since this is a transversal study.

5. Conclusions

In conclusion, we believe that the study is relevant, since the exploration of health and consumption patterns can serve as a reference for the planning of sustainable preventive occupational health policies, both in labor and health institutions and in companies. These programs should focus, at least, on the unemployed, those who belong to the most vulnerable occupational social classes and considering the gender differences described. Specifically, two patterns of health erosion have been identified as a result of high rates of job insecurity. On the one hand, the most vulnerable people (unemployed and manual workers) suffer with a higher prevalence of depression, chronic anxiety, hypnosedative use and tobacco consumption, and therefore active employment policies should be promoted to reduce the high unemployment rates that still exist in Spain. On the other hand, more qualified people and, above all, managers have reported greater work stress and alcohol consumption. The problem of these groups does not lie so much in sustaining employment, but rather in the deregulation of working conditions which has led to an increase in the intensification of employment, which is a determining factor in the increase of work-related stress and alcohol consumption. To all this, we should add another series of policies to reconcile work and family life (for example, reducing working hours and establishing schedules compatible with reproductive tasks), since, as we have seen, it affects working women in particular in a negative way. It seems reasonable, therefore, to call for the revival of social dialogue for the implementation of sustainable measures to improve the quantity and quality of employment, since neoliberal policies for the management of the economic crisis have caused a serious public health problem. However, it should be remembered that this study is of an exploratory nature, and therefore, rather than directly suggesting courses of action, it highlights the need to increase research into labor relations and occupational health, and then, on that basis, to implement specific labor and health policies.

Author Contributions: Conceptualization, R.P.C. and P.J.B.C.; methodology, R.P.C.; formal analysis, R.P.C.; research, R.P.C.; curatorship of data, R.P.C.; preparation of the original draft of the manuscript, R.P.C.; review and editing of the manuscript, P.J.B.C.; supervision, P.J.B.C. All authors have read and agreed to the published version of the manuscript.

Funding: This research was funded by the Spanish Ministry of Education, Culture and Sports, grant number FPU2016/04591.

Acknowledgments: The authors would like to thank the Ministry of Health, Consumer Affairs and Social Welfare for providing the microdata from the National Health Survey in Spain, 2017.

Conflicts of Interest: The authors declare no conflict of interest.

Appendix A

Table A1. Relationship between self-perceived health and health problems.

Pathologies	Self-Perceived Ill Health N° (%) [a]	Good Self-Perceived Health N° (%) [a]	p–Value [b]
High blood pressure	6047 (32)	313 (7.5)	0.000
Myocardial infarction	529 (2.8)	17 (0.4)	0.000
Angina pectoris	504 (2.7)	11 (0.3)	0.000
Other heart diseases	1535 (8.1)	51 (1.2)	0.000
Varicose veins in the legs	3298 (17.5)	219 (5.2)	0.000
Arthrosis	5304 (28.2)	155 (3.7)	0.000
Back pain (cervical)	4007 (21.2)	130 (3.1)	0.000
Back pain (lumbar)	5199 (27.5)	190 (4.5)	0.000
Chronic allergy	3447 (18.3)	469 (11.2)	0.000
Asthma	1280 (6.8)	139 (3.3)	0.000
Bronchitis	1152 (6.1)	34 (0.8)	0.000
Diabetes	2214 (11.7)	61 (1.5)	0.000
Stomach ulcer	1040 (5.5)	42 (1)	0.000
Urinary incontinence	1422 (7.5)	43 (1)	0.000
High cholesterol	5207 (27.6)	323 (5.8)	0.000
Cataracts	2881 (15.3)	126 (3)	0.000
Skin problems	1371 (7.3)	126 (3)	0.000
Chronic constipation	1123 (5.9)	33 (0.8)	0.000
Liver dysfunction	336 (1.8)	12 (0.3)	0.000
Ictus	498 (2.6)	10 (0.2)	0.000
Frequent headaches	2450 (13)	166 (6.3)	0.000
Hemorrhoids	1830 (9.7)	136 (3.2)	0.000
Malignant tumors	1130 (6)	53 (1.3)	0.000
Osteoporosis	1177 (6.2)	40 (1)	0.000
Thyroid problems	(1526 (8.1)	122 (2.9)	0.000
Kidney problems	1145 (6.1)	35 (0.8)	0.000

[a] n = Number; % = Percentage over the total sample; [b] p value = Sex differences calculated using a chi-squared test, with 95% confidence level.

Table A2. Relationship between self-perceived health and health problems.

	Dependent Variables							
Selection Regressors	Self-Perceived Health Status	Visits to the Family Doctor	Depression	Chronic Anxiety	Work Stress	TRANQUILIZERS	Antidepressants, Stimulants	Smoking	Alcohol
	Selection Variable: Labor Market Participation Reference Category = Participates								
	Coefficients (Standard Errors)								
Const	0.580308 ***	0.58030 ***	0.58663 ***	0.57940 ***	0.55839 ***	−0.0696068	−0.0605752	0.59434 ***	0.5837 ***
	(0.144644)	(0.144644)	0.144724	(0.144529)	(0.149458)	(0.162769)	(0.163026)	(0.143625)	0.144749
Age	−0.127013 ***	−0.1270 ***	−0.1279 ***	−0.1232 ***	−0.1216 ***	−0.04986 **	−0.0517226 **	−0.1272 ***	−0.1275 ***
	(0.0181994)	(0.018199)	(0.0182110)	(0.018443)	(0.020210)	(0.020718)	(0.0207184)	(0.018069)	0.0182146
Nationality	0.0539992	0.0539992	0.0505017	0.0388518	0.0587547	0.0539741	0.0474748	0.032670	0.0568324
	(0.0521977)	(0.052197)	(0.052265)	(0.052780)	(0.052681)	(0.057980)	(0.0585688)	(0.052608)	0.0208021
Marital status	0.0560410 ***	0.05604 ***	0.05636 ***	0.05985 ***	0.05703 ***	0.07197 ***	0.0745274 ***	0.06513 ***	−0.5189 ***
	(0.0207951)	(0.020795)	(0.0207978)	(0.020785)	(0.020811)	(0.022819)	(0.0231137)	(0.020811)	0.0320898
Education level	0.168384	−0.5175 ***	−0.5178 ***	−0.5217 ***	−0.5183 ***	0.47523 ***	−0.472219 ***	−0.5169 ***	−0.5189 ***
	(0.0513444)	(0.032069)	(0.0320754)	(0.032004)	(0.032044)	(0.035425)	(0.0356332)	(0.032019)	0.0320898
Type of family life	−0.095654 ***	−0.0956 ***	−0.0960 **	−0.0946 ***	−0.0970	−0.0805 ***	−0.0868289 ***	−0.0996 ***	−0.0952 ***
	(0.0269741)	(0.026974)	(0.0269798)	(0.026908)	(0.0270509)	(0.029962)	(0.0303375)	(0.026802)	0.0269854
Family care work	0.168384 ***	0.16838 ***	0.16905 ***	0.17170 ***	0.16852 ***	0.18299 ***	0.186160 ***	0.16628 ***	0.1694 ***
	(0.0513444)	(0.051344)	(0.0513490)	(0.051159)	(0.051284)	(0.055725)	(0.0557636)	(0.051045)	0.0513535
Rho	0.061416	−0.024296	0.0190499	−0.014888	0.077386	−0.026900	−0.022732	−0.024091	−0.017310

*** Significant at 99% confidence; ** Significant at 95% confidence.

References

1. Rigby, M.; García-Calavia, M.Á. Institutional resources as a source of trade union power in Southern Europe. *Eur. J. Ind. Relat.* **2018**, *24*, 129–143. [CrossRef]
2. Barranco, O.; Molina, Ó. Sindicalismo y crisis económica: Amenazas, retos y oportunidades. *Kultur Rev. Interdisc. Sobre Cult. Ciutat* **2014**, *1*, 171–194. [CrossRef]
3. Benner, M. *Before and Beyond the Global Economic Crisis*; Edward Elgar: Cheltenham, UK, 2013.
4. Gago, A. Crisis, cambio en la UE y estrategias sindicales: El impacto de la condicionalidad en el repertorio estratégico de los sindicatos españoles durante la crisis de la eurozona. *Rev. Esp. Cienc. Polít.* **2016**, *42*, 45–68. [CrossRef]
5. Beneyto, P.J.; Alós, R.; Jódar, P.; Vidal, S. La afiliación sindical en la crisis Estructura, evolución y trayectorias. *Sociol. Trab.* **2016**, *87*, 25–44.
6. Lehndorff, S. Acting in different worlds. Challenges to transnational trade union cooperation in the eurozone crisis. *Transf. Eur. Rev. Labour Res.* **2015**, *21*, 157–170. [CrossRef]
7. Stuckler, D.; Basu, S.; Suhrcke, M.; Coutts, A.; McKee, M. The public health effect of economic crises and alternative policy responses in Europe: An empirical analysis. *Lancet* **2009**, *374*, 315–323. [CrossRef]
8. Stuckler, D.; King, L.; McKee, M. Mass Privatisation and the Post-Communist Mortality Crisis: A Cross-National Analysis. *Lancet* **2009**, *373*, 399–407. [CrossRef]
9. Bacigalupe, A.; Martín, U.; Font, R.; González-Rábago, Y.; Bergantiños, N. Austeridad y privatización sanitaria en época de crisis: ¿existen diferencias entre las comunidades autónomas? *Gac. Sanit.* **2016**, *30*, 47–51. [CrossRef]
10. Cabrera-León, A.; Codina, A.D.; Mateo, I.; Arroyo-Borrell, E.; Bartoll, X.; Bravo, M.J.; Domínguez-Berjón, M.F.; Renart, G.; Álvarez-Dardet, C.; Marí-Dell'Olmo, M.; et al. Indicadores contextuales para evaluar los determinantes sociales de la salud y la crisis económica española. *Gac. Sanit.* **2017**, *31*, 194–203. [CrossRef]
11. Del Pozo-Rubio, R.; Pardo-García, I.; Escribano-Sotos, F. El copago de dependencia en España a partir de la reforma estructural de 2012. *Gac. Sanit.* **2017**, *31*, 23–29. [CrossRef]
12. Ferrando, J.; Palència, L.; Gotsens, M.; Puig-Barrachina, V.; Marí-Dell'Olmo, M.; Rodríguez-Sanz, M.; Bartoll, X.; Borrell, C. Trends in cancer mortality in Spain: The influence of the financial crisis. *Gac. Sanit.* **2019**, *33*, 229–234. [CrossRef] [PubMed]
13. Porthé, V.; Vargas, I.; Ronda, E.; Malmusi, D.; Bosch, L.; Vázquez, M.L. Has the quality of health care for the immigrant population changed during the economic crisis in Catalonia (Spain)? Opinions of health professionals and immigrant users. *Gac. Sanit.* **2018**, *32*, 425–432. [CrossRef] [PubMed]
14. Benavides, F.G.; Delclós, J.; Serra, C. Estado de bienestar y salud pública: El papel de la salud laboral. *Gac. Sanit.* **2018**, *32*, 377–380. [CrossRef]
15. Sverke, M.; Hellgren, J.; Näswall, K. No Security: A Meta-Analysis and Review of Job Insecurity and Its Consequences. *J. Occup. Health Psychol.* **2002**, *7*, 242–264. [CrossRef] [PubMed]
16. Valenzuela, H.C. Precariedad, precarización y trabajo precario. *Polis* **2015**, *40*, 313–329.
17. Shoss, M.K. Job insecurity: An integrative review and agenda for future research. *J. Manag.* **2017**, *43*, 1911–1939. [CrossRef]
18. Green, F. *Demanding Work: The Paradox of Job Quality in the Affluent Economy*; Princeton University Press: Oxford, UK, 2006.
19. Büssing, A. Can Control at Work and Social Support Moderate Psychological Consequences of Job Insecurity? Results from a Quasi-experimental Study in the Steel Industry. *Eur. J. Work. Organ. Psychol.* **1999**, *8*, 219–242. [CrossRef]
20. Green, F. Unpacking the misery multiplier: How employability modifies the impacts of unemployment and job insecurity on life satisfaction and mental health. *J. Health Econ.* **2011**, *30*, 265–276. [CrossRef]
21. Green, F.; Mostafa, T. *Trends in Job Quality in Europe*; Publications Office of the European Union: Luxembourg, 2012.
22. Greenhalgh, L.; Rosenblatt, Z. Job Insecurity: Toward Conceptual Clarity. *Acad. Manag. Rev.* **1984**, *9*, 438. [CrossRef]
23. Stock, R. *Socio-Economic Security, Justice and the Psychology of Social Relationships*; International Labour Office: Geneva, Switzerland, 2001.

24. Klandermans, B.; Hesselink, J.K.; van Vuuren, T. Employment status and job insecurity: On the subjective appraisal of an objective status. *Econ. Ind. Democr.* **2010**, *31*, 557–577. [CrossRef]
25. De Witte, H.; Näswall, K. "Objective" vs "Subjective" Job Insecurity: Consequences of Temporary Work for Job Satisfaction and Organizational Commitment in Four European Countries. *Econ. Ind. Democr.* **2003**, *24*, 149–188. [CrossRef]
26. Benach, J.; Vives, A.; Amable, M.; Vanroelen, C.; Tarafa, G.; Muntaner, C. Precarious Employment: Understanding an Emerging Social Determinant of Health. *Annu. Rev. Public Health* **2014**, *35*, 229–253. [CrossRef] [PubMed]
27. Ferrie, J.E.; Westerlund, H.; Virtanen, M.; Vahtera, J.; Kivimäki, M. Flexible labor markets and employee health. *SJWEH* **2008**, *6*, 98–110.
28. Dickerson, A.; Green, F. Fears and realisations of employment insecurity. *Labour Econ.* **2012**, *19*, 198–210. [CrossRef]
29. Chung, H. Dualization and subjective employment insecurity: Explaining the subjective employment insecurity divide between permanent and temporary workers across 23 European countries. *Econ. Ind. Democr.* **2016**, *40*, 700–729. [CrossRef]
30. De Cuyper, N.; De Witte, H. Temporary Employment and Perceived Employability: Mediation by Impression Management. *J. Career Dev.* **2010**, *37*, 635–652. [CrossRef]
31. Heponiemi, T.; Elovainio, M.; Pentti, J.; Virtanen, M.; Westerlund, H.; Virtanen, P.; Oksanen, T.; Kivimäki, M.; Vahtera, J. Association of Contractual and Subjective Job Insecurity with Sickness Presenteeism among Public Sector Employees. *J. Occup. Environ. Med.* **2010**, *52*, 830–835. [CrossRef]
32. Virtanen, M.; Kivimäki, M.; Elovainio, M.; Vahtera, J.; Ferrie, J. From insecure to secure employment: Changes in work, health, health related behaviours, and sickness absence. *Occup. Environ. Med.* **2003**, *60*, 948–953. [CrossRef]
33. López-Gómez, M.A.; Durán, X.; Zaballa, E.; Sanchez-Niubo, A.; Delclos, G.L.; Benavides, F.G. Cohort profile: The Spanish WORKing life Social Security (WORKss) cohort study. *BMJ Open* **2016**, *6*, e8555. [CrossRef]
34. Serra, L.; López-Gómez, M.A.; Sanchez-Niubo, A.; Delclos, G.L.; Benavides, F.G. Application of latent growth modeling to identify different working life trajectories: The case of the Spanish WORKss cohort. *Scand. J. Work. Environ. Health* **2016**, *43*, 42–49. [CrossRef]
35. Kivimäki, M.; Vahtera, J.; Pentti, J.; Ferrie, J. Factors underlying the effect of organisational downsizing on health of employees: Longitudinal cohort study. *BMJ* **2000**, *320*, 971–975. [CrossRef] [PubMed]
36. Vahtera, J.; Kivimäki, M.; Pentti, J.; Linna, A.; Virtanen, M.; Virtanen, P.; Ferrie, J. Organisational downsizing, sickness absence, and mortality: 10-town prospective cohort study. *BMJ Clin. Res. Ed.* **2004**, *328*, 555. [CrossRef]
37. Marler, J.H.; Woodard-Barringer, M.; Milkovich, G.T. Boundaryless and traditional contingent employees: Worlds apart. *J. Organ. Behav.* **2002**, *23*, 425–453. [CrossRef]
38. Cano, E. La extensión de la precariedad laboral como norma social. *Soc. Y Utopía Rev. De Cienc. Soc.* **2007**, *29*, 117–138.
39. Katz, L.F.; Krueger, A.B. The Rise and Nature of Alternative Work Arrangements in the United States, 1995–2015. *ILR Rev.* **2018**, *72*, 382–416. [CrossRef]
40. Aronsson, G.; Gustafsson, K.; Dallner, M. Work environment and health in different types of temporary jobs. *Eur. J. Work. Organ. Psychol.* **2002**, *11*, 151–175. [CrossRef]
41. Fiori, F.; Rinesi, F.; Spizzichino, D.; Di Giorgio, G. Employment insecurity and mental health during the economic recession: An analysis of the young adult labour force in Italy. *Soc. Sci. Med.* **2016**, *153*, 90–98. [CrossRef]
42. Hammarström, A. Health consequences of youth unemployment—Review from a gender perspective. *Soc. Sci. Med.* **1994**, *38*, 699–709. [CrossRef]
43. Granado, A.E. Crisis económica, políticas, desempleo y salud (mental). *Rev. Asoc. Esp. Neuropsiquiatr.* **2014**, *34*, 385–404. [CrossRef]
44. Serrano-Rosa, M.A.; Baena, S.; Molins-Correa, F. Diferencias entre empleabilidad, inseguridad laboral y salud en trabajadores y desempleados. *Acción Psicológica* **2018**, *15*, 87–102. [CrossRef]
45. Berntson, E.; Marklund, S. The Relationship Between Perceived Employability and Subsequent Health. *Work Stress* **2007**, *21*, 279–292. [CrossRef]

46. Vanhercke, D.; De Cuyper, N.; Peeters, E.; De Witte, H. Defining Perceived Employability: A Psychological Approach. *Pers. Rev.* **2014**, *43*, 592–605. [CrossRef]
47. de Grip, A.; van Loo, J.; Sanders, J. The Industry Employability Index: Taking Account of Supply and Demand Characteristics. *Int. Labour Rev.* **2004**, *143*, 211–233. [CrossRef]
48. Allebeck, P. Health Effects of the Crisis: Challenges for Science and Policy. *Eur. J. Public Health* **2013**, *23*, 721. [CrossRef] [PubMed]
49. Bernal, J.L.; Gasparrini, A.; Artundo, C.M.; McKee, M. The Effect of the Late 2000s Financial Crisis on Suicides in Spain: An Interrupted Time-Series Analysis. *Eur. J. Public Health* **2013**, *23*, 732–736. [CrossRef]
50. Salvador-Carulla, L.; Roca, M. Mental Health Impact of the Economic Crisis in Spain. *Int. J. Psychiatry* **2013**, *10*, 8–10.
51. Urbanos-Garrido, R.; López-Valcárcel, B.G. The influence of the economic crisis on the association between unemployment and health: An empirical analysis for Spain. *Eur. J. Health Econ.* **2014**, *16*, 175–184. [CrossRef]
52. Bartoll, X.; Palència, L.; Malmusi, D.; Suhrcke, M.; Borrell, C. The evolution of mental health in Spain during the economic crisis. *Eur. J. Public Health* **2013**, *24*, 415–418. [CrossRef]
53. Sirviö, A.; Ek, E.; Jokelainen, J.; Koiranen, M.; Järvikoski, T.; Taanila, A. Precariousness and discontinuous work history in association with health. *Scand. J. Public Health* **2012**, *40*, 360–367. [CrossRef]
54. Benavides, F.G.; Ruiz-Forès, N.; Delclós, G.; Domingo-Salvany, A. Consumo de alcohol y otras drogas en el medio laboral en España. *Gac. Sanit.* **2013**, *27*, 248–253. [CrossRef]
55. Arias-Uriona, A.M.; Ordóñez, J.C. Factores de precariedad laboral y su relación con la salud de trabajadores en Bolivia. *Rev. Panam. Salud Pública* **2018**, *42*, e98. [CrossRef] [PubMed]
56. García-Díaz, V.; Fernández-Feito, A.; Arias, L.; Lana, A. Consumo de tabaco y alcohol según la jornada laboral en España. *Gac. Sanit.* **2015**, *29*, 364–369. [CrossRef] [PubMed]
57. Colell, E.; Sanchez-Niubo, A.; Benavides, F.G.; Delclos, G.L.; Domingo-Salvany, A. Work-related stress factors associated with problem drinking: A study of the Spanish working population. *Am. J. Ind. Med.* **2014**, *57*, 837–846. [CrossRef] [PubMed]
58. Colell, E.; Sanchez-Niubo, A.; Ferrer, M.; Domingo-Salvany, A. Gender differences in the use of alcohol and prescription drugs in relation to job insecurity. Testing a model of mediating factors. *Int. J. Drug Policy* **2016**, *37*, 21–30. [CrossRef] [PubMed]
59. Colell, E.; Sánchez-Niubò, A.; Domingo-Salvany, A.; Delclos, G.; Benavides, F.G. Prevalencia de consumo de hipnosedantes en población ocupada y factores de estrés laboral asociados. *Gac. Sanit.* **2014**, *28*, 369–375. [CrossRef]
60. Arias de la Torre, J.; Molina, A.J.; Fernández-Villa, T.; Artazcoz, L.; Martín, V. Mental health, family roles and employment status inside and outside the household in Spain. *Gac. Sanit.* **2019**, *33*, 235–241. [CrossRef]
61. Virtanen, M.; Honkonen, T.; Kivimäki, M.; Ahola, K.; Vahtera, J.; Aromaa, A.; Lönnqvist, J. Work stress, mental health and antidepressant medication findings from the Health 2000 Study. *J. Affect. Disord.* **2007**, *98*, 189–197. [CrossRef]
62. Wang, J. Work stress as a risk factor for major depressive episode(s). *Psychol. Med.* **2004**, *35*, 865–871. [CrossRef]
63. Romelsjö, A.; Stenbacka, M.; Lundberg, M.; Upmark, M. A population study of the association between hospitalization for alcoholism among employees in different socio-economic classes and the risk of mobility out of, or within, the workforce. *Eur. J. Public Health* **2004**, *14*, 53–57. [CrossRef]
64. Artazcoz, L.; Cortès, I.; Borrell, C.; Escribà-Agüir, V.; Cascant, L. Social inequalities in the association between partner/marital status and health among workers in Spain. *Soc. Sci. Med.* **2011**, *72*, 600–607. [CrossRef]
65. Arcas, M.M.; Novoa, A.M.; Artazcoz, L. Gender inequalities in the association between demands of family and domestic life and health in Spanish workers. *Eur. J. Public Health* **2012**, *23*, 883–888. [CrossRef] [PubMed]
66. Krieger, N. Genders, sexes, and health: what are the connections—And why does it matter? *Int. J. Epidemiol.* **2003**, *32*, 652–657. [CrossRef] [PubMed]
67. Messing, K.; Mager Stellman, J. Sex, gender and women's occupational health: The importance of considering mechanism. *Environ. Res.* **2006**, *101*, 149–162. [CrossRef]
68. Hankivsky, O.; Christoffersen, A. Intersectionality and the determinants of health: A Canadian perspective. *Crit. Public Health* **2008**, *18*, 271–283. [CrossRef]
69. Hankivsky, O. Women's health, men's health, and gender and health: Implications of intersectionality. *Soc. Sci. Med.* **2012**, *74*, 1712–1720. [CrossRef]

70. Ministerio De Sanidad Consumo Y Bienestar Social. Encuesta Nacional de Salud 2017. ENSE 2017 Metodología. 2017. Available online: https://www.ine.es/metodologia/t15/t153041917.pdf11 (accessed on 24 March 2020).
71. Henares-Montiel, J.; Ruiz-Pérez, I.; Sordo, L. Salud mental en España y diferencias por sexo y por comunidades autónomas. *Gac. Sanit.* **2020**, *34*, 114–119. [CrossRef]
72. Beneyto, P.J.; Payá, R. Mercado de trabajo y estructura ocupacional. In *Estructura Social Contemporánea*; Perelló, S., Ed.; Tirant lo Blanch: Valencia, Spain, 2019; pp. 169–204.
73. Croezen, S.; Burdorf, A.; Van Lenthe, F.J. Self-perceived health in older Europeans: Does the choice of survey matter? *Eur. J. Public Health* **2016**, *26*, 686–692. [CrossRef]
74. Gumà, J.; Arpino, B.; Solé-Auró, A. Determinantes sociales de la salud de distintos niveles por género: Educación y hogar en España. *Gac. Sanit.* **2019**, *33*, 127–133. [CrossRef]
75. De Bruin, A.; Picavet, H.S.J.; Nossikov, A. *Health Interview Surveys. Towards Interna-Tional Harmonization of Methods and Instruments*; WHO Regional Office for Europe: Copenhagen, Denmark, 1996.
76. Simó-Noguera, C.; Hernández-Monleón, A.; Muñoz-Rodríguez, D.; González-Sanjuán, M.E. El efecto del estado civil y de la convivencia en pareja en la salud. *Rev. Española Investig. Sociológicas* **2015**, *151*, 141–166. [CrossRef]
77. Teixidó-Compañó, E.; Espelt, A.; Sordo, L.; Bravo, M.J.; Sarasa-Renedo, A.; Indave, B.I.; Bosque-Prous, M.; Brugal, M.T. Differences between men and women in substance use: The role of educational level and employment status. *Gac. Sanit.* **2018**, *32*, 41–47. [CrossRef]
78. Wittchen, H.U.; Jacobi, F.; Rehm, J.; Gustavsson, A.; Svensson, M.; Jönsson, B.; Olesen, J.; Allgulander, C.; Alonso, J.; Faravelli, C.; et al. The size and burden of mental disorders and other disorders of the brain in Europe 2010. *Eur. Neuropsychopharmacol.* **2011**, *21*, 655–679. [CrossRef] [PubMed]
79. Bosque-Prous, M.; Espelt, A.; Borrell, C.; Bartroli, M.; Guitart, A.M.; Villalbi, J.R.; Brugal, T. Gender differences in hazardous drinking among middle-aged in Europe: The role of social context and women's empowerment. *Eur. J. Public Health* **2015**, *25*, 698–705. [CrossRef] [PubMed]
80. Mäkelä, P.; Gmel, G.; Grittner, U.; Kuendig, H.; Kuntsche, S.; Bloomfield, K.; Room, R. Drinking patterns and their gender differences in Europe. *Alcohol Alcohol. Suppl.* **2006**, *41*, i8–i18. [CrossRef] [PubMed]
81. Eurofound. European Working Conditions Survey 2015. Available online: https://www.eurofound.europa.eu/data/european-working-conditions-survey (accessed on 1 April 2020).
82. Barros, A.R.R.; Griep, R.H.; Rotenberg, L. Self-medication among nursing workers from public hospitals. *Rev. Latinoam. Enferm.* **2010**, *17*, 1015–1022. [CrossRef]
83. Sobradiel, N.; García-Vicent, V. Consumo de tabaco y patología psiquiátrica. *Trastor. Adict.* **2007**, *9*, 31–38. [CrossRef]
84. Benavides, F.G.; Benach, J.; Román, C. Tipos de empleo y salud: Análisis de la segunda Encuesta Europea de Condiciones de Trabajo. *Gac. Sanit.* **1999**, *13*, 425–430. [CrossRef]
85. Castillo, J.J.Y.; Agulló, I. *Trabajo y Vida en la Sociedad de la Información. Un Distrito Tecnológico en el Norte de Madrid*; La Catarata: Madrid, Spain, 2012.
86. Sánchez, A.L. La participación de los trabajadores en la calidad total: Nuevos dispositivos disciplinarios de organización del trabajo. *Rev. Española Investig. Sociológicas* **2004**, *106*, 63. [CrossRef]
87. Pérez-Zapata, O.; Alvarez-Hernández, G.; Castaño-Collado, C.; Lahera-Sánchez, A. Sostenibilidad y calidad del trabajo en riesgo: La intensificación del trabajo del conocimiento. *Rev. Minist. Empl. Y Segur. Soc.* **2015**, *116*, 175–214.
88. Pinilla, J. La intensificación del esfuerzo de trabajo en España. *Cuad. Relac. Labor.* **2004**, *22*, 117–135.
89. García, F.J.P.; López-Peláez, A. La intensificación del trabajo en España (2007–2011): Trabajo en equipo y flexibilidad. *Rev. Española Investig. Sociológicas* **2017**, *160*, 79–94. [CrossRef]
90. Schieman, S.; Whitestone, Y.K.; van Gundy, K. The Nature of Work and the Stress of Higher Status. *J. Health Soc. Behav.* **2006**, *47*, 242–257. [CrossRef] [PubMed]
91. Bøggild, H.; Knutsson, A. Shift work, risk factors and cardiovascular disease. *Scand. J. Work. Environ. Health* **1999**, *25*, 85–99. [CrossRef] [PubMed]

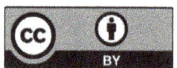

© 2020 by the authors. Licensee MDPI, Basel, Switzerland. This article is an open access article distributed under the terms and conditions of the Creative Commons Attribution (CC BY) license (http://creativecommons.org/licenses/by/4.0/).

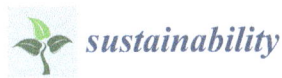

Article

COVID-19: A Relook at Healthcare Systems and Aged Populations

Thanh-Long Giang [1,2,*], Dinh-Tri Vo [2,3] and Quan-Hoang Vuong [4,5,*]

1. Faculty of Economics, National Economics University (NEU), Hanoi 11616, Vietnam
2. IPAG Lab, IPAG Business School, 75006 Paris, France; tri.vo@ipag.fr
3. School of Finance, University of Economics Hochiminh City (UEH), Ho Chi Minh City 724000, Vietnam
4. Centre for Interdisciplinary Social Research, Phenikaa University, Hanoi 100803, Vietnam
5. Centre Emile Bernheim, Université Libre de Bruxelles, B-1050 Brussels, Belgium
* Correspondence: longgt@neu.edu.vn (T.-L.G.); hoang.vuongquan@phenikaa-uni.edu.vn or qvuong@ulb.ac.be (Q.-H.V.)

Received: 21 April 2020; Accepted: 16 May 2020; Published: 20 May 2020

Abstract: Using data from the WHO's Situation Report on the COVID-19 pandemic from 21 January 2020 to 30 March 2020 along with other health, demographic, and macroeconomic indicators from the WHO's Application Programming Interface and the World Bank's Development Indicators, this paper explores the death rates of infected persons and their possible associated factors. Through the panel analysis, we found consistent results that healthcare system conditions, particularly the number of hospital beds and medical staff, have played extremely important roles in reducing death rates of COVID-19 infected persons. In addition, both the mortality rates due to different non-communicable diseases (NCDs) and rate of people aged 65 and over were significantly related to the death rates. We also found that controlling international and domestic travelling by air along with increasingly popular anti-COVID-19 actions (i.e., quarantine and social distancing) would help reduce the death rates in all countries. We conducted tests for robustness and found that the Driscoll and Kraay (1998) method was the most suitable estimator with a finite sample, which helped confirm the robustness of our estimations. Based on the findings, we suggest that preparedness of healthcare systems for aged populations need more attentions from the public and politicians, regardless of income level, when facing COVID-19-like pandemics.

Keywords: COVID-19; healthcare systems; aged populations

1. Introduction

The rapid COVID-19 outbreak since late February 2020 has posed critical challenges for public health, politics, and medical communities [1,2]. Although old lessons (such as quarantine, isolation, social distancing, and travel restrictions) are still helpful, the roles of hospital beds, medical staff (i.e., nurses and physicians) and aging population on the severity of this pandemic has not yet been studied systematically.

Is the number of deaths related to COVID-19 the consequence of overwhelmed healthcare systems and aging populations? In Europe and USA, the healthcare systems have been restructured toward centralization and budget cutoff. Aged populations are a clear evidence of this in these countries. Since the outbreak of COVID-19, several studies found that the fatality rate has been significantly higher with an increasing profile of age [3,4]. Furthermore, concerns about the healthcare systems in such countries as Italy, Spain, France, UK, and USA currently have been a hot topic on public media. The importance of the healthcare systems has been emphasized by [5,6] and [7].

Given these concerns, this study aims to examine the factors associated with the death rates of the COVID-19 infected people, in which we emphasize healthcare systems and aged populations along with other covariates. In the next section, we present a literature review on healthcare systems, aged populations, and important factors supposed to have direct correlations with the death rate from COVID-19 and some previous epidemics. We then introduce data, research methods, and discussed empirical results. Finally, we conclude and share our perspectives on healthcare systems and aged populations.

2. Literature Review

2.1. Health Systems and Pandemics

Discussing about the roles of human resources and healthcare infrastructure, [7] argued that staffing and supplies should be critically and carefully planned because COVID-19 patients should be discharged only to designated facilities or to those already caring for such patients. Practically, however, it might be that non-institutional care systems (such as home-based) were not capable to deal with a large number of discharged patients. In addition, since healthcare workers and supplies were critically important in mitigating the outbreak, it would be also crucial to prepare supplies protecting health workers who work with infected patients, and this in turn would help reduce infection and death rates.

Reviewing the history of pandemics in 1918, 1957, and 1968 [8] showed that, in recent flu seasons, hospital emergency departments faced limits in emergency rooms and inpatient beds when the number of patients increased substantially. For the US healthcare system in pandemic, one of the most concerning issue was human resources at institutional care facilities because home-care and community-care settings did not have enough experienced nurses and managers when facing a surge of patients at communities. Healthcare workers are extremely important for fighting outbreak. In pandemics with an increasing number of patients, hospital intensive care unit (ICU) beds and ventilators would not be useful if there are inadequate numbers and types of healthcare personnel.

Also discussed the US healthcare system, [9] argued that only 15 states could be able to respond fully to emergency, while others would run out of beds or face a shortage of nurses in similar situations. More critically at national level, if the country faces a 1918-like pandemic, hospital beds would increase about twice and patients in the intensive care unit (ICU) would increase about 4.6 times. Staff shortages would exacerbate the pandemic situation because it was also possible that some healthcare workers might expose themselves to infectious patients. At the same time, facing drained resources, healthcare workers would have to make important and difficult decisions about allocating limited resources while prioritizing and triaging patients.

Developing computational models with data collected from the 2014–2015 Ebola outbreak in Guinea, Liberia, and Sierra Leone, [10] estimated the repercussions of the outbreak on the populations at risk for three diseases (malaria, HIV/AIDS, and tuberculosis). They showed that accessibility to healthcare services is important to reduce the number of deaths. The simulated results indicated that if there was a 50% reduction in access to healthcare services, the Ebola outbreak would have exacerbated malaria, HIV/AIDS, and tuberculosis mortality rates by additional death counts of 6269 in Guinea, 1535 in Liberia, and 2819 in Sierra Leone.

Using observations from various data sources and reports, [11] reviewed how countries responded to COVID-19 by combining containment and mitigation activities along with delaying major surges of patients and levelling the demand for hospital beds. This proposition was also supported by [5,6]. The success of South Korea in controlling the COVID-19 with high detection rate, which required the readiness of healthcare systems, should be a guiding reference [12]. This view was also supported by [13].

Health care workers and supplies would be critically essential in mitigating the outbreak. Preparing supplies, such as N95 respirator masks and other personal protective equipment, is important to protect health workers while working with infected patients. This in turn would help reduce infection and death rates. More importantly, the emergency need of Intensive Care Units (ICU) could collapse the healthcare system [14].

2.2. Aged Population, Health Conditions and Fatality in COVID-19

Using demographic and health-related data of 191 COVID-19 adult inpatients (aged 18 and over) from Jinyintan Hospital and Wuhan Pulmonary Hospital in Wuhan, of which 137 were discharged and 54 died in hospital by 31 January 2020, [4] explored risk factors associated with in-hospital death. They found that 91 patients (48% of the studied sample) had a comorbidity, in which hypertension was the most common, and then diabetes and coronary heart disease. Multivariable regression showed increasing odds of in-hospital death associated with older age, higher Sequential Organ Failure Assessment (SOFA) score, and d-dimer greater than 1 g/mL on admission. The authors concluded that those risk factors could help clinicians to identify patients with poor prognosis at an early stage.

Similarly, extracting data and analyses from other studies, [11] emphasized that older people (particularly those aged 80 and over) and people with comorbidities (such as cardiac disease, respiratory disease, and diabetes) were at the highest risk of serious disease and death. As shown in the US, the authors were concerned that individuals in aged care facilities were at particular risk of serious disease when the healthcare system faced a surge in COVID-19 patients.

Exploring data from 13 January to 12 February 2020 in China, [15] analyzed data on 799 patients with confirmed COVID-19 who were transferred to or admitted in Tongji Hospital. As of 28 February 2020, 113 of the 799 patients died (a mortality rate of 14.1%) and 161 patients recovered and were discharged. The statistics showed that the median age of deceased patients was 68, which was significantly older than that of recovered patients, with a median age of 51. Of these patients, 71 persons (or 63% of patients who died) and 62 persons (or 39% of patients who recovered) had at least one chronic medical condition. Among deceased patients, hypertension, cardiovascular disease, and cerebrovascular disease were much more frequent than the other diseases.

Doing similar research with data from 138 patients with confirmed COVID-19 hospitalized at Zhongnan Hospital from 1 January to 28 January 2020 and followed-up by 3 February 2020, [16] described epidemiological and clinical characteristics of those patients. The median age was 56 years, and 54.3% were men. A total of 36 patients (26.1%) were transferred to the ICU because of complications, including acute respiratory distress syndrome, arrhythmia, and shock. Compared with patients not treated in ICU, those treated in ICU were older (median age 51 for the former vs 66 for the latter) and were more likely to have underlying comorbidities (72.2% vs 37.3%). Such a medical situation suggests that age and comorbidity might be risk factors for poor outcome. There was no difference in the proportion of men and women between ICU patients and non-ICU patients.

2.3. Travelling and Other Control Measures in COVID-19

To estimate COVID-19 outbreak size in Italy, [17] used data on non-residential travelers and their average length of stay with an assumption that the epidemic began in late January 2020. They found that the COVID-19 case exportations from Italy were larger than the official case counts.

For the case of China, [18] showed that, up to mid-January 2020, more than 95% of the daily exposing risk of CoV-19 was due to international travel. The authors also showed that the travel restrictions decreased the daily rate of exportation.

With data from 28 countries which imported COVID-19 cases, [19] argued that travel restrictions were not effective enough to prevent the global spread of COVID-19 in most airports. Their study highlighted the need to strengthen local capacities for disease monitoring and control rather than controlling the importation of COVID-19 at national borders via the airline network. Similarly, [20] argued that a lock-down along with nationwide traffic restrictions and a stay-at-home movement had a determining effect on the spread of COVID-19.

3. Study Data and Methods

3.1. Data

We manually downloaded the situation reports from the World Health Organization (WHO) from Report no.1 (21 January 2020) to Report no.70 (30 March 2020). With the extracted data, we then combined them with data from the World Bank's Development Indicators and the WHO's Application Programming Interface (API) for the selected variables. Due to the availability from data source, we took the value of the most recent year. The description of variables is presented in Table 1.

Table 1. Description of variables.

Explanatory Variable	Definition	Source
Death rate	Total deaths/total cases, calculated by daily report	WHO reports on COVID-19
Hospital beds	Hospital beds (per 1000 citizens)	World Bank Development Indicator (WDI)
HR (Human Resources)	Sum of physicians (per 1000 citizens) and nurses and midwives (per 1000 citizens)	WDI
DoC (Death due to non-communicable diseases)	Probability (%) of dying between age 30 and exact age 70 from any of cardiovascular disease, cancer, diabetes, or chronic respiratory disease	WHO
Population 65	Proportion of population aged 65 and above in the total population (%)	WDI
GDP capita	GDP per capita (constant 2010 US$)	WDI
Air passengers	Air transport, passengers carried (1000)	WDI

In the following step, we computed the death rate from each report and selected a sample of countries that had more than 100 confirmed cases (so we had 95 countries in the studied sample). The final panel data set consisted of 70 points of observation, in which the least minimum country-time observation of variable was 3447 (Table 2). In this table, n is the number of country-report observations; other values are at country level (such as the highest cases of 122,653 was of the US at the 70th report). At the date of the 70th report, the country with the highest confirmed number of cases was the US with 122,653 cases, and the country with the highest number of deaths was Italy with 10,781 cases. The average death rate for the whole sample was 1.44%.

Table 2. Descriptive statistics.

Explanatory Variable	n	mean	sd	min	max	se
Total cases	3529	2458	11,315	1	122,653	190.54
Total deaths	3530	97	584	0	10,781	9.82
Death_rate	3529	0.0144	0.0444	0	1	0.0007
Hospital_beds	3515	38.3772	27.942	3	134	0.4713
HR	3530	8.6846	5.3958	0	22.478	0.0908
DoC	3515	15.6049	5.4477	8.4	29.8	0.0919
Population_65	3467	12.77	6.63	1.09	27.58	0.11
GDP capita	3447	25,858.96	23,168.084	563.82	110,742.31	394.61
Air passengers	3530	68,978	156,841	0	889,202	2639.81

Note: HR: sum of physicians (per 1000 citizens) and nurses and midwives (per 1000 citizens); DoC: probability (%) of dying between age 30 and exact age 70 from any of cardiovascular disease, cancer, diabetes, or chronic respiratory disease. Source: Authors' calculations from the collected data.

On average, countries in the sample had 38.38 hospital beds per 1000 citizens and 8.68 medical staff (including nurses and physicians) per 1000 citizens. The average proportion of people aged 65 and over for the whole studied sample was 12.77%.

3.2. Methods

We first estimated three models with pooled estimator. Then, we compared our interested model by employing pooled, fixed-effects (FE) and between-estimator methods.

As different countries at various income levels have different healthcare systems and aged populations, for further analysis, we divided the sample into two sub-samples according to the income classification by [21]: high income countries (HICs) and middle- & low-income countries (MLICs).

We also employed Pesaran's cross section dependence (CD) test to detect cross-sectional dependence. As the results suggested the possibility of the problem, we applied Robust Covariance Matrix Estimators to check the standard errors. With the properties of a finite sample, the method provided in [22] was the most suitable estimator, compared with the White method [23].

Finally, we compared the results for the pooled estimation without and with Robust Standard Errors.

4. Empirical Results

4.1. Main Results

In Table 3, we present the results obtained from different estimations. In all models, four variables (hospital beds, human resources (HR), death due to non-communicable diseases (DoC), and population 65) showed their consistent impacts on the death rate of COVID-19 infected persons. In regard to health systems, variables "hospital beds" and "HR" implied that the better the healthcare infrastructure and human resources, the lower the death rate. Such a situation is clearly illustrated in the case of Italy, Spain, and the US during the studied period, as reported in [24].

Table 3. Pooled estimations with baseline and extended models.

Explanatory Variable	Dependent Variable: Death_Rate		
	(1)	(2)	(3)
Hospital beds	−0.00004	−0.0002***	−0.0002***
	(0.00003)	(0.00004)	(0.00005)
HR	−0.0003***	−0.001***	−0.001***
	(0.0002)	(0.0003)	(0.0003)
DoC	0.001***	0.002***	0.003***
	(0.0002)	(0.0002)	(0.0002)
Population_65		0.001***	0.002***
		(0.0002)	(0.0002)
Log(GDP per capita)			0.004***
			(0.001)
Log(Air passengers)			0.003***
			(0.0004)
Constant	−0.004	−0.019***	−0.108***
	(0.004)	(0.004)	(0.014)
Observation	3220	3210	3032
R^2	0.050	0.066	0.091
Adjusted R^2	0.049	0.065	0.089
F Statistic	55.87***	56.42***	50.47***

Note: * $p < 0.1$; ** $p < 0.05$; *** $p < 0.01$. HR: sum of physicians (per 1000 citizens) and nurses and midwives (per 1000 citizens); DoC: probability (%) of dying between age 30 and exact age 70 from any of cardiovascular disease, cancer, diabetes, or chronic respiratory disease. Source: Own calculations.

Factors representing demographic ("population 65") and health ("DoC") aspects also reflected the real situations: older people accounted for the majority of deaths, and most of those had various comorbidities, particularly non-communicable diseases (such as cancer, diabetes, or chronic respiratory disease) [15].

When adding logarithm of real GDP per capita (Model 2 in Table 3), its coefficient was positive and statistically significant, meaning that, given other demographic and healthcare system conditions, higher income countries experienced higher death rates than did those at lower income levels. This has been true in practice where both the number of deaths and the death rates in such high-income countries as the US, UK, Italy, and Spain were much higher than those of lower income countries.

One of the key channels for spreading out the COVID-19 pandemic has been domestic and international travels. The results from Model 3 with an addition of the variable showing the rate of passengers carried by air indicated that the countries which had a higher rate of passengers experienced higher rate of deaths. This finding reflected the real situation that the virus is transmitted from human to human, and the countries where a lot of people moving in and out for various purposes like businesses, travelling, and visiting, like Italy, Spain, the US, the UK, and China (especially in the spring holiday season), had an increasing number of people infected during the studied period. The recent social distancing and isolation in many countries and their regions have proved that less travelling and movement helped reduce the infection rates, and thus—to some extent—reduced the death rates [15,20].

A new approach in this paper was to apply the between-estimator estimation in order to explore the relationships of the model. In recent years, this method has been a new edge in evaluating the long-run effects of macroeconomic factors (see, for instance, [25–28]). This methodology, using the time-averaged data, was suitable with the dataset of this study since all independent variables were collapsed at one time.

Table 4 presents the results from pooled, fixed-effects (FE) and between-estimator methods. The results clearly showed the confirmation on the sign and significance of variables "hospital beds", "HR" and "population 65". More importantly, the R^2 was at 0.599, meaning that the model was better than the other. It is worth noting, however, that we could not apply this estimator when splitting the sample for further analyses since we had limited observations.

Table 4. Different estimation methods.

Explanatory Variable	Dependent Variable: Death_Rate		
	Pooled	FE	Between
Hospital beds	−0.0002***	−0.0002***	−0.002***
	(0.00005)	(0.00005)	(0.0003)
HR	−0.001***	−0.001***	−0.012***
	(0.0003)	(0.0003)	(0.003)
DoC	0.003***	0.003***	0.004
	(0.0002)	(0.0002)	(0.002)
Population_65	0.002***	0.002***	0.011***
	(0.0002)	(0.0002)	(0.002)
Log(real GDP per capita)	0.004***	0.003**	0.037***
	(0.001)	(0.001)	(0.021)
Log(Air passengers)	0.003***	0.003***	−0.006***
	(0.0004)	(0.0004)	(0.003)
Constant	−0.108***		−0.282
	(0.014)		(0.202)
Observation	3032	3032	70
R^2	0.091	0.091	0.599
Adjusted R^2	0.089	0.068	0.561
F Statistic	50.47*** (df = 6;3025)	49.52*** (df = 6;2956)	15.70*** (df = 6;63)

Note: * $p < 0.1$; ** $p < 0.05$; *** $p < 0.01$. HR: sum of physicians (per 1000 citizens) and nurses and midwives (per 1000 citizens); DoC: probability (%) of dying between age 30 and exact age 70 from any of cardiovascular disease, cancer, diabetes, or chronic respiratory disease. Source: Own calculations.

4.2. Further Results

Since countries at different income levels have different healthcare systems and strategies to deal with COVID-19 pandemic, we were interested in exploring how the aforementioned factors influenced the death rates of the COVID-19 infected persons in those different countries. Table 5 shows the results estimated for two groups of countries by income levels: high-income countries (HICs) and middle- & low-income countries (MLICs).

These results were different from those in the FE models for all countries as presented in Table 4. The negative coefficient for HICs was kept, meaning that healthcare system infrastructure was important to reduce the death rates of COVID-19 infected people in these countries.

Regardless of income levels, the coefficients for variable "HR" were negative and statistically significant in both groups of countries, meaning that the number of medical staff available in the pandemic has been extremely important for reducing death rates.

Except for HI countries, the coefficient of variable "DoC" for MLICs was positive and statistically significant, and this could be explained with the same reason discussed in the FE models in Table 4.

The coefficient for variable "Population 65" was positive and statistically significant in HICs, while it was not the case for MLICs. Such results could be elucidated the same as in FE models in Table 4. HICs had a higher rate of older people, who have been at highest risk of death under COVID-19.

In both groups of countries, coefficients for variable "real GDP per capita" were positive and statistically significant, meaning that higher income countries had higher death rates than those at lower income levels in the same group. This could be explained by various facts, including a higher proportion of people aged 65 and over and a higher number of air passengers—among others—in higher income countries.

Table 5. Estimations for two groups of income.

Explanatory Variable	Dependent Variable: Death_Rate	
	HICs	MLICs
Hospital beds	0.00004 *	0.0002
	(0.00002)	(0.0002)
HR	−0.001 ***	−0.008 ***
	(0.0002)	(0.001)
DoC	0.0001	0.005 ***
	(0.0002)	(0.0004)
Population_65	0.001 ***	0.0003
	(0.0001)	(0.001)
Log(real GDP per capita)	0.007 ***	0.026 ***
	(0.002)	(0.003)
Log(Air passengers)	0.002 ***	0.0003
	(0.0002)	(0.001)
Observation	1604	1428
R^2	0.211	0.132
Adjusted R^2	0.172	0.084
F Statistic	67.915 *** (df = 6;1528)	34.406 *** (df = 6;1352)

Note: * $p < 0.1$; ** $p < 0.05$; *** $p < 0.01$. HR: sum of physicians (per 1000 citizens) and nurses and midwives (per 1000 citizens); DoC: probability (%) of dying between age 30 and exact age 70 from any of cardiovascular disease, cancer, diabetes, or chronic respiratory disease. Source: Own calculations.

For the variable showing travelling impact (i.e., "Air passengers"), the coefficient for HICs was positive and statistically significant, showing the fact that these countries experienced huge flows of immigrants and emigrants during the studied period, and thus have experienced more infected people and more deaths. In contrast, MLICs started quarantine at the early stage of COVID-19 spreading so that they could limit the number of infected people via international and domestic travelling flows.

To check the robustness for all above estimations, we conducted different methods to see whether the standard errors of the same variables were significantly different. The results are presented in Table 6. We could see clearly a small difference in the standard errors of the same variables between estimations. These results confirmed that the main results in Table 4 were robust; that is, the correlations between the death rate and important explanatory variables (such as number of hospital beds, number of medical staffs, DoC, aged population, and air passengers) were significant strongly. Furthermore, there was only one difference in the significance but not the sign of the variable "real GDP per capita". This implied that we could not confirm strongly the correlation between real GDP per capital and the death rate. Meanwhile, among countries with different income levels, the heterogeneity did exist in some variables.

Table 6. Robust covariance matrix estimators.

Explanatory Variable	Dependent Variable: Death_Rate		
	FE	Driscoll-Kraay	White
Hospital beds	−0.0002***	−0.0002***	−0.0002
	(0.00005)	(0.0001)	(0.0002)
HR	−0.001***	−0.001***	−0.001*
	(0.0003)	(0.0002)	(0.001)
DoC	0.003***	0.003***	0.003
	(0.0002)	(0.001)	(0.002)
Population_65	0.002***	0.002***	0.002***
	(0.0002)	(0.0002)	(0.001)
Log(GDP per capita)	0.003***	0.003*	0.003
	(0.001)	(0.002)	(0.006)
Log(Air passengers)	0.003***	0.003***	0.003***
	(0.0004)	(0.0002)	(0.0002)
Observation	3032		
R^2	0.091		
Adjusted R^2	0.068		
F Statistic	49.522***		

Note: * $p < 0.1$; ** $p < 0.05$; *** $p < 0.01$. HR: sum of physicians (per 1000 citizens) and nurses and midwives (per 1000 citizens); DoC: probability (%) of dying between age 30 and exact age 70 from any of cardiovascular disease, cancer, diabetes, or chronic respiratory disease. Source: Own calculations.

5. Concluding Remarks

In this paper, we used the daily statistics on the death rates of the COVID-19 infected people in various countries which had more than 100 infected cases from 21 January 2020 to 30 March 2020, and explored their possible associated factors. Although the results were different when we controlled for various factors (such as income levels), we still found consistent results that healthcare system conditions, particularly the number of hospital beds and the number of medical staff, played extremely important roles in reducing death rates of COVID-19 infected persons. In addition, both mortality rates due to different non-communicable diseases (NCDs) and the rate of people aged 65 and over were significantly related to the death rates in all countries, meaning that aged populations along with prevalent NCDs would exacerbate the situation of death under any pandemics related to pneumonia like COVID-19. We also found that controlling international and domestic travelling by air along with increasingly popular anti-COVID-19 actions (i.e., quarantine and social distancing) helped reduce the death rates in all countries. Last but not least, the danger of COVID-19 has made clear that the preparedness of healthcare systems and aged populations needs more attention from public and politicians, regardless of income level, when facing COVID-19-like pandemics. In any country, timely and strong cooperation between government, civil society, and private individuals are important in building up the trust in fighting public health crisis like COVID-19 [29].

Given the nature of global research with cross-sectional data, this study could not avoid some key limitations, as follows. First, we could not disaggregate the data on death by sex and age groups since the used statistics did not cover these important indicators for all countries in the studied sample. Second, some non-health and non-demographic factors such as culture and living styles could not explore due to unavailable data; those could be studied at a country-specific level. Third, due to limited timeline for the study (up to 30 March 2020), the impact of various measures coping with COVID-19 such as social distancing and lock-down could not be explored. We hope to integrate these factors in the coming studies with a specific group of countries or a single country.

Author Contributions: T.-L.G. checked data analysis, drafting, editing and finalizing the article. D.-T.V. was in charge of data collection and calculations as well as drafting the article. Q.-H.V. provided comments to revise drafts. The final version was completed and agreed by all authors. All authors have read and agreed to the published version of the manuscript.

Funding: This research received no external funding.

Conflicts of Interest: The authors declare no conflict of interest.

References

1. Fauci, A.S.; Lane, H.C.; Redfield, R.R. Covid-19—Navigating the Uncharted. *N. Engl. J. Med.* **2020**, *382*, 1268–1269. [CrossRef] [PubMed]
2. McCloskey, B.; Heymann, D.L. SARS to novel coronavirus–Old lessons and new lessons. *Epidemiol. Infect.* **2020**, *148*, e22. [CrossRef] [PubMed]
3. Verity, R.; Okell, L.C.; Dorigatti, I.; Winskill, P.; Whittaker, C.; Imai, N.; Cuomo-Dannenburg, G.; Thompson, H.; Walker, P.G.T.; Fu, H.; et al. Estimates of the severity of coronavirus disease 2019: A model-based analysis. *Lancet Infect. Dis.* **2020**, *3099*, 1–9. [CrossRef]
4. Zhou, F.; Yu, T.; Du, R.; Fan, G.; Liu, Y.; Liu, Z.; Xiang, J.; Wang, Y.; Song, B.; Gu, X.; et al. Clinical course and risk factors for mortality of adult inpatients with COVID-19 in Wuhan, China: A retrospective cohort study. *Lancet* **2020**, *395*, 1054–1062. [CrossRef]
5. Gates, B. Responding to Covid-19—A Once-in-a-Century Pandemic? *N. Engl. J. Med.* **2020**, *382*, 1677–1679. [CrossRef] [PubMed]
6. Gilbert, M.; Pullano, G.; Pinotti, F.; Valdano, E.; Poletto, C.; Boëlle, P.-Y.; D'Ortenzio, E.; Yazdanpanah, Y.; Eholie, S.P.; Altmann, M.; et al. Preparedness and vulnerability of African countries against importations of COVID-19: A modelling study. *Lancet* **2020**, *395*, 871–877. [CrossRef]
7. Hick, J.L.; Biddinger, P.D. Novel Coronavirus and Old Lessons—Preparing the Health System for the Pandemic. *N. Engl. J. Med.* **2020**, *382*, e55. [CrossRef]
8. Levin, P.J.; Gebbie, E.N.; Qureshi, K. Can the Health-Care System Meet the Challenge of Pandemic Flu? Planning, Ethical, and Workforce Considerations. *Public Health Rep.* **2007**, *122*, 573–578. [CrossRef]
9. Hampton, T. Pandemic Flu Planning Falls Short. *JAMA* **2007**, *297*, 1177. [CrossRef]
10. Parpia, A.S.; Ndeffo-Mbah, M.L.; Wenzel, N.S.; Galvani, A.P. Effects of Response to 2014–2015 Ebola Outbreak on Deaths from Malaria, HIV/AIDS, and Tuberculosis, West Africa. *Emerg. Infect. Dis.* **2016**, *22*, 433–441. [CrossRef]
11. Bedford, J.; Enria, D.; Giesecke, J.; Heymann, D.L.; Ihekweazu, C.; Kobinger, G.; Lane, H.C.; Memish, Z.; Oh, M.-D.; Sall, A.A.; et al. COVID-19: Towards controlling of a pandemic. *Lancet* **2020**, *395*, 1015–1018. [CrossRef]
12. Tang, B.; Xia, F.; Bragazzi, N.L.; McCarthy, Z.; Wang, X.; He, S.; Sun, X.; Tang, S.; Xiao, Y.; Wu, J. Lessons drawn from China and South Korea for managing COVID-19 epidemic: Insights from a comparative modeling study. *Bull World Health Organ.* **2020**. [CrossRef]
13. Wang, Z.; He, T.; Zhu, L.; Sheng, H.; Huang, S.; Hu, J. Active quarantine measures are the primary means to reduce the fatality rate of COVID-19. *Bull World Health Organ.* **2020**. [CrossRef]
14. Van Wees, J.-D.; Osinga, S.; Van Der Kuip, M.; Tanck, M.; Hanegraaf, M.; Pluymaekers, M.; Leeuwenburgh, O.; Van Bijsterveldt, L.; Zindler, J.; Van Furth, M.T. Forecasting hospitalization and ICU rates of the COVID-19 outbreak: An efficient SEIR model. *Bull World Health Organ.* **2020**. [CrossRef]
15. Chen, T.; Wu, D.; Chen, H.; Yan, W.; Yang, D.; Chen, G.; Ma, K.; Xu, D.; Yu, H.; Wang, H.; et al. Clinical characteristics of 113 deceased patients with coronavirus disease 2019: Retrospective study. *BMJ* **2020**, *368*, m1091. [CrossRef] [PubMed]
16. Wang, D.; Hu, B.; Hu, C.; Zhu, F.; Liu, X.; Zhang, J.; Wang, B.; Xiang, H.; Cheng, Z.; Xiong, Y.; et al. Clinical Characteristics of 138 Hospitalized Patients With 2019 Novel Coronavirus–Infected Pneumonia in Wuhan, China. *JAMA* **2020**, *323*, 1061. [CrossRef]
17. Tuite, A.R.; Ng, V.; Rees, E.; Fisman, D.N. Estimation of COVID-19 outbreak size in Italy. *Lancet Infect. Dis.* **2020**, *20*, 537. [CrossRef]
18. Wells, C.R.; Sah, P.; Moghadas, S.M.; Pandey, A.; Shoukat, A.; Wang, Y.; Wang, Z.; Meyers, L.A.; Singer, B.H.; Galvani, A.P. Impact of International Travel and Border Control Measures on the Global Spread of the Novel 2019 Coronavirus Outbreak. Available online: https://www.pnas.org/content/117/13/7504 (accessed on 10 April 2020).
19. Shi, S.; Tanaka, S.; Ueno, R.; Gilmour, S.; Tanoue, Y.; Kawashima, T.; Nomura, S.; Miyata, H.; Yoneoka, D. Impact of travel restrictions on importation of novel coronavirus infection: An effective distance approach. *Bull World Health Organ.* **2020**. [CrossRef]

20. Yuan, Z.; Xiao, Y.; Dai, Z.; Huang, J.; Chen, Y. A simple model to assess Wuhan lock-down effect and region efforts during COVID-19 epidemic in China Mainland. *Bull World Health Organ.* **2020**. [CrossRef]
21. World Bank. World Development Indicators. Available online: http://datatopics.worldbank.org/world-development-indicators/ (accessed on 10 March 2020).
22. Driscoll, J.C.; Kraay, A.C. Consistent Covariance Matrix Estimation with Spatially Dependent Panel Data. *Rev. Econ. Stat.* **1998**, *80*, 549–560. [CrossRef]
23. Hoechle, D. Robust Standard Errors for Panel Regressions with Cross-Sectional Dependence. *Stata J.: Promot. Commun. Stat. Stata* **2007**, *7*, 281–312. [CrossRef]
24. Worldometer. Coronavirus, Confirmed Cases and Deaths by Country, Territory, or Conveyance. 2020. Available online: https://www.worldometers.info/coronavirus/ (accessed on 10 April 2020).
25. Csereklyei, Z. Price and income elasticities of residential and industrial electricity demand in the European Union. *Energy Policy* **2020**, *137*, 111079. [CrossRef]
26. Hauk, W.R.; Wacziarg, R. A Monte Carlo study of growth regressions. *J. Econ. Growth* **2009**, *14*, 103–147. [CrossRef]
27. Woo, J.; Kumar, M.S. Public Debt and Growth. *Economica* **2015**, *82*, 705–739. [CrossRef]
28. Stern, D.I. Between estimates of the emissions-income elasticity. *Ecol. Econ.* **2010**, *69*, 2173–2182. [CrossRef]
29. La, V.-P.; Pham, T.-H.; Ho, T.M.; Nguyen, M.-H.; Nguyen, K.-L.P.; Vuong, T.-T.; Nguyen, H.-K.T.; Tran, T.; Van Khuc, Q.; Ho, T.M.; et al. Policy Response, Social Media and Science Journalism for the Sustainability of the Public Health System Amid the COVID-19 Outbreak: The Vietnam Lessons. *Sustainability* **2020**, *12*, 2931. [CrossRef]

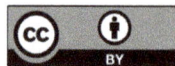

© 2020 by the authors. Licensee MDPI, Basel, Switzerland. This article is an open access article distributed under the terms and conditions of the Creative Commons Attribution (CC BY) license (http://creativecommons.org/licenses/by/4.0/).

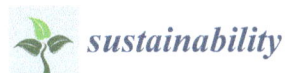

Article

Policy Response, Social Media and Science Journalism for the Sustainability of the Public Health System Amid the COVID-19 Outbreak: The Vietnam Lessons

Viet-Phuong La [1,2], Thanh-Hang Pham [3,4,*], Manh-Toan Ho [1,2,*], Minh-Hoang Nguyen [1,2], Khanh-Linh P. Nguyen [1,2], Thu-Trang Vuong [5], Hong-Kong T. Nguyen [1,2], Trung Tran [6], Quy Khuc [7], Manh-Tung Ho [1,2] and Quan-Hoang Vuong [1,8,*]

[1] Centre for Interdisciplinary Social Research, Phenikaa University, Yen Nghia Ward, Ha Dong District, Hanoi 100803, Vietnam; phuong.laviet@phenikaa-uni.edu.vn (V.-P.L.); hoang.nguyenminh@phenikaa-uni.edu.vn (M.-H.N.); linh.nguyenphuckhanh@phenikaa-uni.edu.vn (K.-L.P.N.); htn2107@caa.columbia.edu (H.-K.T.N.); tung.homanh@phenikaa-uni.edu.vn (M.-T.H.)
[2] A.I. for Social Data Lab, Vuong & Associates, 3/161 Thinh Quang, Dong Da District, Hanoi 100000, Vietnam
[3] Faculty of Management and Tourism, Hanoi University, Km9, Nguyen Trai Road, Thanh Xuan, Hanoi 100803, Vietnam
[4] School of Business, RMIT Vietnam University, Hanoi 100000, Viet Nam
[5] Sciences Po Paris, 27 Rue Saint-Guillaume, 75007 Paris, France; thutrang.vuong@sciencespo.fr
[6] Vietnam Academy for Ethnic Minorities, Hanoi 100000, Vietnam; trungt1978@gmail.com
[7] Faculty of Economics and Finance, Phenikaa University, Yen Nghia Ward, Ha Dong District, Hanoi 100803, Vietnam; quy.khucvan@phenikaa-uni.edu.vn
[8] Centre Emile Bernheim, Université Libre de Bruxelles, 1050 Brussels, Belgium
[*] Correspondence: hangpt@hanu.edu.vn (T.-H.P.); toan.homanh@phenikaa-uni.edu.vn (M.-T.H.); hoang.vuongquan@phenikaa-uni.edu.vn or qvuong@ulb.ac.be (Q.-H.V.)

Received: 22 March 2020; Accepted: 4 April 2020; Published: 7 April 2020

Abstract: Having geographical proximity and a high volume of trade with China, the first country to record an outbreak of the new Coronavirus disease (COVID-19), Vietnam was expected to have a high risk of transmission. However, as of 4 April 2020, in comparison to attempts to containing the disease around the world, responses from Vietnam are seen as prompt and effective in protecting the interests of its citizens, with 239 confirmed cases and no fatalities. This study analyzes the situation in terms of Vietnam's policy response, social media and science journalism. A self-made web crawl engine was used to scan and collect official media news related to COVID-19 between the beginning of January and April 4, yielding a comprehensive dataset of 14,952 news items. The findings shed light on how Vietnam—despite being under-resourced—has demonstrated political readiness to combat the emerging pandemic since the earliest days. Timely communication on any developments of the outbreak from the government and the media, combined with up-to-date research on the new virus by the Vietnamese science community, have altogether provided reliable sources of information. By emphasizing the need for immediate and genuine cooperation between government, civil society and private individuals, the case study offers valuable lessons for other nations concerning not only the concurrent fight against the COVID-19 pandemic but also the overall responses to a public health crisis.

Keywords: coronavirus; COVID-19; SARS-CoV-2; pandemic; policy response; social media; science journalism; public health system; Vietnam

1. Introduction

"Dans les champs de l'observation le hasard ne favorise que les esprits préparés."
—Louis Pasteur (1822–1895)

As China grappled to contain the outbreak of the novel coronavirus disease (COVID-19), caused by the virus officially named Severe Acute Respiratory Syndrome Coronavirus 2 (SARS-CoV-2), in the first few months of 2020, Vietnam, which shares a border of 1281 kilometers and a high volume of trade with the northern giant [1], was bracing itself for a high risk of cross-border infections. Within more than two months from January 23 when the first case of COVID-19 was detected in Vietnam, there have been 239 confirmed cases with zero deaths [2]. During the same period, the number of infections in China had skyrocketed from 600 people, with 17 deaths to 82,526 cases with 3330 deaths [3].

Despite the differences in their domestic contexts, such abysmal contrast between the two neighbors could raise questions as to how Vietnam, a populous but less-resourced nation of nearly 100 million people, has managed to contain the spread of the new disease. This feat merits in-depth studies, especially in light of the World Health Organization's (WHO) declaration of COVID-19 as a pandemic on March 11th [4] and the chaotic self-quarantine and lockdown in various countries in Europe and America.

Vietnam was among the first countries to have confirmed cases of COVID-19, with the first two patients (both Chinese) detected on January 23 [5]. This study identifies four periods of disease outbreak in Vietnam, namely (i) pre-January 23, (ii) between January 23 and February 26 when the first batch of sixteen patients were tested and treated till their discharge, (iii) between February 27 and March 5 when there was no new case and (iv) and post-March 6 when the 17th patient was detected and led a new wave of infections from incoming tourists and returning travelers [6].

As Figure 1 shows, compared to other countries, the infection rate in Vietnam was evidently much lower than that in China, Italy, South Korea, the United Kingdom and the United States. All these countries, except China, had the first cases announced in January [3]. In the period from January 23 to February 25, the rise in cases in Vietnam was comparable to that in the United States, United Kingdom and Germany. From late February to March 5, the situation in Vietnam appeared under control with no new cases while cases in South Korea and Italy soared to 5766 and 3089, respectively [3]. From March 6 onward, the steep upward trend was seen in much of Europe and the United States, which as of March 30 was ranked first with 122,653 cases [3].

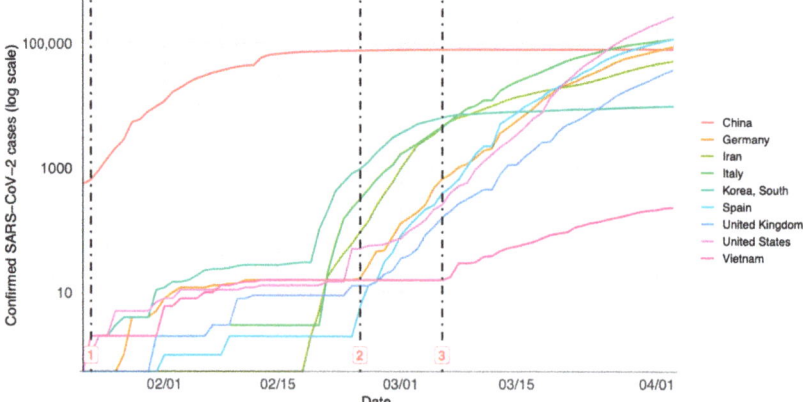

Figure 1. The rise of new Coronavirus disease (COVID-19) cases in selected countries (as of April 4, 2020). Note: ① is the first case in Vietnam; ② is when the patient 16 recovered, ended the 1st outbreak; ③ is the 17th case in Vietnam, also the beginning of the 2nd phase of the outbreak.

While Vietnam also saw an uptick in new cases during March, its response to COVID-19, which is a combination of political readiness, timely communication and scientific journalism, offers valuable lessons in dealing with situations of epidemics on a state level. As of April 4, the number of COVID-19 infections in Vietnam was 239, in which 90 patients had recovered, 149 are being treated and no deaths recorded (See Figure 1).

The study, though in its preliminary and subject to changes as the disease progresses, may nonetheless be instructive and helpful for other countries to better understand the role of policy response, social media and science journalism in maintaining public health. The case of Vietnam provides empirical evidence for assessing the efficacy of specific measures in fighting the pandemic.

2. Literature Review

Within the first three months of the new decade, the novel coronavirus, officially named SARS-CoV-2—and the corresponding disease COVID-19—has spread from Wuhan city in China's central province of Hubei to 201 other countries and territories. Over 1,123,024 people have been infected with over 59,140 lives lost as of April 4, 2020, according to the Global COVID-19 Tracker Map at John Hopkins University [7]. The rapid contagion and severity of the new disease has prompted WHO to update its statement, from classifying the outbreak as a "Public Health Emergency of International Concern" on January 30 to a "Pandemic" on March 11 [4].

Given the urgency of this outbreak, the international academic community is mobilizing ways to accelerate the development of disease detection and intervention. A statement by the research-charity based Wellcome Trust in London has gathered more than 100 signatories to ensure access to data and research findings on the disease could better inform the public and save lives. These include leading publishers such as Springer Nature, Elsevier or Taylor and Francis as well as prestigious journals such as *The Journal of the American Medical Association*, *The British Medical Journal*, the *Lancet* and *New England Journal of Medicine* [8]. In these leading journals, editorials echoed a call for researchers to "keep sharing, stay open" [9]. In *Nature Medicine*, the editorial also stated that "communication, collaboration and cooperation can stop the 2019 coronavirus" [10]. Editors in the leading medical journal BMJ asserted that "while scientists and public health professionals are working non-stop to contain the novel coronavirus, political scientists, economists and sociologists should also ready themselves for rapid response" [11].

Complementing the clinical research on COVID-19 are studies that integrate social sciences in the outbreak response. Social sciences research is expected to produce rich and detailed insights into the social, behavioral and contextual aspects of the communities, societies and populations affected by infectious disease epidemics. The overarching aim is to bring together social sciences knowledge and biomedical understanding of the COVID-19 epidemic. Such connection would strengthen the response at international, regional, national and local levels to stop the spread of COVID-19 and mitigate its social and economic impacts [12].

Among countries affected by the pandemic, Vietnam, with its geographical proximity with China, faces a high likelihood of being severely affected by the spread of the disease. Moreover, although the Vietnamese healthcare system is under-resourced and has inherent weaknesses [13–17], especially concerning health insurance and patient welfare [17,18], the Vietnamese response to urgent situations has been commendable. It is likely that the Vietnamese government has learnt from its experiences in the past, especially in dealing with the Severe Acute Respiratory Syndrome (SARS) epidemic in 2003. Vietnam's success in the effective control of SARS for the first time in the world was achieved by "complete isolation of patients and implementation of nosocomial infection control from an early stage of epidemic" [19]. The lesson is clear for Vietnam: early risk management requires taking adequate actions from the early stage of the disease.

The few studies on the outbreak in Vietnam have largely focused on the clinical aspects [20], with the exception of [21], which is on public risk perception. This piece analyzes the government's response in terms of public health measures and policy implementation, as well as the mobilization of citizens' collaboration in containing the disease have been very limited. This shall be a subtle call to action for researchers in Vietnamese social sciences.

3. Materials and Methods

This paper reviews Vietnamese policy response, news and science journalisms related to COVID-19 recently. Findings were derived from the analysis of a database of recent policies, articles and the credibility of data sources in Vietnam. Extensive coverage was given to the pandemic in both the official press and academic journals as well as through reports, briefs and presentations by members of concerned organizations (e.g., WHO).

A Python-powered web crawler engine was used to scan the data from online newspapers in Vietnam, such as *Tuổi Trẻ, Thanh Niên, VnExpress* or *Kênh 14*, to name a few. Then, the scanned data were saved into a news analysis system, which is developed by.NET Core, for storage and future analysis. The data structure contains three main components:

- Projects & Data Sources: Settings for projects and news sources.
- Data Logging: Log of the data collection process
- News & Filters: Collected news with filters.

Examples of Python code are as follows (Figure 2):

```python
def parseDetail(self, response):
    projectId = response.meta.get('projectId')
    projectSourceId = response.meta.get('projectSourceId')
    sourceId = response.meta.get('sourceId')
    sourceUrl = response.meta.get('sourceUrl')
    projectCfg = response.meta.get('projectCfg')
    crawlCfg = response.meta.get('crawlCfg')
    parseCfg = response.meta.get('parseCfg')
    pageId = response.meta.get('pageId')

    keyGroup = response.meta.get('keyGroup')

    if self.existNewsUrl(projectId, response.url):
        return(None)

    #print(keyGroup)
    newsTitle = NewsParser.extractText(NewsParser.parseItem(response, parseCfg["TitleCfg"]))
    print(newsTitle)

    newsDate = NewsParser.parseDate(response, parseCfg["DateCfg"])
    print(newsDate)

    if projectCfg["UpToDate"]:
        upToDate = datetime.strptime(projectCfg["UpToDate"], "%Y-%m-%dT%H:%M:%S")
        if upToDate > newsDate:
            if projectSourceId not in self.completed:
                self.completed.append(projectSourceId)
            return(None)

    newsSapo = ""
    if "SapoCfg" in parseCfg:
        parseSapo = NewsParser.parseItem(response, parseCfg["SapoCfg"])
        newsSapo = NewsParser.extractText(parseSapo)
        #print(newsSapo)
```

Figure 2. Examples of Python code.

Using this system, we can set up sources and keywords. Furthermore, all tools and datasets will be maintained for future mining. We expect the dataset to keep growing over time, presenting us with new opportunities to extract deeper and more valuable insights.

In this article, using five keywords related to COVID-19, namely: *covid, ncov, corona, viem phoi* (Vietnamese for pneumonia, which has some symptoms in common with COVID-19), *sars-cov*, between January 9 and April 4, the tool has collected 14,952 news reports on the topic of concern, as presented in Table 1.

Table 1. List of online news sources (as of April 4, 2020).

Sources	Start Date	News
kenh14.vn	15/01/2020	2132
vtc.vn	17/01/2020	909
suckhoedoisong.vn	09/01/2020	929
cafef.vn	12/01/2020	804
tuoitre.vn	12/01/2020	1196
chinhphu.vn	09/01/2020	441
Zing.vn	17/01/2020	1360
dantri.com.vn	10/02/2020	1838
plo.vn	23/01/2020	400
vnexpress.net	23/01/2020	917
vov.vn	27/02/2020	1748
nld.vn	28/02/2020	577
rfa.org	10/02/2020	248
thanhnien.vn	18/02/2020	1453

Raw data were manually cleaned then categorized based on its characteristics, such as the timeline of COVID-19 cases, the timeline of international events regarding COVID-19, media reports and policy response from the Vietnamese government. Regarding the social media aspect, due to technical limitations, we could not scan information from Facebook. Thus, we used the remediation of social media on news outlets as a proxy to explore the social media aspect. Keywords that uniquely fit with the aspect, including 'mạng xã hội' (social media), 'cư dân mạng' (netizens), Facebook and Zalo, were used to search within the collected dataset. Furthermore, the data of the VN INDEX, which represents the changes in the Vietnamese stock market's prices during the COVID-19 pandemic, was also added to complete the dataset. Finally, we store the cleaned data as a comprehensive dataset in excel files.

The dataset (updated as of April 4, 2020) is available at Open Science Framework (OSF) (URL: https://osf.io/4w9ef/; DOI: 10.17605/OSF.IO/4W9EF) [22]. Having organized the dataset, we then calculated descriptive statistics to illustrate how the Vietnamese government, news and science journalism respond to COVID-19.

4. Results

4.1. Chronology

Figure 3 presents a timeline of the spread of COVID-19 in Vietnam, tracing from the first identified patient in on January 23 to the most recent case on March 31. At this time, the number of cases in Vietnam exceeded 200 and for the sake of better presentation of data, we decided to cut off the data on this day. The most updated version of the chronology as well other data can be accessed from OSF [22].

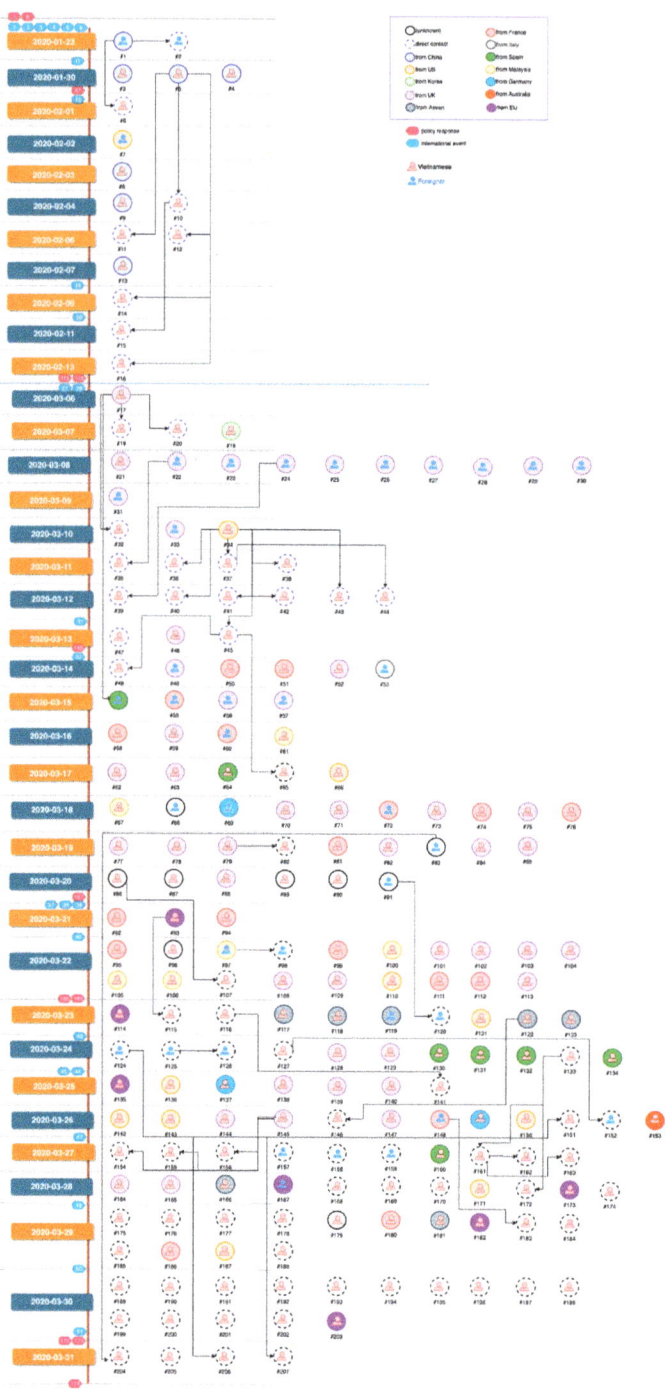

Figure 3. Chronology of COVID-19 in Vietnam (as of March 31, 2020).

Based on this timeline, four main periods of the COVID-19 outbreak in Vietnam are identified in Table 2.

Table 2. Four periods of the COVID-19 outbreak in Vietnam.

Period	Date	Event
1	Before January 23	No confirmed case in Vietnam
2	January 23–February 26	First confirmed case in Vietnam–16th infected case discharged from hospital (Figure 4)
3	February 27–March 5	No new case in Vietnam
4	March 6–present [April 4]	17th infected case confirmed and more reported afterward

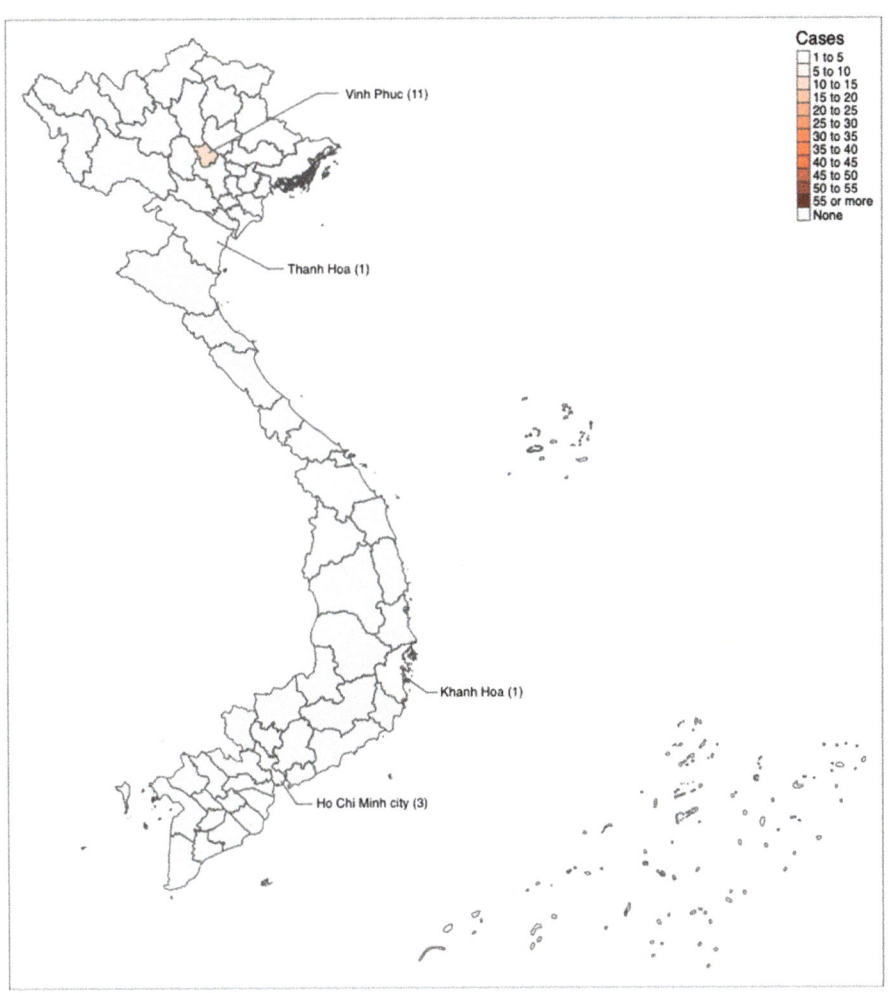

Figure 4. Locations of the first outbreak (16 cases) of COVID-19 in Vietnam.

4.2. Policy Response

We have manually extracted news reports regarding the government's actions following the outbreak. We have identified 173 official instructions, guidelines, plans, dispatch, policies and direct actions from the government, which were categorized as follows (Table 3):

Table 3. Categories of Vietnamese government policy response.

Category	Count	Enacted in
Fake news prevention	10	Periods 2,4
Assessment of the prevention	5	Periods 1,2
Assessment of the threat	4	Periods 1,2
Education	15	Periods 2,3,4
Emergency response	30	Periods 2,4
Guidelines and plans	10	Periods 1–4
Innovation	1	Period 3
Market control	18	Periods 2,3,4
National funding	1	Period 4
National Pandemic announcement	1	Period 4
Outbreak-is-over announcement	1	Period 2
Preventive action	35	Periods 2,3,4
Reward	1	Period 1
Social distancing announcement	1	Period 4
Citizen support	16	Period 2,4
Travel restrictions	24	Periods 2,3,4

4.2.1. Period 1: Before January 23, 2020

In this period before the first case was confirmed, the policy response focused on the assessment of the threat, together with developing guidelines and plans as preventive measures for the coming combat for the newly detected disease. As early as January 3, even before the first fatal case in China [12] and only a few days after China confirmed the outbreak of a new coronavirus [23], the Ministry of Health (MOH) had issued a directive on tightening quarantine at the Vietnam-China border [24]. On January 10, the Public Health Emergency Operation Center under the MOH followed up with a meeting to evaluate the disease situation and suggest preventive and treatment measures.

From January 16 to 20, the MOH issued two decisions (No. 125/QĐ-BYT and No. 156/QĐ-BYT) to provide guidelines and plans to prevent spread of the new coronavirus [25]. One urgent official dispatch (62/KCB-NV) to hospitals and local health departments stresses the importance of early disease prevention and detection [26].

4.2.2. Period 2: January 23, 2020–February 26, 2020

After the first confirmed case of COVID-19 infection, the policies focused both on minimizing risks from inbound travelers and containing the disease domestically. The policies include emergency responses, preventive actions, travel restrictions and market control.

During this period, because the hotspot of the disease was in China, attempts to control the spread from other countries focused on China-originated sources of infection. Vietnam started with strict screening on passengers from China at airports, seaports and land crossings, followed with isolating passengers suspected of infection, and entirely restricting flights to Wuhan and other affected areas in China [27]. On February 3 when the number of cases in China had shot up to 20,400, the Vietnamese government heightened quarantine to cover all travelers who have come from or transited through the COVID-19 affected areas in China [28]. In the last days of the period, with Daegu, South Korea becoming the latest COVID-19 hotspot, the MOH added health declaration for all passengers from or transiting through South Korea and imposed isolation for those with symptoms [29].

At the same time, a series of emergency responses and preventive actions were made from the central to local governments. These included calls for increased cooperation among localities as well as specific tasks for multiple ministries and agencies [30,31]. With Deputy Prime Minister Vu Duc Dam appointed as the head of the steering committee for COVID-19 combat, intra-governmental cooperation is formalized and government officials are held to the highest accountability.

When the sixth COVID-19 case—also the first case of domestic transmission—was confirmed on February 1, the government declared the epidemic of a new coronavirus-caused infectious disease in Vietnam [32]. What followed were strict measures to prevent the virus from spreading, including quarantine, isolation of suspected virus carriers and voluntary isolation at the community [30]. This period was marked by a 20-day lockdown of a commune of 10,600 people in the northern province of Vinh Phuc after ten people tested positive to the new virus [33].

In response to potential public hoarding of certain goods, from February 1, the government had worked with relevant authorities to inspect pharmacies nationwide and withdraw business licenses of those which increased prices of face masks, hand sanitizers and medical gloves [34]. Within three days, more than 1200 drug stores were penalized and over 313,000 face masks were seized [35].

Another action taken by the government was the introduction of technological platforms, including the website http://ncov.moh.gov.vn and the NCOVI and Vietnam Health apps, to provide updated information about the epidemic, including testing data, advice on precautionary measures and live chat for questions related to COVID-19 [36].

However, there were two mistakes during this period. In the first case, the Vietnam National Administration of Tourism had attempted to promote a campaign called "Vietnam—Safe Haven" while the spread of COVID-19 was still at the early stage [37]. The campaign aimed to attract foreign tourists on the ground that Vietnam has managed this public health crisis well; consequently, 41% of the COVID-19 cases since patient 17—effectively a "patient zero" of the second cluster of the outbreak in Vietnam—are foreign tourists [38].

In the second case, the Ministry of Education and Training (MOET) had made three significant mistakes when school shutdowns began [39]. First, given the uncertain nature of the pandemic, it was a bad decision to close schools for one week at a time and then extend such shutdown week-by-week, leaving students and parents hanging every week and burdening their household decision-making. Second, because the ministry failed to provide educational guidelines timely, a longer break right after the Vietnamese national Tet holidays left the false impression of an extended vacation for families. This meant many families take the weeks off to travel, instead of staying home to minimize exposure and transmission. Third, the ministry's decisions on which groups of students (i.e., elementary and secondary) stay home and what universities should do (i.e., self-determination) were erratic and lacking scientific basis. When no age group has been proven "safe" from virus transmission, and young people could be asymptomatic carriers of the virus, letting them back to school could turn them into transmission vectors and threatened immunocompromised members of their own family, such as grandparents. Only after protest from the public did the ministry decree all school buildings to be shut down and all students to stay home.

Despite these few blunders, all confirmed cases were discharged from hospitals at the end of this period. Deputy Prime Minister Vu Duc Dam had declared that Vietnam "won the first battle against the epidemic" [40].

4.2.3. Period 3: February 27, 2020–March 5, 2020

Between February 26 and March 4, with no new patients detected, Vietnam entered a pause in the timeline of the outbreak. By contrast, the world, from Asia to Latin America and Sub-Saharan Africa, was seeing a rapid spread of the disease [41,42], with two new coronavirus hotspots emerging outside China. As of March 5, the number of infected patients in South Korea had hit 6284 and in Italy 3858 [3].

The pause in Vietnam, however, does not mean any changes to existing disease prevention and control policies. The government continued to impose stricter travel restrictions, such as halting visa exemption for citizens of severely affected countries, including South Korea and Italy, and ask schools and universities nationwide to keep closing. Pandemic combat remains a top priority. An army simulation exercise in response to the outbreak was held on March 4.

Yet, there were signs of imprudence. Deputy Prime Minister Vu Duc Dam, the leader of Vietnam National Steering Committee for COVID-19, had hastily announced on March 4 that: "If another week passes without new cases, Vietnam will announce the end of the epidemic" [43]. This leads to lax regulations among frontline guards against the disease and may have contributed to the outbreak after case 17.

4.2.4. Period 4: March 6, 2020–Current

After 22 days of having no new confirmed case of COVID-19, on March 6, the 17th patient was confirmed. This marked the second outbreak of Vietnam with the source of infection evaluated as much more complicated rather than just China or Korea (See Figure 5). The new cases in this period were mainly tourists and Vietnamese citizens coming back from European countries as well as people who had direct contact with the infected patients. On March 30, as the number of cases climbed every day, the Prime Minister declared the COVID-19 outbreak as a nationwide pandemic [44]. This declaration heightened alert over disease prevention, especially following the first cases of cross-infection to healthcare workers from a cluster at a tier-one hospital in Hanoi. As of March 31, there were 34 infected cases related to Bach Mai Hospital [45].

In response, the Vietnamese government imposed many rigorous measures [46], including a temporary suspension of visa issuance to all foreigners for 30 days effective on March 18 [47], obligated 14-day quarantine at centralized facilities from March 21 and ultimately, temporary suspension of entry to all foreigners on March 22 [48] (See Table 4).

Table 4. The halting of visa issuance to foreign countries.

Country	Date Issued	Number of Cases in Vietnam (as of the announcement)
All countries	March 18	66
The United Kingdom and Schengen	March 15	53
Italy	March 3	17
South Korea	February 29	16
China	February 2	7

At the domestic level, the government has implemented urgent measures in multiple domains.

All schools have closed across the country and are likely expected to stay closed for a long period of time [49]. Large-scale quarantine and isolation of suspected cases persisted; and self-isolation for people with high risks of infection was carried out. All religious organizations are asked to stop holding mass gatherings from March 21 while all cultural, sports and entertainment activities in public places are prohibited from March 28 to April 15 [50,51]. The biggest change yet is, effective April 1, Vietnam enforced a "15-day nationwide social distancing" in which every household, village, commune, district and province would go into self-isolation [52]. Meanwhile, incoming flights to Vietnam are halted, while traveling within the country has also been restricted [53].

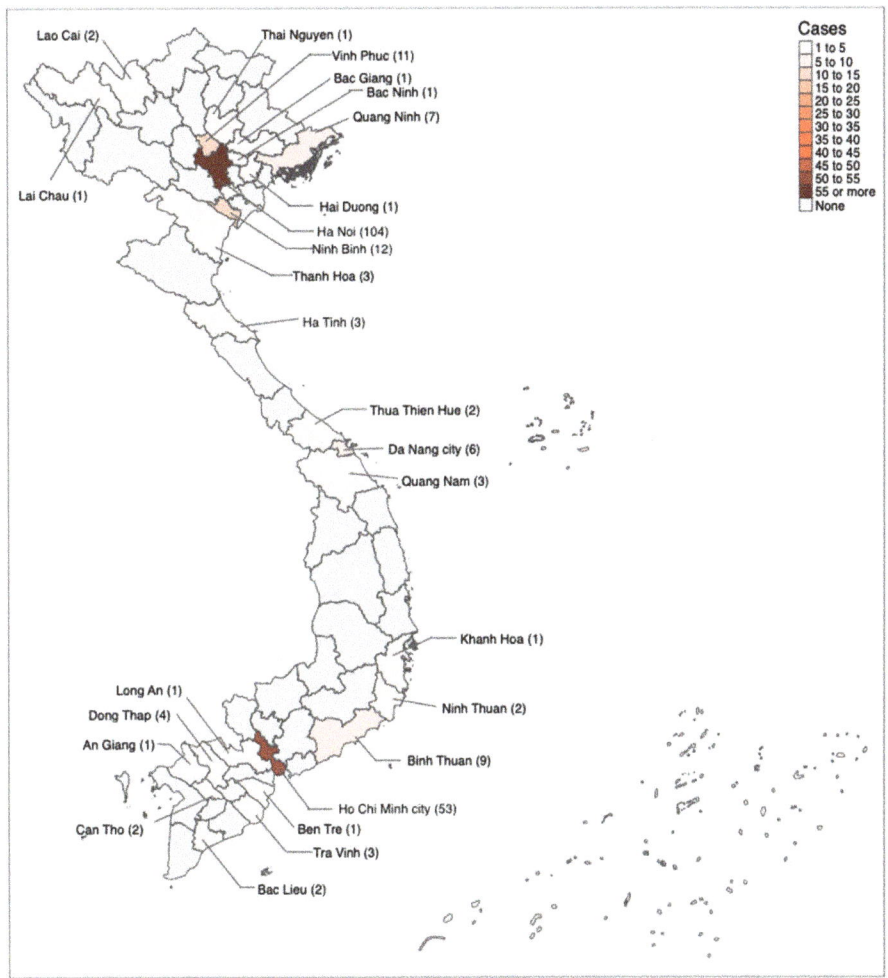

Figure 5. Locations of the second outbreak of COVID-19 in Vietnam (as of April 4, 2020).

Since the beginning of COVID-19 outbreak in Vietnam, the government has been focusing on hospital management policies to make sure the medical system is ready for the combat. In fact, the government issued several instructions about hospital management early on in late January, for example how to screen patients in hospital visits or specific distribution of responsibility to each level of hospital [54]. Since February, temporary hospitals have been set up to cure COVID-19 patients, for example the 300-bed field hospital in Vinh Phuc in the first outbreak [55] or two field hospitals to quarantine up to 1000 people in Hanoi [56]. From another perspective, two hospitals in Hanoi, namely Hong Ngoc and Saint Paul, used to be suspended or have a number of healthcare workers quarantined because of direct contact with COVID-19 patients without proper prevention measures. After these incidents, the city's authorities asked all medical centers to learn from these experiences and Hanoi Department of Health to conduct more effective training for healthcare workers as well as monitoring the process of taking care of infected patients to prevent the outbreak within hospitals [57]. In the second outbreak, the Vietnamese policy response related to hospitality management focused on Bach Mai Hospital as the biggest COVID-19 cluster in the country [58]. On March 28, Bach Mai hospital, which is Hanoi's largest leading hospital, was completely blocked after twelve infected cases related to this medical center were confirmed. More than 5000 health care workers, patients and food workers in the hospital were tested for the virus and another 40,000 people who were at the hospital have been tracked down and asked to self-quarantine at home for 14 days [59]. During that night, a temporary hospital was set up within Bach Mai hospital to prepare for the worst scenario. However, two days later, the Ministry of Health announced that Bach Mai hospital cannot stop receiving and curing patients with serious and complex medical conditions from provincial hospitals, 80% of whom may lose their lives without proper treatment [60].

Overall, amid COVID-19 outbreak, the hospital management policies imposed by the government have been well followed by all-level hospitals—and as an encouragement—Prime Minister Nguyen Xuan Phuc acknowledged and praised the contribution of "soldiers in white blouse" in a letter sent to frontline doctors and nurses on March 26 [61].

Regarding economic activities, to assure the public over supply of essential goods, following the short panic-buying of Hanoi citizens when the 17th case was detected, officials across the country immediately worked with suppliers and distributors [62–64]. After the declaration of the nationwide social distancing on March 31, the government made sure to reassure people of the maintained transportation network for essential goods, especially food.

In addition, the State Bank of Vietnam, the country's central bank, on March 12 drafted a circular which would support credit organizations to restructure debt payment deadlines and cut borrowing interest rate and exemption for enterprises heavily affected by the pandemic. It was stated that over 44,000 customers with a total debt of VND222 trillion (US$9.51 billion) would benefit from this program [65]. Furthermore, on March 31, the government has discussed a welfare measure according to which all poor households would receive an aid of 1,000,000 VND per person per month [66].

In terms of technological application, the Vietnamese government opened a system to record electronic health declaration form for overseas travelers entering the country for the purpose of case monitoring and surveillance [67]. In addition, the Hanoi Smart City app was also activated to provide a risk assessment tool, consultation on prevention measurements, contact reports and live updates for Hanoi citizens [68].

The prompt and effective measures undertaken by the Vietnamese government to date have been highly regarded by international organizations [69]. Domestically, the results from global public research focusing on people's perception of their government's reaction by Dalia Research revealed that Vietnamese people have the most confidence in their government's response to the COVID-19 pandemic among 45 countries surveyed [70]. About 62% of the Vietnamese respondents think that the government is doing the "right amount' in response to the situation [71].

4.3. Media Communication

4.3.1. Official Press

Prior to the first case of COVID-19 in Vietnam, news on a "strange pneumonia" in China had circulated on Vietnamese media as early as the beginning of January 2020. Our dataset suggests news regarding this "strange pneumonia" first appeared on *Báo Chính phủ* (chinhphu.vn), *Vietnam Government Portal* and *Sức Khỏe và Đời Sống* [Health and Life] (suckhoedoisong.vn), the official news channel of the Ministry of Health, on January 9 [72,73].

According to the article written by the Public Health Emergency Operation Center on *Sức Khỏe và Đời Sống* [73], public health experts expected high risk of having an outbreak in Vietnam because it was near the Tet holidays (or Chinese New Year). The following preventive measures had been proposed:

- Monitoring information from WHO and other sources
- Communicating the information clearly to the citizen
- Increasing disease surveillance at the border

- Maintaining the alertness of the Public Health Emergency Operation Center and four Institutes of Hygiene and Epidemiology.
- Planning prevention and control measures.

It should be noted that other news outlets such as *Tuổi Trẻ, Thanh Niên* or *Quân Đội Nhân Dân* even shared the information to public earlier, from as early as January 3 [74,75]. Thus, the timely attention from newspapers and news media and afterward, social media, has played a crucial role in disseminating information to the public.

Since then, thousands of articles have been written updating Vietnamese people about the outbreak in the country and globally. Data from 14 online newspapers only generated nearly 15,000 articles published from January 9 to April 4. This helps considerably in raising public awareness about the disease as well as informing people on disease prevention and protection.

As can be seen from Figure 6, the amount of media communication to the public remained high at around 150 to 190 articles daily. However, there were days when newspapers appeared to pay attention to other events, and this number of articles dropped to below 100 in the third period. Overall, the flow of news and information to the public was on-going and rather substantial during the outbreaks.

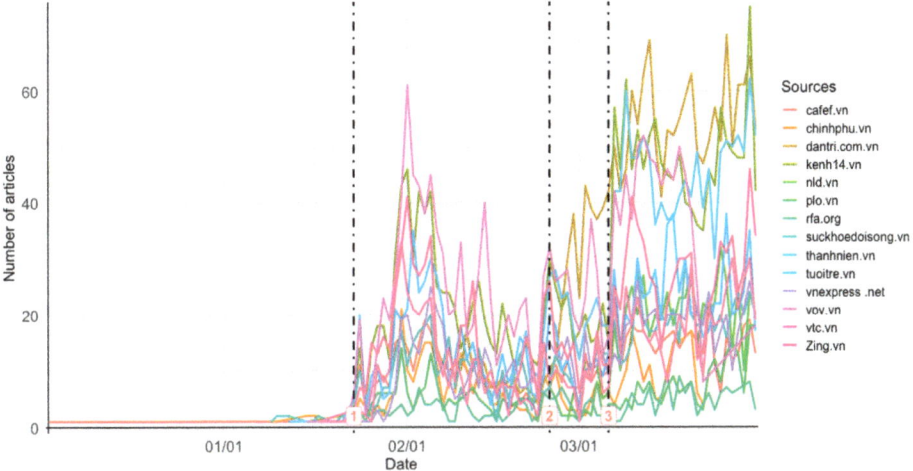

Figure 6. Number of articles about coronavirus in major newspapers.

4.3.2. Social Media

One particular characteristic of social media in Vietnam is the widespread use of Facebook (57.34% of the population [76]) and the local app Zalo (100 million users) [77]. These social media channels provide additional room for the government, particularly the Ministry of Health, to communicate coronavirus-related information to its citizens in a timely manner.

As Figure 7 suggests, the number of articles, including keywords such as Facebook or '*mạng xã hội*' (social media) in Vietnamese newspapers is high. As the information has been disseminated through social media on an hourly basis, as well as the update from influencers or reporters, the newspapers had to remediate these contents. In the first and fourth periods, as many as 50 to 60 articles were circulated in each period. Meanwhile, 'Zalo' and '*cư dân mạng*' (netizen) received less attention.

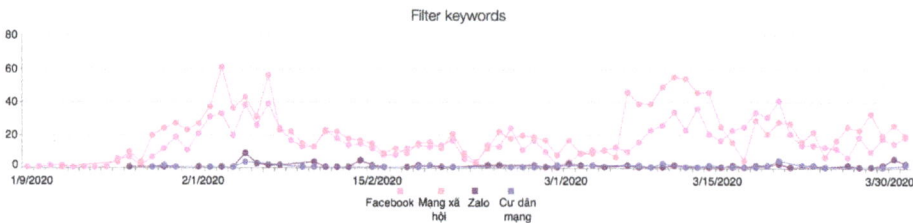

Figure 7. Number of articles about social media and coronavirus on major Vietnamese newspapers.

During the fourth period, information density proved to be an essential aspect of dealing with pandemic. There exists a stereotype of students and expatriates coming back from developed countries as being more informed and better behaved given their higher level of education. However, recent events have shown that stereotypes remain stereotypes. Patient 17 in Vietnam is a notable illustration: a well-educated upper-middle-class person who acted in an extremely ignorant manner, refused to self-quarantine for 14 days, and thus had likely spread the virus to many other cases afterward.

Media communication created both positive and negative impacts on public awareness and attention during this period. On the one hand, individual effort in supporting public awareness and protection against the virus was praised by social media. For example, Vietnamese dancer Quang Dang with the handwashing song, known as "*Ghen Co Vy*," went viral globally and attracted thousands of views, and many people around the world are posting their own covers [78]. Some Youtubers with a large number of subscribers have also contributed interesting and diverse perspectives about the pandemic, for instance the 16-year-old YouTuber named Melly Vuong [79]. In quarantine areas, people update about their life on social media, which spread a positive review of the facilities and healthcare system. For example, the well-known local fashionista Chau Bui made videos of her quarantine period, all of which amassed nearly one million views [80]. Famous artists are reported on social media for their donations to the healthcare facilities in Vietnam [81]. Social media also reacted vividly to cases of confirmed patients or quarantined people. For example, Patient 17, who returned from Europe and did not provide accurate health status declaration, got serious criticism from social media.

However, the negative side of rapid social media response is a strong emergence of fake news. The problem was most acute during the early days of critical events such as the confirmed case of the first or 17th patient with the involvement of celebrities and famous people. Responses to combat such mis/dis-information were made in both periods 2 and 4 (Table 3), formalized in a government decree in which anyone spreading fake news could be fined between (US$430-860), around 3–6 months' worth of basic salary in Vietnam [81].

4.3.3. Science Journalism

In the fight against coronavirus, science journalism plays a crucial role in informing the global research community as well as providing reliable information to the public. Vietnamese hospitals have contributed very promptly to the call for sharing knowledge and data about the disease [38] on January 28th, 2020, even before the call from Nature editors to all COVID-19 researchers [10]. Since then, there have been several significant works contributed by Vietnamese authors to the scientific community (see Table 5).

These efforts of Vietnamese scientists were also reported on the official press, for example, Vnexpress on January 30th posted an article entitled, "The first case of nCoV in Vietnam on the world's "medical bible"" [82], introducing the work by [38].

Table 5. Articles about COVID-19 published by Vietnamese authors.

No.	Title	Authors	Journal/Source	Date
1	Importation and Human-to-Human Transmission of a Novel Coronavirus in Vietnam	Phan, Lan T., Nguyen, Thuong V., Luong, Quang C., Nguyen, Thinh V. Nguyen, Hieu T., Le, Hung Q., Nguyen, Thuc T., Cao, Thang M. Pham, Quang D.	The New England Journal of Medicine	January 28, 2020
2	Outbreak investigation for COVID-19 in northern Vietnam	Hai Nguyen Thanh, Truong Nguyen Van, Huong Ngo Thi Thu, Binh Nghiem Van, Binh Doan Thanh, Ha Phung Thi Thu,	The Lancet Infectious Diseases	March 4, 2020
3	Duration of viral detection in throat and rectum of a patient with COVID-19	Le Van Tan, Nghiem My Ngoc, Bui Thi Ton That, Le Thi Tam Uyen, Nguyen Thi Thu Hong, Nguyen Thi Phuong Dung, Le Nguyen Truc Nhu, Tran Tan Thanh, Dinh Nguyen Huy Man, Nguyen Thanh Phong, Tran Tinh Hien, Nguyen Thanh Truong, Guy Thwaites, Nguyen Van Vinh Chau	medRxiv	March 16, 2020
4	The COVID-19 risk perception: A survey on socioeconomics and media attention	Toan Luu Duc Huynh	Economics Bulletin	March 25, 2020

Regarding initiatives of science journalism, the use of preprints to speed up the publishing process has been a focus in the combat against COVID-19 [83,84], for example [20]. This shows the positive signal of the Vietnamese scientific community to move forward with these global trends. The findings from Vietnamese hospitals and authors can, therefore, contribute to the database of global knowledge and expertise and may help to curtail this outbreak and prepare for future outbreaks.

On April 3, one of the leading universities in Vietnam, the National Economic University, also released a report titled "Assessment of COVID-19 impacts on the economy and policy recommendations," which has been heavily covered on the media [85]. Therefore, it appeared that researchers from hospitals and universities, rather than other types of institutions, have published more on COVID-19. This is consistent with the findings from [86] that university-affiliated authors in Vietnam tend to have higher research productivity than institution-affiliated peers.

Additionally, scientific publications and information also play a critical role in debunking myths on the disease and quickly communicating reliable information to the public, for instance, pushing back against a steady stream of rumors and conspiracy theories about the origin of the coronavirus outbreak [87]. This source may be used by newspapers and social media to disseminate information more widely to the general public (for example [88]). In Vietnam, various scientists have frequently updated scientific knowledge and perspectives on their personal Facebook accounts to inform the community. For instance, the Facebook posts by Tran Xuan Bach—an Associate Professor of John Hopkins University based in Hanoi—had attracted nearly 13,000 views and hundreds of shares from the public [89]. Furthermore, interviews with doctors and scientists were also conducted both in written form and in live form, for example, the live consultation session on the topic "Information about Coronavirus and respiratory diseases—How to prevent and treat" broadcasted on VTV News Newspaper [90].

In terms of scientific advancement, Vietnam has successfully produced test kits to diagnose COVID-19 infection in just one hour. The kit was stated to meet the WHO and the U.S. Center for Disease Control and Prevention Standards, and 20 countries were negotiating to buy these products [91]. Besides this, several scientific projects are being conducted to produce similar rapid testing kits to meet the increasing demand worldwide, for example, those by Hanoi University of Science and Technology or Vietnam Academy of Science and Technology [91]. On March 3, the Vietnam Academy of Science and Technology officially announced the successful manufacturing of SARS-CoV-2 Virus Diagnostic Kit [92].

Besides scientific publications, university websites and various information-sharing magazines also contributed to enhancing the awareness of COVID-19. For instance, Phenikaa University has posted instructions to prevent the coronavirus up-to-date and donated more than 8000 liters of hand sanitizer to residential areas, Hanoi Youth Union, Departments of Education and hundreds of schools in Vietnam Northern provinces [93]. Similarly, more than 20 universities across the country have produced sanitizers and provided them free for their communities [94].

On March 31, 10 COVID-19 testing kiosks have been set up all around Hanoi, prioritizing the areas around Bach Mai hospital which was one of the largest recent outbreak hotspot [95]. Five thousand quick test kits—which give results after 10 minutes of testing—were distributed by the Ministry of Health to these testing kiosks, and were ready immediately on March 31st morning [96]. This is an important development, as Vietnam has so far relied on suboptimal methods such as self-report via declaration of medical status and targeting high-risk populations. Mass testing is a proactive measure that aims to directly inspect the entire population, leading to early detection and thus minimizing spread [97]. This was a lesson explicitly learned from South Korea, as not only the test kits were Korean-developed but the help of Korean experts was also enlisted in implementing mass testing in Vietnam. The importance of cross-border lesson learning underlines the significance of science journalism, especially when disease containment has to be coordinated on an international level.

4.3.4. Socioeconomic Aspects

While imposing strict directives to prevent the dissemination of the novel coronavirus, adverse impacts on the socio-economic situations in Vietnam are observable as consequences. For instance, the number of international visitors to Vietnam in the first three months of 2020 was expected to decline by 800,000 compared to last year [98]. However, as stated by Prime Minister Nguyen Xuan Phuc: "the government is willing to sacrifice economic benefits in the short term for the health of people," Vietnam government acknowledges the adverse consequences of preventive measures. The acknowledgment is also reflected through the simultaneous reduction of interest rate by the State Bank of Vietnam [99].

In the economic domain, for the stock market (Figure 8), before the detection of the first COVID-19 case in Vietnam, in period 1, the information for the disease in China appeared to have little impact on the market. During period 2, from January 23 to February 26, the market started the downward trend and lost more than 6.6%, from 959.58 points to 895.97 points. In period 3, the VN-Index experienced a minimal decrease from 895.97 on February 26 to 893.31 on March 5, 2020. During period 4, between confirmation of the 17th case in Vietnam on March 6 and the 207th case on March 31, the stock market suffered severely, with its benchmark VN-Index recording a sharp loss of nearly 229 points, or 25.7%.The weak market sentiment and force-sell pressure in Vietnam are predicted to persist, given the complicated developments in stock markets around the world.

While Vietnam is no longer a centrally planned economy [100,101], in the face of a public health crisis and national emergency as this one, the government was quick to control any sudden spikes in prices of consumer goods, and thus, effectively preventing price speculation and gouging. In the very first day of Period 4 of COVID-19 detection and intervention in Vietnam, there was an initial wave of panic stockpiling of food among local consumers [102]. However, within two days, the government met and discussed measures not only to cope with the disease outbreak but also to stabilize the domestic market [103]. By comparison, elsewhere around the globe, even in developed nations such as Australia [104] and the United States [105], consumers were reported to hoard a massive amount of food, toilet papers, hand sanitizer and anti-bacterial wipes; some were doing it so as to profit off the public's panic buying. While there is insufficient data for comparing prices before and after the outbreak among countries, it appears that the situation in Vietnam is kept relatively better under control than in other countries. This is evidenced by the fact that the government, in conjunction with producers and supermarkets, was prompt to assure the public of food security as well as price stabilization.

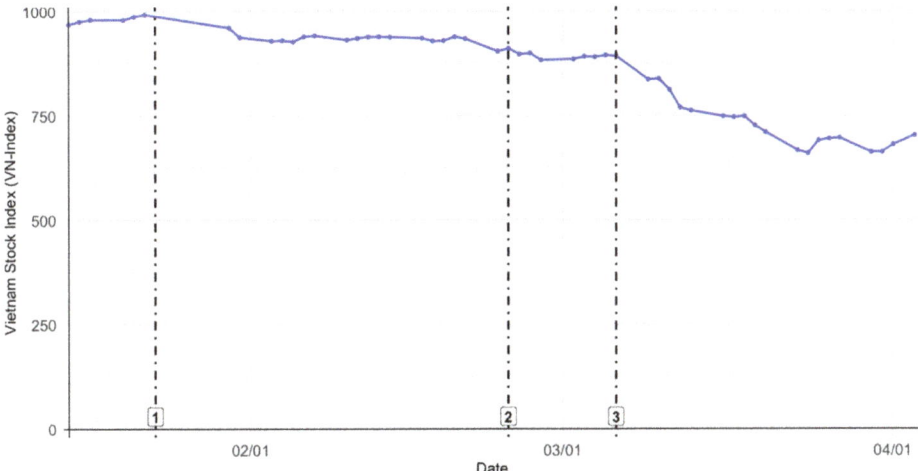

Figure 8. The changes in the benchmark VN-Index of Vietnam's stock market during the COVID-19 outbreak (As of April 4, 2020). Note: ① is the first case in Vietnam; ② is when the patient 16 recovered, ended the 1st outbreak; ③ is the 17th case in Vietnam, also the beginning of the 2nd outbreak.

In the social domain, during the early days after the first infected case, there had been rumors that the Vietnamese government was hiding information about the novel coronavirus, which caused some confusion and insecurity for the public [106]. To respond to this information, the authorities and mainstream media promptly reassured the citizens that transparency is the fundamental principle of the country in preventing the spread of the virus [107]. Government officials further explained that data and information from four Public Health Emergency Operation Centers of Vietnam were directly connected to the Centers for Disease Control and Prevention USA and, therefore, shared openly to the global database [107].

In the later periods, the emergence of strong political leaders such as Deputy Prime Minister Vu Duc Dam had a significant and positive influence on public perception of the Vietnamese government as well as the consensus and trust in Vietnam's efforts to fight against the pandemic. On social media, images and quotes of Deputy PM Dam appeared extensively on citizen's posts, which created a sense of solidarity and the belief in governments' efforts. Recently, the call from Prime Minister Nguyen Xuan Phuc on the whole nation's joint efforts in COVID-19 combat attracted public attention and support from individual citizens [108]. Responding to this call, one can easily see many images of bank transfer to the Vietnamese Fatherland Front on social media of Vietnamese people to support the government in the combat. On a larger scale, many enterprises, regardless of their size, also contributed to the national combat by donating their products such as masks, rice or milk, by donating their hotels for isolation wards—or most popularly—by donating cash [109].

The social response can also be seen from various groups, including residential, work-related and informal groups. Since the early days of the outbreak, residential groups played a central role in transferring information to individual citizens by means of public announcements, leaflets, posters or standees [110]. In big cities, apartment buildings as well as office buildings took measures to prevent the spread of the virus, for instance by sanitizing the whole building or checking people's temperatures before entering together with putting sanitizers in public spaces [111]. In daily transactions such as food shipping (see Figure 9), safety measures are being enforced by citizens. The image, once again, reminds old people of how daily transactions were secretly conducted in the centrally planned economy period. In the digital space, multiple groups have been formed, especially on social media, to share information about the pandemic and collaborate efforts to help fight against it.

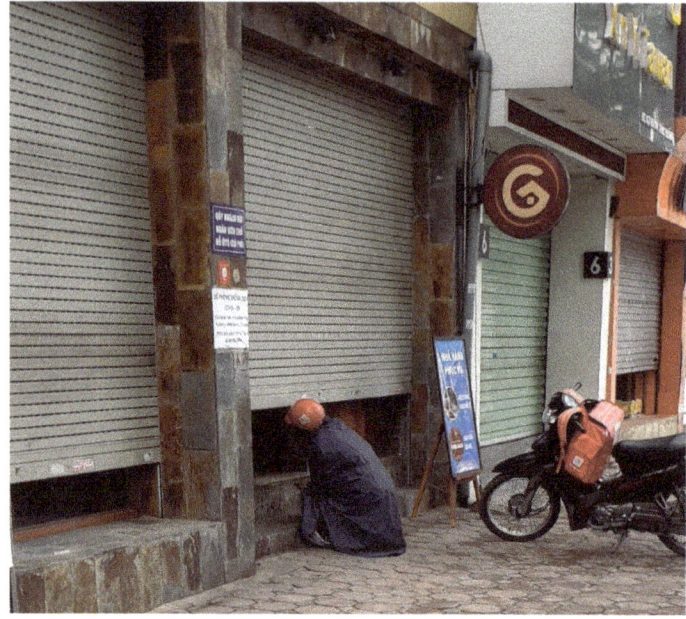

Figure 9. Safe business transaction in the COVID-19 time. ©2020 photo courtesy: Dam Thu Ha.

Several other social aspects of Vietnamese citizens had significant impacts on their reactions to the pandemic. Since the very early days, the Vietnamese people have paid close attention to the information through mass media and social media about the "strange pneumonia" from the neighboring country, China. This helped them to have preparedness and readiness to act very early on. This process of gradually distilling information also contributed to the fact that most of the time, the people responded to the situation without panicking. In addition, in the Vietnamese culture characterized by adoption of new ideas [112], the act of wearing masks has been seen as normal and as a way to protect oneself, not as a source of risks and infection for surrounding people as in some countries. Therefore, the habit of using face masks, after being encouraged by the government as an effective measure for protection, has been reinforced among the public.

5. Discussion and Conclusions

First of all, the early risk assessment and immediate action of the Vietnam government, as well as the seamless coordination between government and citizens, are some of the main contributors to the prompt and effective reaction vis-à-vis the COVID-19 pandemic, which is caused by the corona virus officially named SARS-CoV-2, in Vietnam up till now. To date, Vietnam has managed to keep the situation under control in several regards. All patients who tested positive either have recovered or were recovering; there has been zero death. In terms of prevention, the Vietnamese government has maintained rather impressive cooperation with citizens and measures such as mandatory mask-wearing, systemic health status declarations and checks and self-quarantine have all been swiftly and smoothly implemented. Despite having made certain missteps or near-missteps as have been analyzed in the above sections, the government had been sensible enough to perceive warnings and recognize said mistakes.

The early policy response for preventive and treatment measures before the first case appearing in Vietnam is a highlight because Vietnam obtains a comparatively long shared borderline with China, and that was during the Tet holiday—the traditional new year of both Vietnam and China when the mobility rate was substantially high. The later simultaneous responses of the government presented through continuous directives of the Prime Minister according to the COVID-19 situation provide public health measures (school closure, public health quarantine, social distancing, etc.) and maintain the supply of fundamental goods for preventing the dissemination of the disease. Besides that, the effective control of the infected case number is also greatly influenced by the fluent coordination among governmental agencies. To achieve smooth national coordination during the harsh time, a whole-of-government pandemic prevention drill was held during the period when no newly infected cases were found. These efforts of Vietnam all met the suggestions by WHO for responding to community spread of COVID-19 [113] and implied the high awareness and integration of Vietnam government, which are two out of five main factors of a resilient health system proposed by [114]. Indeed, the government learned from its previous experience during the SARS 2003 epidemic and established a public health response mechanism that has proven to be effective to date.

Despite the optimistic results of the measures that have been taken to prevent the spread of COVID-19, one must not deny the mistake that may have intensified the severe consequences of the second outbreak. The Ministry of Education and Training was responsible for lack of guidelines for students as well as indecisive policies regarding school shutdowns during the early phases of the pandemic. The Ministry of Culture, Sports and Tourism had also taken missteps in underestimating the spread of the diseases and falling lax in controlling cross-borders contamination. It highlights a certain disconnect between the declaration of the PM to prioritize the health of citizens above economic concerns: indeed, the Ministry had thought to take advantage of a global pandemic to promote tourism, and Vietnam had paid dearly.

As has been suggested by Leach, et al. [115], governments often preferred to frame disease outbreaks as acute, thus relying on temporary, short-term measures of public intervention; an alternative to this framing would be to consider infectious diseases as endemic and long-present in the locality, thus adapting the entire community's lifestyle to deal with it. As COVID-19 is a novel disease, the Vietnamese government has indeed responded to it as an epidemic outbreak; however, it could also be observed that the rapid response itself owed to the fact that Vietnam had had a history of dealing with epidemics and pandemics, namely SARS in 2003 and H5N1 flu in 2008; as well as A/H1N1 in 2009, the disease continued to make its reappearance in smaller outbreaks in years to come, such as in 2018 [116]. For this reason, one may be able to have a positive outlook on Vietnam's sustainability, at least in terms of efficient decision-making, in the continuing battle against the spread of COVID-19.

Sustainability in terms of resources, however, merited a closer look. In view of the phenomenon of pre-lockdown panic-buying, particularly reported in the United States, but also in certain other countries such as France or Germany, food insecurity and commodity shortage have become legitimate concerns. In certain circles on social media, certain pictures of Vietnam and the US have been posted alongside to highlight the contrast between the quite adequate food distribution in Vietnam as well as the free meals provided in quarantine hospitals on one hand, and the empty shelves of not only food but also sanitary products (toilet rolls, hand sanitizer, soap, etc.) due to hoarding in certain places in the United States on the other. In addition, one could not discuss resource drainage in the face of a pandemic without evoking labor. It goes without saying that the medical personnel was on the frontline, but other than medical professions, it should be noted that manual laborers who uphold the infrastructure, such as store staff, garbage collectors, deliverers, etc. This aspect of resource merits as much attention from governments and planning as any other.

With regard to resources required to sustain prevention measures, there are positive signs. it is worth noting that Vietnam is efficient enough in the production of test kits for both domestic use and export deals. This would be comparable to South Korea's testing ability, which had been put to use with remarkable success in curbing the spread of the disease as the country became the world's second-largest outbreak. [117]. However, as the second outbreak continued to spread, the efficiency of current preventive methods grew questionable. The demand for capable healthcare infrastructure to accommodate new cases thus remained pressing. Considering the fact that Vietnamese central hospitals suffered from chronic overpopulation in yearly minor outbreaks, this issue should very much concern policymakers. A suggestion would be to immediately devise plans to restrict mobility between provinces—both to prevent disease spread and to avoid overloading central hospitals—as well as to upgrade and equip regional hospitals and encourage infected citizens to utilize medical facilities in their proximity.

Concerning communication and information dissemination in the face of the pandemic, we have observed a pattern in the official press. Journalists have indeed picked up on the vocabulary used by officials in public speeches. As such, articles reporting on measures against COVID-19 employed rhetoric often associated to wars, such as: "fight the enemy" (*đánh giặc*, in which the word *giặc* connotes the illegitimacy of said enemy, a nuance difficult to translate), "leave nobody behind" (*không bỏ lại ai phía sau*; as if in a battle march), "grand solidarity" (*đại đoàn kết*, alluding to the two Indochina wars against France and the US), etc. This sort of highly combative language was, in fact, not new, as it has been used in official narratives for a good number of national media campaigns. On the other hand, technical terminologies seemed to be much less abundant in Vietnamese media reports.

Influential political leaders and experienced teams of officials were quick to recognize the crisis and implemented rigorous strategies to address the emerging outbreak. The media response has also helped in promoting public awareness about the disease and how people can protect themselves and the communities around them. Science journalism equally played a crucial role in communicating effectively and prompt information to the public and global research communities.

The three pillars of society's responses have contributed majorly to the situation of Vietnam, in which the community has responded quickly to a crisis and protect the interests of its citizens. It also reveals valuable lessons for other nations in the concurrent fight against the COVID-19 pandemic, namely an emphasis on mobilizing citizens' awareness of disease prevention without spreading panic, via fostering genuine cooperation between government, civil society and private individuals.

6. Limitations of the Study and Future Research Directions

We fully acknowledge the shortcomings of this paper. As the pandemic is still spreading and the situation continues to move rapidly at the time of writing, we are faced with a shortage of backing in the extant literature. While we have tried our best with rigorous methodology and technical tools—namely, using a web crawler to gather data *en masse* from news sites—there remain certain arbitrary choices that we had had to make as researchers, such as the choice of which news sites to consider, and which to exclude, from our analysis.

In terms of data curation and flexibility of analysis, our methodology also shows several limitations. It should be noted that news articles on online news sites were quite often reposted from one location to another, thus inflating the number of articles reporting on COVID-19 compared to the substantial information being disseminated. Rather than an error, we believe this phenomenon of media communication to be interesting in itself. However, we do not believe ourselves to be sufficiently equipped for analysis thereof, nor do we believe such an analysis would fit within the scope of our article. We would welcome any contribution, related or not to this point.

Author Contributions: conceptualization, V.-P.L. and Q.-H.V.; data curation, V.-P.L. and M.-H.N.; formal analysis, V.-P.L. and T.-H.P.; investigation, T.H.P., M.-T.H., K.-L.P.N., H.-K.T.N. and M.-T.H.; methodology, V.-P.L., M.-T.H., T.T. and Q.H.V.; project administration, M.-T.H.; resources, T.T. and Q.K.; software, V.-P.L. and Q.-H.V.; supervision, T.T. and Q.-H.V.; validation, M.-H.N., H.-K.T.N., M.-T.H., T.T., Q.K. and Q.-H.V.; Visualization, V.-P.L. and M.-T.H.; writing—original draft, T.H.P., K.-L.P.N. and T.-T.V.; writing—review & editing, T.H.P., M.-T.H., M.-H.N., K.-L.P.N., T.-T.V., H.-K.T.N., M.-T.H. and Q.K. All authors have read and agreed to the published version of the manuscript.

Funding: This research received no external funding.

Acknowledgments: We would like to dedicate this work to our homeland, Vietnam, to our government and to the Vietnamese people for all that we have done together as a nation in the combat against COVID-19. Our thoughts are with the people affected and all the brave and selfless healthcare workers who are helping those most in need. We hope that this difficult time for the whole humanity will end soon.

Conflicts of Interest: The authors declare no conflict of interest.

References

1. Central Intelligence Agency. The World Facebook—Vietnam. Available online: https://www.cia.gov/library/publications/the-world-factbook/geos/vm.html (accessed on 16 March 2020).
2. Ministry of Health. Information Page about COVID-19 Respiratory Disease Outbreak. Available online: https://ncov.moh.gov.vn/ (accessed on 31 March 2020).
3. World Health Organization. Situation reports. Available online: https://www.who.int/emergencies/diseases/novel-coronavirus-2019/situation-reports/ (accessed on 31 March 2020).
4. World Health Organization. General's Opening Remarks at the Media Briefing on COVID-19—11 March 2020. Available online: https://www.who.int/dg/speeches/detail/who-director-general-s-opening-remarks-at-the-media-briefing-on-covid-19---11-march-2020 (accessed on 16 March 2020).
5. Ministry of Health. *Công văn số 358/BYT-DP ngày 26/01/2020 Vv phối hợp tuyên truyền, giám sát và điều tra ổ dịch viêm đường hô hấp cấp do nCoV [Official Dispatch Number 358/BYT-DP on 26 Jan 2020 about Cooperation in Communication, Surveillance, and Investigation of an Outbreak of Acute Respiratory Infection Caused by nCoV]*; Ministry of Health: Hanoi, Vietnam, 2020.
6. Anh, L.; Long, X.; Tue, C.; Dieu, T. Hà Nội có 1 ca dương tính nCoV, là ca thứ 17 ở Việt Nam [Hanoi had a First Positive Case of nCoV, the 17th of Vietnam]. Available online: https://tuoitre.vn/ha-noi-co-1-ca-duong-tinh-ncov-la-ca-thu-17-o-viet-nam-20200306221140631.htm (accessed on 17 March 2020).
7. CSSE. Coronavirus COVID-19 Global Cases by the Center for Systems Science and Engineering (CSSE) at Johns Hopkins. Available online: https://coronavirus.jhu.edu/map.html (accessed on 1 April 2020).
8. Wellcome Trust. *Sharing Research Data and Findings Relevant to the Novel Coronavirus (COVID-19) outbreak*; Wellcome Trust: London, UK, 2020.
9. Nature. Calling all Coronavirus Researchers: Keep Sharing, Stay Open. Available online: https://www.nature.com/articles/d41586-020-00307-x (accessed on 16 March 2020).
10. Editorial. Communication, collaboration and cooperation can stop the 2019 coronavirus. *Nat. Med.* **2020**, *26*, 151. [CrossRef] [PubMed]
11. Kickbusch, I.; Leung, G. Response to the emerging novel coronavirus outbreak. *BMJ* **2020**, *368*, m406. [CrossRef] [PubMed]
12. World Health Organization. *A Coordinated Global Research Roadmap*; World Health Organization: Geneva, Switzerland, 2020.
13. Vuong, Q.-H. The (ir)rational consideration of the cost of science in transition economies. *Nat. Hum. Behav.* **2018**, *2*, 5. [CrossRef] [PubMed]
14. Vuong, Q.H. Be rich or don't be sick: Estimating Vietnamese patients' risk of falling into destitution. *SpringerPlus* **2015**, *4*, 529. [CrossRef] [PubMed]
15. Vuong, Q.-H.; Ho, T.-M.; Nguyen, H.-K.; Vuong, T.-T. Healthcare consumers' sensitivity to costs: A reflection on behavioural economics from an emerging market. *Palgrave Commun.* **2018**, *4*, 70. [CrossRef]
16. Nguyen, V.A.T.; Nguyen, N.Q.H.; Khuat, T.H.; Nguyen, P.T.T.; Do, T.T.; Vu, X.T.; Tran, K.; Ho, M.T.; Vuong, T.T.; Vuong, Q.H. Righting the Misperceptions of Men Having Sex with Men: A Pre-Requisite for Protecting and Understanding Gender Incongruence in Vietnam. *J. Clin. Med.* **2019**, *8*, 105. [CrossRef] [PubMed]
17. Vuong, Q.-H.; Vu, Q.-H. Learning healthcare needs when the body speaks: Insights from a 2016 Vietnamese survey on general physical examinations. *Indian J. Community Health* **2017**, *29*, 101–107.
18. Vuong, Q.-H. Sociodemographic factors influencing Vietnamese patient satisfaction with healthcare services and some meaningful empirical thresholds. *Iran. J. Public Health* **2018**, *47*, 119. [PubMed]
19. Ohara, H. Experience and review of SARS control in Vietnam and China. *Trop. Med. Health* **2004**, *32*, 235–240. [CrossRef]

20. Thanh, H.N.; Van, T.N.; Thu, H.N.T.; Van, B.N.; Thanh, B.D.; Thu, H.P.T.; Kieu, A.N.T.; Viet, N.N.; Marks, G.B.; Fox, G.J. Outbreak investigation for COVID-19 in northern Vietnam. *Lancet Infect. Dis.* **2020**. [CrossRef]
21. Phan, L.T.; Nguyen, T.V.; Luong, Q.C.; Nguyen, T.V.; Nguyen, H.T.; Le, H.Q.; Nguyen, T.T.; Cao, T.M.; Pham, Q.D. Importation and Human-to-Human Transmission of a Novel Coronavirus in Vietnam. *N. Engl. J. Med.* **2020**, *382*, 872–874. [CrossRef] [PubMed]
22. Tan, L.V.; Ngoc, N.M.; That, B.T.T.; Uyen, L.T.T.; Hong, N.T.T.; Dung, N.T.P.; Nhu, L.N.T.; Thanh, T.T.; Man, D.N.H.; Phong, N.T.; et al. Duration of viral detection in throat and rectum of a patient with COVID-19. *medRxiv* **2020**. [CrossRef]
23. Huynh, T.L. The COVID-19 risk perception: A survey on socioeconomics and media attention. *Econ. Bull.* **2020**, *40*, 758–764.
24. Vuong, Q.-H.; La, V.-P.; Hoang, N.M.; Linh, N.P.K.; Pham, T.-H.; Ho, T.M. *COVID-19-AISDL*; OSF: Peoria, IL, USA, 2020. [CrossRef]
25. Lanese, N. A New, Unidentified Virus Is Causing Pneumonia Outbreak in China, Officials Say. Available online: https://www.livescience.com/china-mystery-pneumonia-is-not-sars.html (accessed on 17 March 2020).
26. Hue, B. Bộ Y tế chỉ đạo kiểm soát chặt, tránh nguy cơ lây virus qua cửa khẩu [MOH: Tightening Quarantine at the Border to Prevent the Transmission of Any New Viruses]. Available online: https://news.zing.vn/bo-y-te-chi-dao-kiem-soat-chat-tranh-nguy-co-lay-virus-qua-cua-khau-post1032354.html (accessed on 22 March 2020).
27. Ministry of Health. Các văn bản về công tác chẩn đoán điều trị, kiểm soát nhiễm khuẩn bệnh viêm phổi cấp do chủng vi rút Corona mới (nCoV). [Documents about Diagnosis, Treatment and Infection Control of Acute Pneumonia Caused by New Strain of Corona Virus (nCoV)]. Available online: https://kcb.vn/cac-van-ban-ve-cong-tac-chan-doan-dieu-tri-kiem-soat-nhiem-khuan-benh-viem-phoi-cap-do-chung-vi-rut-corona-moi-ncov.html (accessed on 17 March 2020).
28. Hiep, P. Cảnh báo Việt Nam có nguy cơ cao lây nhiễm viêm phổi cấp do nCoV. [Warning Vietnam's High Risk for Acute Pneumonia Infection Caused by nCoV]. Available online: https://suckhoedoisong.vn/phat-hien-som-va-chuan-bi-tot-viec-phong-chong-benh-dich-viem-phoi-cap-do-corona-virut-moi-n168063.html (accessed on 17 March 2020).
29. Giang, H. Coronavirus Update: Gov't Demands High Sense of Responsibility for nCoV Combat. Available online: news.chinhphu.vn/Home/Coronavirus-update-Govt-demands-high-sense-of-responsibility-for-nCoV-combat/20201/38614.vgp (accessed on 22 March 2020).
30. Giang, H. VN to Quarantine all Travellers from Coronavirus-Affected Areas. Available online: http://news.chinhphu.vn/Home/VN-to-quarantine-all-travellers-from-coronavirusaffected-areas/20202/38646.vgp (accessed on 22 March 2020).
31. General Department of Preventive Medicine. Công văn số 868/BYT-DP về Hướng dẫn cách ly đối với người về từ Hàn Quốc. [Decree No. 868/BYT-DP about Instructrions for Isolation for People Coming from South Korea]. Available online: vncdc.gov.vn/vi/phong-chong-dich-benh-viem-phoi-cap-ncov/11872/huong-dan-cach-ly-doi-voi-nguoi-ve-tu-han-quoc (accessed on 22 March 2020).
32. Anh, K. Gov't Demands Measures to Prevent Outbreak of Infectious Coronavirus. Available online: http://news.chinhphu.vn/Home/Govt-demands-measures-to-prevent-outbreak-of-infectious-Coronavirus/20201/38592.vgp (accessed on 19 March 2020).
33. van, N. Gov't Issues Directive on Novel Coronavirus Prevention and Control. Available online: news.chinhphu.vn/Home/Govt-issues-directive-on-novel-coronavirus-prevention-and-control/20201/38600.vgp (accessed on 22 March 2020).
34. Minh, Q. Fighting nCoV Epidemic is Top Task Now, Says Deputy PM. Available online: news.chinhphu.vn/Home/Fighting-nCoV-epidemic-is-top-task-now-says-Deputy-PM/20202/38632.vgp (accessed on 22 March 2020).
35. Tuoi Tre News. Vietnam Seals off Commune of 10,600 to Control COVID-19. Available online: https://tuoitrenews.vn/news/society/20200213/vietnam-seals-off-commune-of-10600-to-control-covid19/52973.html (accessed on 22 March 2020).
36. VOV. Deputy PM Urges Control of Face Mask Numbers in Light of nCoV. Available online: https://english.vov.vn/society/deputy-pm-urges-control-of-face-mask-numbers-in-light-of-ncov-409494.vov (accessed on 23 March 2020).

37. Mai, N. 1,220 Drug Stores in Vietnam Fined for Making Use of nCoV. Available online: http://hanoitimes.vn/vietnam-authority-fines-1221-drug-stores-for-raising-prices-of-medical-equipment-300938.html (accessed on 22 March 2020).
38. Thuy, B. Bộ Y tế ra mắt hai kênh thông tin về dịch bệnh do nCoV. [Ministry of Health Introduces Two Information Channels about the nCoV Outbreak]. Available online: http://dangcongsan.vn/thoi-su/bo-y-te-ra-mat-hai-kenh-thong-tin-ve-dich-benh-do-ncov-548197.html (accessed on 19 March 2020).
39. Mai, H. Kích hoạt Việt Nam - Điểm đến an toàn. [Activate Vietnam—Safety destination]. Available online: https://thanhnien.vn/tai-chinh-kinh-doanh/kich-hoat-viet-nam-diem-den-an-toan-1185443.html (accessed on 16 March 2020).
40. Van, K. Bộ trưởng Phùng Xuân Nhạ gửi công văn "Hỏa tốc" đề nghị kéo dài thời gian nghỉ học đến hết tháng 02/2020. [Minister Phung Xuan Nha Sent an Official "Fire Speed" Documentary to Propose to Extend the Period of Absence from School to the End of February 2020]. Available online: http://toquoc.vn/bo-truong-phung-xuan-nha-gui-cong-van-hoa-toc-de-nghi-keo-dai-thoi-gian-nghi-hoc-den-het-thang-02-2020-20200214221816515.htm (accessed on 16 March 2020).
41. Nga, L. Vietnam Wins First Round of Coronavirus Fight: Deputy PM. Available online: https://e.vnexpress.net/news/news/vietnam-wins-first-round-of-coronavirus-fight-deputy-pm-4060132.html (accessed on 20 March 2020).
42. Paraguassu, L.; Mandl, C. Brazil Confirms First Coronavirus Case in Latin America. Available online: https://uk.reuters.com/article/uk-china-health-brazil/brazil-confirms-first-coronavirus-case-in-latin-america-source-idUKKCN20K1FL (accessed on 17 March 2020).
43. Burke, J.; Rourke, A. Nigeria Confirms First Coronavirus Case in Sub-Saharan Africa. Available online: https://www.theguardian.com/world/2020/feb/28/coronavirus-found-in-sub-saharan-africa-as-who-says-spread-could-get-out-of-control (accessed on 17 March 2020).
44. Minh, Q. PM Agrees to Declare COVID-19 Outbreak as Nationwide Pandemic. Available online: http://news.chinhphu.vn/Home/PM-agrees-to-declare-COVID19-outbreak-as-nationwide-pandemic/20203/39466.vgp (accessed on 1 April 2020).
45. Vietnamnet. Residents around Bach Mai Hospital's COVID-19 Cluster to be Given Quick Tests. Available online: https://vietnamnet.vn/en/society/residents-around-bach-mai-hospital-s-covid-19-cluster-to-be-given-quick-tests-629562.html (accessed on 1 April 2020).
46. Dung, T. Steering Committee Calls for Accelerating COVID-19 Responses as Situation Getting Worse Swiftly. Available online: http://news.chinhphu.vn/Home/Steering-Committee-calls-for-accelerating-COVID19-responses-as-situation-getting-worse-swiftly/20203/39262.vgp (accessed on 19 March 2020).
47. Minh, Q. BREAKING: VN Halts visa Issuance to Foreigners to Staunch COVID-19 Spread. Available online: http://news.chinhphu.vn/Home/BREAKING-VN-halts-visa-issuance-to-foreigners-to-staunch-COVID19-spread/20203/39226.vgp (accessed on 17 March 2020).
48. Minh, Q. BREAKING: VN to Halt Entry to All Foreigners Since March 22 due to COVID-19. Available online: http://news.chinhphu.vn/Home/BREAKING-VN-to-halt-entry-to-all-foreigners-since-March-22-due-to-COVID19/20203/39326.vgp (accessed on 19 March 2020).
49. Ha, M. Bộ GD&ĐT công bố chương trình đã tinh giản [MOET Announced a Streamlined Curriculum]. Available online: https://dantri.com.vn/giao-duc-khuyen-hoc/bo-gddt-cong-bo-chuong-trinh-da-tinh-gian-20200331170632835.htm (accessed on 4 April 2020).
50. Tuan, V. Vietnam to Cancel Religious Events in Coronavirus Counter Measure. Available online: https://e.vnexpress.net/news/news/vietnam-to-cancel-religious-events-in-coronavirus-counter-measure-4072652.html (accessed on 22 March 2020).
51. van, N. Gov't Bans Sports and Entertainment Activities until April 15. Available online: http://news.chinhphu.vn/Home/Govt-bans-sports-and-entertainment-activities-until-April-15/20203/39415.vgp (accessed on 1 April 2020).
52. An, N. Thực hiện cách ly toàn xã hội từ 0h ngày 1-4 [Social Distancing from 0h, April 1st]. Available online: https://tuoitre.vn/thuc-hien-cach-ly-toan-xa-hoi-tu-0h-ngay-1-4-20200331115839.htm (accessed on 1 April 2020).
53. Trang, P. Dừng toàn bộ vận tải hành khách đường bộ [Suspend all Road Passenger Transport]. Available online: http://baochinhphu.vn/Hoat-dong-Bo-nganh/Dung-toan-bo-van-tai-hanh-khach-duong-bo/391552.vgp (accessed on 1 April 2020).

54. Ministry of Health. Bộ Y tế phân tuyến điều trị bệnh nCoV. [Ministry of Health: Screening Patients for nCOV Treatment]. Available online: https://www.moh.gov.vn/web/guest/thong-tin-chi-dao-dieu-hanh/-/asset_publisher/DOHhlnDN87WZ/content/bo-y-te-phan-tuyen-ieu-tri-benh-ncov?inheritRedirect=false&redirect=https%3A%2F%2Fwww.moh.gov.vn%3A443%2Fweb%2Fguest%2Fthong-tin-chi-dao-dieu-hanh%3Fp_p_id%3D101_INSTANCE_DOHhlnDN87WZ%26p_p_lifecycle%3D0%26p_p_state%3Dnormal%26p_p_mode%3Dview%26p_p_col_id%3Drow-0-column-2%26p_p_col_count%3D1 (accessed on 4 April 2020).
55. Nguyen, Q.; Chau, M. Vietnam Province Isolates 10,600 People Amid Virus: Tuoi Tre. Available online: https://www.bloomberg.com/news/articles/2020-02-13/vietnam-province-isolates-10-600-people-amid-virus-tuoi-tre (accessed on 4 April 2020).
56. Vo, H. Hanoi Plans Two Field Hospitals in Case nCoV Infections Rise. Available online: https://e.vnexpress.net/news/news/hanoi-plans-two-field-hospitals-in-case-ncov-infections-rise-4050012.html (accessed on 4 April 2020).
57. Vu, H. Hà Nội: 2 bệnh nhân Covid-19 đến khám, 31 nhân viên y tế bị cách ly. [Hanoi: After two COVID-19 Patients Visits, 31 Health Care Workers Isolated]. Available online: https://thanhnien.vn/thoi-su/ha-noi-2-benh-nhan-covid-19-den-kham-31-nhan-vien-y-te-bi-cach-ly-1195553.html (accessed on 4 April 2020).
58. Minh, Q. Deputy PM Asks for Steering Resources to Control COVID-19 Cluster in Bach Mai Hospital. Available online: http://news.chinhphu.vn/Home/Deputy-PM-asks-for-steering-resources-to-control-COVID19-cluster-in-Bach-Mai-Hospital/20203/39440.vgp (accessed on 4 April 2020).
59. Boudreau, J.; Nguyen, X.Q. Hanoi's Largest Hospital Locked Down on Virus Outbreak Fears. Available online: https://www.bloomberg.com/news/articles/2020-03-28/hanoi-s-largest-hospital-locked-down-on-virus-outbreak-fears (accessed on 4 April 2020).
60. Ministry of Health. Bệnh viện Bạch Mai không thể dừng tiếp nhận, cứu người. [Bach Mai Hosppital Cannot Stop Receiving and Curing Patients]. Available online: https://moh.gov.vn/tin-tong-hop/-/asset_publisher/k206Q9qkZOqn/content/benh-vien-bach-mai-khong-the-dung-tiep-nhan-cuu-nguoi (accessed on 4 April 2020).
61. Ha, H. Gov't Chief Stimulates 'Warriors' in COVID-19 Combat. Available online: http://news.chinhphu.vn/Home/Govt-chief-stimulates-warriors-in-COVID19-combat/20203/39389.vgp (accessed on 4 April 2020).
62. The Saigon Times Daily. Hanoi Officials Take Quick Action following First Covid-19 Case in City. Available online: https://english.thesaigontimes.vn/75243/hanoi-officials-take-quick-action-following-first-covid-19-case-in-city.html (accessed on 22 March 2020).
63. VNA/VLLF. PM Orders Food Security 'under any Circumstance'. Available online: http://vietnamlawmagazine.vn/pm-orders-food-security-\T1\textquoteleftunder-any-circumstance-27088.html (accessed on 22 March 2020).
64. Viet Nam News. Ministry to Ensure Supply of Goods during COVID-19 Pandemic. Available online: https://vietnamnews.vn/economy/653882/ministry-to-ensure-supply-of-goods-during-covid-19-pandemic.html (accessed on 22 March 2020).
65. Loan, K. Banks Cut Interest Rates to Support Businesses Amidst COVID-19 Outbreak. Available online: news.chinhphu.vn/Home/Banks-cut-interest-rates-to-support-businesses-amidst-COVID19-outbreak/20203/39131.vgp (accessed on 22 March 2020).
66. Tuan, D. Thủ tướng: Hỗ trợ trực tiếp người nghèo, người lao động gặp khó khăn do COVID-19 [PM: Fully Support Poor People and Workers Who are Struggle during COVID-19]. Available online: http://baochinhphu.vn/Tin-noi-bat/Thu-tuong-Ho-tro-truc-tiep-nguoi-ngheo-nguoi-lao-dong-gap-kho-khan-do-COVID19/391536.vgp (accessed on 1 April 2020).
67. Vietnamnet. COVID-19: Compulsory e-Health Declaration for all Passengers Entering Vietnam. Available online: https://vietnamnet.vn/en/society/covid-19-compulsory-e-health-declaration-for-all-passengers-entering-vietnam-622401.html (accessed on 19 March 2020).
68. PV. Hà Nội: Kích hoạt hệ thống giám sát cộng đồng bằng GPS theo dõi dịch COVID-19. [Hanoi: Activate Community Monitoring System by GPS to track COVID-19 Outbreak]. Available online: https://vtv.vn/suc-khoe/ha-noi-kich-hoat-he-thong-giam-sat-cong-dong-bang-gps-theo-doi-dich-covid-19-20200320012959468.htm (accessed on 1 April 2020).
69. Dung, T. WHO Speaks Highly VN's Approach to COVID-19 Combat. Available online: http://news.chinhphu.vn/Home/WHO-speaks-highly-VNs-approach-to-COVID19-combat/20203/39182.vgp (accessed on 19 March 2020).

70. Research, D. Global Study about COVID-19: Dalia Assesses How the world Ranks Their Governments' Response to the Pandemic. Available online: https://daliaresearch.com/blog/dalia-assesses-how-the-world-ranks-their-governments-response-to-covid-19/ (accessed on 7 April 2020).
71. VNS. Vietnamese Confident in Government's Response to COVID-19: International Survey. Available online: https://vietnamnews.vn/society/654401/vietnamese-confident-in-governments-response-to-covid-19-international-survey.html (accessed on 1 April 2020).
72. Minh, H. Đề xuất phương án phòng dịch viêm phổi cấp từ Trung Quốc [Plans to Prevent a New Pneumonia from China]. Available online: http://baochinhphu.vn/Suc-khoe/De-xuat-phuong-an-phong-dich-viem-phoi-cap-tu-Trung-Quoc/384647.vgp (accessed on 17 March 2020).
73. PHOEC. Có 2 trường hợp mắc viêm phổi cấp ở Trung Quốc đã hồi phục hoàn toàn [2 Cases of Pneumina in China Fully Recovered]. Available online: https://suckhoedoisong.vn/da-co-2-truong-hop-bi-viem-phoi-cap-o-trung-quoc-hoi-phuc-hoan-toan-n167676.html (accessed on 17 March 2020).
74. Nguyen, B. Bùng phát dịch viêm phổi lạ ở Trung Quốc [Outbreak of a Strang Pneumonia in China]. Available online: https://www.qdnd.vn/thoi-su-quoc-te/doi-song-quoc-te/bung-phat-dich-viem-phoi-la-o-trung-quoc-606920 (accessed on 17 March 2020).
75. Long, P. Bệnh viêm phổi lạ Trung Quốc đã lây lan: Hong Kong phát hiện 16 trường hợp [Strange Pneumonia in China: Hong Kong Detected 16 New Case]. Available online: https://tuoitre.vn/benh-viem-phoi-la-trung-quoc-da-lay-lan-hong-kong-phat-hien-16-truong-hop-2020010714555464.htm (accessed on 17 March 2020).
76. Lan, M. Hơn 57% người dân Việt Nam sử dụng Facebook và sẽ tiếp tục gia tăng. [More than 57% of Vietnamese People Use Facebook and will Continue to Increase]. Available online: https://cafebiz.vn/hon-57-nguoi-dan-viet-nam-su-dung-facebook-va-se-tiep-tuc-gia-tang-20190624085831031.chn (accessed on 16 March 2020).
77. Anh, T. Zalo cán mốc 100 triệu người dùng [Zalo has 100 Million Users]. Available online: https://news.zing.vn/zalo-can-moc-100-trieu-nguoi-dung-post844537.html (accessed on 16 March 2020).
78. Cost, B. Coronavirus Spawns viral TikTok Dance about Washing Your Hands. Available online: https://nypost.com/2020/03/04/coronavirus-spawns-viral-tiktok-dance-about-washing-your-hands/ (accessed on 16 March 2020).
79. Vuong, M. Artists during the Quarantine/Lockdown be Like. Available online: https://www.youtube.com/watch?v=RMuXcrj2YpY&pbjreload=10 (accessed on 4 April 2020).
80. Ly, M. Châu Bùi: 'Đi cách ly, tưởng không may thành may không tưởng!'. [Chau Bui: 'Go Quarantined, Unfortunate Turned into Fortunate]. Available online: https://tuoitre.vn/chau-bui-di-cach-ly-tuong-khong-may-thanh-may-khong-tuong-20200311164253829.htm (accessed on 16 March 2020).
81. Tuoi Tre News. Vietnam Introduces Hefty Fines for Spreading Fake News. Available online: https://tuoitrenews.vn/news/society/20200205/vietnam-introduces-hefty-fines-for-spreading-fake-news/52863.html (accessed on 16 March 2020).
82. Le, P. Ca bệnh nCoV đầu tiên ở Việt Nam lên 'kinh thánh y khoa' thế giới. [The first case of nCoV in Vietnam on the World's "Medical Bible"]. Available online: https://vnexpress.net/dich-viem-phoi-corona/ca-benh-ncov-dau-tien-o-viet-nam-len-kinh-thanh-y-khoa-the-gioi-4047805.html (accessed on 19 March 2020).
83. Kupferschmidt, K. 'A Completely New Culture of Doing Research.' Coronavirus Outbreak Changes how Scientists Communicate. Available online: https://www.sciencemag.org/news/2020/02/completely-new-culture-doing-research-coronavirus-outbreak-changes-how-scientists (accessed on 16 March 2020).
84. Vuong, Q.-H. The rise of preprints and their value in social sciences and humanities. *Sci. Ed.* **2020**, *7*, 70–72. [CrossRef]
85. University, N.E. National Economic University Released Report "Assessment of COVID-19 Impacsts on the Economy and Policy Recommendations". Available online: https://neu.edu.vn/vi/ban-tin-neu/truong-dai-hoc-kinh-te-quoc-dan-cong-bo-bao-cao-danh-gia-tac-dong-cua-covid-19-den-nen-kinh-te-va-cac-khuyen-nghi-chinh-sach-2116 (accessed on 4 April 2020).
86. Vuong, Q.-H.; Napier, N.K.; Ho, T.M.; Nguyen, V.H.; Vuong, T.-T.; Pham, H.H.; Nguyen, H.K.T. Effects of work environment and collaboration on research productivity in Vietnamese social sciences: evidence from 2008 to 2017 scopus data. *Stud. High. Educ.* **2019**, *44*, 2132–2147. [CrossRef]
87. Cohen, J. Scientists 'Strongly Condemn' Rumors and Conspiracy Theories about Origin of Coronavirus Outbreak. Available online: https://www.sciencemag.org/news/2020/02/scientists-strongly-condemn-rumors-and-conspiracy-theories-about-origin-coronavirus (accessed on 16 March 2020).

88. Balloux, F. Available online: https://twitter.com/BallouxFrancois/status/1238837158007447558?s=19 (accessed on 7 April 2020).
89. Tran, B. Facebook Account "Bi Ti". Available online: https://www.facebook.com/biti84 (accessed on 19 March 2020).
90. VTV News. Information about Corona Virus and Respiratory Diseases—How to Prevent and Treat. Available online: https://vtv.vn/truc-tuyen/gltt-thong-tin-vhttps://vtv.vn/truc-tuyen/gltt-thong-tin-ve-virus-corona-cac-benh-ho-hap-cach-phong-ngua-va-dieu-tri-20h-31-1-20200130204149031.htme-virus-corona-cac-benh-ho-hap-cach-phong-ngua-va-dieu-tri-20h-31-1-20200130204149031.htm (accessed on 19 March 2020).
91. Le, T. 20 nước đặt mua kít phát hiện Covid-19 của Việt Nam. [20 Countries Order COVID-19 Testing Kit of Vietnam]. Available online: https://nhandan.com.vn/khoahoc-congnghe/item/43654002-20-nuoc-dat-mua-kit-phat-hien-covid-19-cua-viet-nam.html (accessed on 19 March 2020).
92. Vietnam Academy of Science and Technology. Introducing Research Results of Successfully Manufacturing the SARS-COV-2 Virus Diagnostic Kit of Institute of Biotechnology, VAST. Available online: http://www.vast.ac.vn/en/news/science-and-technology-news/1975-introducing-research-results-of-successfully-manufacturing-the-sars-cov-2-virus-diagnostic-kit-of-institute-of-biotechnology-vast (accessed on 4 April 2020).
93. Linh, T. Trường Phenikaa pha chế hơn 5.000 lít nước rửa tay tặng các trường học và cư dân. [Phenikaa University Dispenses more than 5,000 Liters of Hand-Washing Liquid to Schools and Residents]. Available online: https://giaoduc.net.vn/giao-duc-24h/truong-phenikaa-pha-che-hon-5000-lit-nuoc-rua-tay-tang-cac-truong-hoc-va-cu-dan-post207000.gd (accessed on 16 March 2020).
94. Mi, N. Họp khẩn cấp phòng chống bệnh viêm phổi 'lạ' ở Trung Quốc xâm nhập vào Việt Nam. [Emergency Meeting to Prevent 'Strange' Pneumonia in China from Entering Vietnam]. Available online: https://thanhnien.vn/suc-khoe/hop-khan-cap-phong-chong-benh-viem-phoi-la-o-trung-quoc-xam-nhap-vao-viet-nam-1170118.html (accessed on 16 March 2020).
95. Xuan, L. Hà Nội bắt đầu xét nghiệm nhanh COVID-19 ngoài cộng đồng, có kết quả trong 10 phút [Hanoi Begins Quick Testing COVID-19 in Public, Results Come in 10 Minutes]. Available online: https://tuoitre.vn/ha-noi-bat-dau-xet-nghiem-nhanh-covid-19-ngoai-cong-dong-co-ket-qua-trong-10-phut-20200330140703285.htm (accessed on 1 April 2020).
96. Ngoc, G. Người Hà Nội cách 2 mét xếp hàng dài, xét nghiệm nhanh Covid -19 trong 10 phút [Citizens of Hanoi Maintain 2m Distance during Line up, Quick Testing COVID-19 in 10 Minutes]. Available online: https://thanhnien.vn/doi-song/nguoi-ha-noi-cach-2-met-xep-hang-dai-xet-nghiem-nhanh-covid-19-trong-10-phut-1203965.html (accessed on 1 April 2020).
97. Beaubien, J. *How South Korea Reined In The Outbreak Without Shutting Everything down*; NPR: Washington, DC, USA, 26 March 2020.
98. Nam, N. Lượng khách quốc tế đến Việt Nam giảm bởi dịch bệnh do COVID-19 [International Tourists to Vietnam Slump due to COVID-19]. Available online: http://baochinhphu.vn/Du-lich/Luong-khach-quoc-te-den-Viet-Nam-giam-boi-dich-benh-do-COVID19/387330.vgp (accessed on 17 March 2020).
99. Xuan, T. Ngân hàng Nhà nước giảm đồng loạt lãi suất điều hành [State Bank of Vietnam Decreases Operating Rate]. Available online: https://thanhnien.vn/tai-chinh-kinh-doanh/ngan-hang-nha-nuoc-giam-dong-loat-lai-suat-dieu-hanh-1196825.html (accessed on 17 March 2020).
100. Vuong, Q.-H. Managers and Management in Vietnam: 25 Years of Economic Renovation (Doi Moi). *Pac. Aff.* **2014**, *87*, 378–380.
101. Vu, D.L.N.; Napier, N.K.; Vuong, Q.-H. Entrepreneurship and creativity in transition turmoil: the case of Vietnam. In Proceedings of the International Conference on Management, Leadership and Governance, Bangkok, Thailand, 7–8 February 2013; Vincent, R., Lugkana, W., Eds.; Academic Conferences and Publishing International Limited: Reading, UK; pp. 329–339.
102. Hang, T. Hàng hóa không thiếu, người Hà Nội vẫn ùn ùn mua hàng tích trữ [Despite Substantial Supply of Goods, People in Hanoi Still Queue to Buy Stocks]. Available online: https://thanhnien.vn/doi-song/hang-hoa-khong-thieu-nguoi-ha-noi-van-un-un-mua-hang-tich-tru-1192257.html (accessed on 18 March 2020).
103. Tuan, D. Thủ tướng Nguyễn Xuân Phúc: Việt Nam sẽ chặn đứng dịch bệnh [Prime Minister Nguyen Xuan Phuc: Vietnam is Going to Stop the Outbreak]. Available online: http://www.hanoimoi.com.vn/tin-tuc/Xa-hoi/960600/thu-tuong-nguyen-xuan-phuc-viet-nam-se-chan-dung-dich-benh (accessed on 18 March 2020).

104. Koziol, M. Revealed: The Sydney Suburbs Stocking up on Toilet Paper. Available online: https://www.smh.com.au/national/nsw/revealed-the-sydney-suburbs-stocking-up-on-toilet-paper-20200305-p547b1.html (accessed on 17 March 2020).
105. Telford, T.; Bhattarai, A. Long lines, low supplies: Coronavirus chaos sends shoppers into panic-buying mode. Available online: https://www.washingtonpost.com/business/2020/03/02/grocery-stores-coronavirus-panic-buying/ (accessed on 17 March 2020).
106. Son, V. Is Vietnam silently hiding COVID outbreak? Available online: https://dantri.com.vn/suc-khoe/viet-nam-co-am-tham-giau-dich-covid-hay-khong-20200225171439082.htm (accessed on 19 March 2020).
107. Huy, Q.; Hang, T. Ministry of Health: Vietnam is not Hiding about COVID-19 Outbreak. Available online: https://news.zing.vn/bo-y-te-viet-nam-khong-giau-thong-tin-ve-dich-covid-19-post1051408.html (accessed on 19 March 2020).
108. Nhu, V. PM Phuc Calls for Nation's Joint Efforts in COVID-19 Combat. Available online: http://news.chinhphu.vn/Home/PM-Phuc-calls-for-nations-joint-efforts-in-COVID19-combat/20203/39232.vgp (accessed on 19 March 2020).
109. eMagazine. COVID 19 Updated List of Enterprises that Contributed in the Outbreak Combat. Available online: https://enternews.vn/covid-19-cap-nhat-danh-sach-doanh-nghiep-chung-tay-phong-chong-dich-168911.html (accessed on 19 March 2020).
110. Linh, T.; Trang, T. Hanoi: Residential Buildings Cooperated in the Combat against Corona Virus. Available online: https://baotainguyenmoitruong.vn/ha-noi-cac-toa-nha-chung-cu-chung-tay-phong-chong-dich-do-virus-corona-298914.html (accessed on 19 March 2020).
111. Hanoimoi. Prevention and Treatment of COVID-19 in Apartment Buildings—Applying Multiple Measures. Available online: www.hanoimoi.com.vn/tin-tuc/Doi-song/958230/phong-chong-dich-benh-do-covid-19-tai-cac-chung-cu-tap-the-cu-trien-khai-nhieu-bien-phap (accessed on 19 March 2020).
112. Vuong, Q.-H.; Bui, Q.-K.; La, V.-P.; Vuong, T.-T.; Nguyen, V.-H.T.; Ho, M.-T.; Nguyen, H.-K.T.; Ho, M.-T. Cultural additivity: Behavioural insights from the interaction of Confucianism, Buddhism and Taoism in folktales. *Palgrave Commun.* **2018**, *4*, 143. [CrossRef]
113. World Health Organization. Responding to Community Spread of COVID-19 - Interim Guidance. Available online: https://www.who.int/docs/default-source/coronaviruse/20200307-responding-to-covid-19-communitytransmission-final.pdf (accessed on 17 March 2020).
114. Kruk, M.E.; Myers, M.; Varpilah, S.T.; Dahn, B.T. What is a resilient health system? Lessons from Ebola. *Lancet* **2015**, *385*, 1910–1912. [CrossRef]
115. Leach, M.; Scoones, I.; Stirling, A. Governing epidemics in an age of complexity: Narratives, politics and pathways to sustainability. *Glob. Environ. Chang.* **2010**, *20*, 369–377. [CrossRef]
116. Nguyen, Q. Swine Flu Claims Eighth Human Victim in Vietnam in 2018. Available online: https://e.vnexpress.net/news/news/swine-flu-claims-eighth-human-victim-in-vietnam-in-2018-3790527.html (accessed on 1 April 2020).
117. Ngoc, B. 20 countries, territories order Covid-19 test kits made in Vietnam. *VNExpress*. Available online: https://e.vnexpress.net/news/news/20-countries-territories-order-covid-19-test-kits-made-in-vietnam-4070785.html (accessed on 17 March 2020).

© 2020 by the authors. Licensee MDPI, Basel, Switzerland. This article is an open access article distributed under the terms and conditions of the Creative Commons Attribution (CC BY) license (http://creativecommons.org/licenses/by/4.0/).

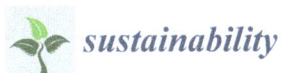

Article

A Scientometric Study on Depression among University Students in East Asia: Research and System Insufficiencies?

Minh-Hoang Nguyen [1,*], Manh-Tung Ho [1,2], Viet-Phuong La [1], Quynh-Yen Thi. Nguyen [3], Manh-Toan Ho [1], Thu-Trang Vuong [4], Tam-Tri Le [5], Manh-Cuong Nguyen [6] and Quan-Hoang Vuong [1,7,*]

1. Centre for Interdisciplinary Social Research, Phenikaa University, Yen Nghia Ward, Ha Dong District, Hanoi 100803, Vietnam; tung.homanh@phenikaa-uni.edu.vn (M.-T.H.); phuong.laviet@phenikaa-uni.edu.vn (V.-P.L.); toan.homanh@phenikaa-uni.edu.vn (M.-T.H.)
2. Institute of Philosophy, Vietnam Academy of Social Sciences, 59 Lang Ha Street, Ba Dinh District, Hanoi 100000, Vietnam
3. College of Asia Pacific Studies, Ritsumeikan Asia Pacific University, Beppu, Oita 874-8577, Japan; thiqng17@apu.ac.jp
4. Sciences Po Paris, 27 Rue Saint-Guillaume, 75007 Paris, France; thutrang.vuong@sciencespo.fr
5. International Cooperation Policy, Graduate School of Asia Pacific Studies, Ritsumeikan Asia Pacific University, Beppu, Oita 874-8577, Japan; letamtri10@gmail.com
6. Faculty of International Studies, Hanoi University, Km9, Nguyen Trai Road, Thanh Xuan, Hanoi 100803, Vietnam; manhcuongvhgd@gmail.com
7. Centre Emile Bernheim, Université Libre de Bruxelles, 1050 Brussels, Belgium
* Correspondence: hoang.nguyenminh@phenikaa-uni.edu.vn (M.-H.N.); qvuong@ulb.ac.be or hoang.vuongquan@phenikaa-uni.edu.vn (Q.-H.V.)

Received: 30 January 2020; Accepted: 15 February 2020; Published: 17 February 2020

Abstract: Given that mental health issues are acute in Asian countries, particularly Japan and Korea, and university students are more vulnerable to depression than the general population, this study aims to examine the landscapes of scientific research regarding depressive disorders among university students and evaluate the effectiveness of international collaboration and funding provision on the scientific impact in Korea, Japan, and China. Based on articles retrieved from the Web of Science database during the period 1992–2018, we found that the number of scientific publications, international collaborations, and allocated funds regarding depressive disorder among university students in China (97 articles, 43 international collaborations, and 52 funds provided, respectively) overwhelmingly surpassed the case of Korea (37 articles, 12 international collaborations, and 15 funds provided, respectively) and Japan (24 articles, 5 international collaborations, and 6 funds provided, respectively). The differences in collaboration patterns (p-value < 0.05) and the proportion of allocated funds (p-value < 0.05) among Korea, Japan, and China were also noted using Fisher's exact test. Based on the Poisson regression analysis, China's associations of scientific impact with international collaboration ($\beta = -0.322$, p-value < 0.01) and funding provision ($\beta = -0.397$, p-value < 0.01) are negative, while associations of the scientific impact and scientific quality with funding provision and international collaboration were statistically insignificant. These findings hint that Korea and Japan lacked scientific output, diversity in research targets, international collaboration, and funding provision, compared to China, but the quality of either China's internationally collaborated or funded articles was contentious. As a result, policymakers in Korea and Japan are suggested to raise the importance of mental health problems in their future policy planning and resource distribution. Moreover, it would be advisable to establish a rigorous system of evaluation for the quality of internationally collaborated and funded studies in order to increase scientific impact and maintain public trust, especially in China.

Keywords: depressive disorder; university student; scientific output; international collaboration; funding; Korea; Japan; China; scientific impact; scientific quality

1. Introduction

There are more than 1.8 billion young people between the ages of 10 and 24 today, which makes our current young generation the largest ever in history [1]. These are the people who will, in time, grow into the role of "the real owners of Agenda 2030 for Sustainable Development" [2]. Young people are expected to become critical thinkers and innovators, driving factors contributing to the resilience of the community and improving human living quality as well as the health of the planet. For them to be able to take on these future tasks as independent, self-sustaining adults, the youth needs not only education but also protection and support in various aspects of their development.

Healthcare is one such aspect, of which mental health care is becoming a more and more pressing issue. Since 2012, when the use of social media became common, the rate of depression among adolescents has risen significantly. It is also reported that the prevalence of the depressive disorder among university students is 30.6%, which is substantially higher than in the general population [3]. A depressive disorder is a common mental illness that currently affects an estimated more than 300 million people around the world. In 2008, WHO listed depressive disorder as the third cause of burden disease and projected that it would become the most substantial cause of burden disease in 2030. Not only is depressive disorder detected as a predictor for many chronic diseases and medical comorbidity [4,5], it is also a strong determinant of suicidal thoughts, self-harming behaviors, and death in many populations [6–8]. As a result, the demand to tackle depressive disorder among adolescents has been critical. With a vision towards improving global mental health and endorsing the sustainable development, in a recent Commission on Global Mental Health and Sustainable Development by *The Lancet* [9], protecting mental health by public policies, additional financial investment, and enhancing research and innovation have been listed as some of the major approaches [10].

An understanding of the state of current research (including scientific output, international collaboration, and funding allocation) regarding depressive disorder among university students is thus necessary to protect the young generation and contribute to the sustainable public health system. Still, few studies related to this issue have been done. Apart from a few bibliometric and scientometric studies on depressive disorder with biological treatments, comorbidity of pain, and artificial intelligence [10–12], no studies have specifically focused on depressive disorder among university students. The current scientometric study aims to fill this gap by examining the publication trends, patterns of collaboration, and funding situations of studies related to depressive disorder among university students in three Asian countries: South Korea, Japan, and China.

There are several reasons for the selection of these countries. Korea, Japan, and China were all among the top 10 countries for scientific research in 2018, according to *Nature Index* [13]. Nonetheless, South Korea and Japan are reported to obtain fewer citations and produce fewer publications than the world average in terms of mental health research [14]. Apart from low scientific production and impact, South Korea and Japan also had the highest and seventh-highest suicide rates among OECD countries in 2017 with 24.6 and 15.2 per 100,000 persons, respectively [15]. Recent news in Japan reported that Japanese people in their 20s accounted for the second-largest share of people seeking advice through the governmental consultation service designed to tackle suicides by young people [16]. Suicide is also the leading cause of death among adolescents in Korea [17]. The deficiencies in scientific works and severity of suicide rates underline the urgent need for a scientometric study regarding depressive disorder among university students in South Korea and Japan. China, with a comparatively lower suicide rate of 9.7 per 100,000 persons in 2016 [18], is selected in this study for comparison purposes, as China, South Korea, and Japan are in the same East Asian cultural sphere.

Given that international collaboration and funding provision are fundamental components of scientific development, besides understanding the current landscapes of the scientific research, identifying the insufficiencies in funding and international collaboration systems might greatly contribute to the advancement of scientific research regarding depression among university students (the primary contributor to the future sustainable development). As a result, the specific research questions in this study are:

- What are the landscapes of scientific research regarding depressive disorder among university students in Japan, Korea, and China?
- What insufficiencies are there in funding and international collaboration systems regarding depressive disorder among university students in Japan, Korea, and China?
- What recommendations can be made for future policy planning to promote scientific development regarding depressive disorder among university students in Japan, Korea, and China?

In the next section, the materials and methods of this study will be thoroughly explained. In the third section, results regarding publication trends, collaborative patterns, funding, and scientific impact will be presented. The results of this studied will eventually be discussed and concluded at the end.

2. Materials and Methods

This study generally follows the structure prescribed by the Preferred Reporting Items for Systematic Review and Meta-Analysis (PRISMA) guidelines. Nonetheless, due to its scientometric nature, several sections in the PRISMA checklist are not suitable for inclusion. The excluded sections are numbers 5, 12–16, and 19–23 in the checklist, which can be addressed in future studies.

2.1. Inclusion and Exclusion Criteria

The current study examined the landscape of research regarding depression among university/college students in Japan, Korea, and China, employing the data downloaded from the Web of Science (WoS) database of Clarivate. Therefore, the inclusion criteria include: (1) Studies conducted in the targeted country (Japan, Korea, and China), (2) studies related to depressive disorder, and (3) studies with university/college students as participants. The exclusion criteria were: (1) Studies that are not research articles, (2) studies after 2018, (3) meta-analysis studies. The meta-analysis study is not directly involved in the data collection from respondents, which is different from the nature of other research articles, such as experimental and observational studies, so we decided not to include a meta-analysis in this study.

2.2. Search Strategy

Articles for this study were retrieved from WOS on 6 August 2019. The WoS database is the most commonly used database by governmental agencies to assess the scientific performance and quality of a nation [19]. The search was restricted to peer-reviewed papers written in English in the Web of Science Core Collection. In other bibliometrics and scientometrics studies regarding depression [10–12], the term "depression" is most commonly selected as a keyword to identify studies related to depression. Given that depression is also called depressive disorder and mood disorder [20], we selected "depression", "depressive disorder", and "mood disorder" as our keywords in this study. In order to target studies on the university/college student population, the term "college student" and "university student" were used. Moreover, as the international student population in university is gaining attention from researchers [21–26], we also include the keyword "international student" in our search queries. The following search queries were employed to search for articles related to depressive disorders among university/college students in three Asian countries: Korea, Japan, and China.

TS = (depression OR depressive disorder OR mood disorder) AND TS = (college student OR university student OR international student) AND TS = Korea
TS = (depression OR depressive disorder OR mood disorder) AND TS = (college student OR university student OR international student) AND TS = Japan
TS = (depression OR depressive disorder OR mood disorder) AND TS = (college student OR university student OR international student) AND TS = China

2.3. Data Extraction

The extraction and curation of data consist of four steps. First, the data were downloaded from the WOS database in .txt format. The data included all bibliographical information on the articles resulting from the search queries, such as authors, titles, keywords, affiliation, citation, abstract, etc. Second, the data files were curated and converted to the xlsx format using the Bibliometrix package in R [27]. Third, two authors independently screened the title and abstract of all papers to select articles that met inclusion criteria and exclude irrelevant research articles. The results were then cross-checked by two authors, and disagreement was resolved through discussion. Discussions also involved a third author where necessary. Finally, data regarding scientific collaboration patterns and funding sources were extracted by an author, and a second author verified the extracted data.

2.4. Category Classification

To comprehensively understand the current collaboration and funding trends in three studying countries, we classified the collaboration pattern and funding source of each article into several categories based on information displayed in the article.

2.4.1. Scientific Collaboration Patterns

Based on the affiliation section of an article, we classified collaboration types into five main categories:

- Domestic solo paper (**DS**): A paper written by one domestic author
- Foreign solo paper (**FS**): A paper written by one foreign paper
- Domestic collaborative paper (**DC**): Paper co-written by domestic authors
- Foreign collaborative paper (**FC**): Paper co-written by foreign authors
- International collaborative paper (**IC**): Paper co-written by domestic and foreign authors

2.4.2. Funding Sources

Based on the acknowledgment and funding sections of an article, we classified funding sources into eight main categories:

- Central government (**CG**): Fund provided by the ministry, central-governmental organizations, foundations, departments, or agencies.
- Local government (**LG**): Fund provided by municipal or provincial organizations, foundations, departments, or agencies.
- Academic institution (**AI**): Fund provided by the university, college, or educational institutes.
- Business (**B**): Fund provided by private sectors, such as enterprises, corporations, etc.
- Non-profit organization (**NPO**): Fund provided by non-profit organizations, foundations, or societies.
- Others (**O**): Fund provided by other types of organizations.
- Foreign government (**FO-G**): Fund provided by the foreign ministry, central-governmental organizations, foundations, departments, or agencies
- Foreign non-governmental organization (**FO-NGO**): Fund provided by non-governmental organizations, foundations, departments, or agencies.

2.5. Statistical Analysis and Procedure

The statistical analysis in this study consists of three tools: Fisher's exact test, Kruskal–Wallis test, and Poisson regression analysis. The Fisher's Exact test was employed to identify the statistically significant difference in the collaboration patterns and funding provision among Korea, Japan, and China, as it is more appropriate for the data type (nominal) and the modest size of the dataset than chi-squared test [28,29]. The Kruskal–Wallis test was utilized to examine the difference in ordinal data among two or more levels in a group [29]. To estimate the associations of scientific impact measured by the number of total citations with international collaboration, funding provision, and the number of co-authors, we utilized the Poisson regression analysis. Poisson regression was developed to cope with count data-dependent variables and non-parametric models [30,31]. The method is thus suitable for the current study since the number of total citations can be considered as count data, and the distributions of the number of total citations among Korea, Japan, and China are skewed.

In this study, two models were examined. Model (1) is estimated without control variable *"Year"*, while model (2) is estimated with control variable *"Year"* to diminish the effect of publication time bias on the total number of citations.

$$\log(ToCitation) = \alpha + \beta_1 InterCollab + \beta_2 Funding + \beta_3 Author + e \quad (1)$$

$$\log(ToCitation) = \alpha + \beta_1 InterCollab + \beta_2 Funding + \beta_3 Author + \beta_4 Year + e \quad (2)$$

where,
- *ToCitation* is the dependent variable,
- α is the intercept,
- β_1-β_4 are coefficients,
- *InterCollab*, *Funding*, and *Author* independent variables. Description of dependent and independent variables are explained in Table 1,
- *e* is the error term.

Table 1. Description of dependent and independent variables.

Variable Type	Variable Name	Data Type	Description
Dependent variable	ToCitaion	Ordinal data	The number of times that an article is cited by other papers
	JIF.Lev	Ordinal data	The impact factor level of the journal in which the article was published
Independent variable	InterCollab	Binomial data (1 – yes vs. 0 – No)	Whether the article represents an international collaboration or not
	Funding	Binomial data (1 – yes vs. 0 – No)	Whether the article is funded or not
	Author	Continuous data	The number of co-author in the article
Control variable	Year	Continuous data	The year in which the article was published

Models (1) and (2) were also applied for the regression against the dependent variable *"JIF.Lev"*. Improving scientific impact and research quality are among the main purposes of funding provision and international collaboration promotion. Thus, through examining the association of *"ToCitation"* and *"JIF.Lev"* dependent variables with *"InterCollab"* and *"Funding"* independent variables, the effectiveness of funding provision, and international collaboration in raising scientific impact and scientific quality can be evaluated.

After curating the data using the Bibliometrix R package, the data were downloaded as .xlsx format and then converted to .csv format. The .csv data file was later imported to R software for

Fisher's exact test and Poisson analysis performing Generalized Linear Models (GLMs). Even though there were articles published before 2008 in Korea, Japan, and China, only the data during 2008-2018 were employed in the statistical analysis, because the publication during this period is more robust and influenced more by the policies than the prior period. The R software version 3.6.2, 'Dark and Stormy Night' was used throughout the analysis. We chose $p < 0.05$ as a required statistical significance.

3. Results

3.1. Description of Studies

After retrieving data from the Web of Science Core Collection, 225 studies in China, 87 studies in Korea, and 66 studies in Japan before 2019 were identified. Utilizing the Bibliometrix R package, 15 studies in China, six studies in Korea, and 1 study in Japan that are not research articles were excluded. After that, the remaining articles' titles and abstracts were screened independently by two authors. One hundred twenty-eight studies in China, 44 studies in Korea, and 41 studies in Japan were excluded because they were not related to depression, not about college/university students, and not conducted in the selected country. Eventually, 97 articles in China, 37 articles in Korea, and 24 articles in Japan were eligible for inclusion in the Scientometrics study (see Figure 1).

3.2. Scientific Performance Overview

3.2.1. Publication Growth Trend

The total number of publications from 1992 to 2018 is presented in Figure 2. During the period between 1992 and 2007, the problem regarding depressive disorder among university was not seriously paid attention in China, Korea, and Japan. Even though the problem was studied very early in Korea at the beginning of the 1990s [32], the next study was only conducted after almost a decade [33]. China and Japan started to pay attention to depressive disorders among university students relatively later than Korea in 1999 and 1998, respectively.

Unlike Korea and China, in which the first study was performed by researchers from the USA [32,34], two first studies in Japan were conducted completely by domestic researchers [35,36]. The proportion of articles in China, Korea, and Japan before 2008 only accounted for 7% (8/115), 13% (5/40), and 14% (4/28) of the total publications produced, respectively.

From 2008 to 2018, China, Korea, and Japan experienced significant growth in the number of publications. The percentage of publications produced during this time accounted for 77% (77/115), 80% (32/40), and 71% (20/28) in China, Korea, and Japan, respectively. Notably, the total publications of China were double the summation of total publications in both Japan and Korea. By raising its number of publications by ten folds in the last ten years, China obtained the clearest surge in terms of publication quantity. Compared to China, despite the increase in the total number of publications, the publication growth rates of Korea and Japan have been relatively fluctuating over time.

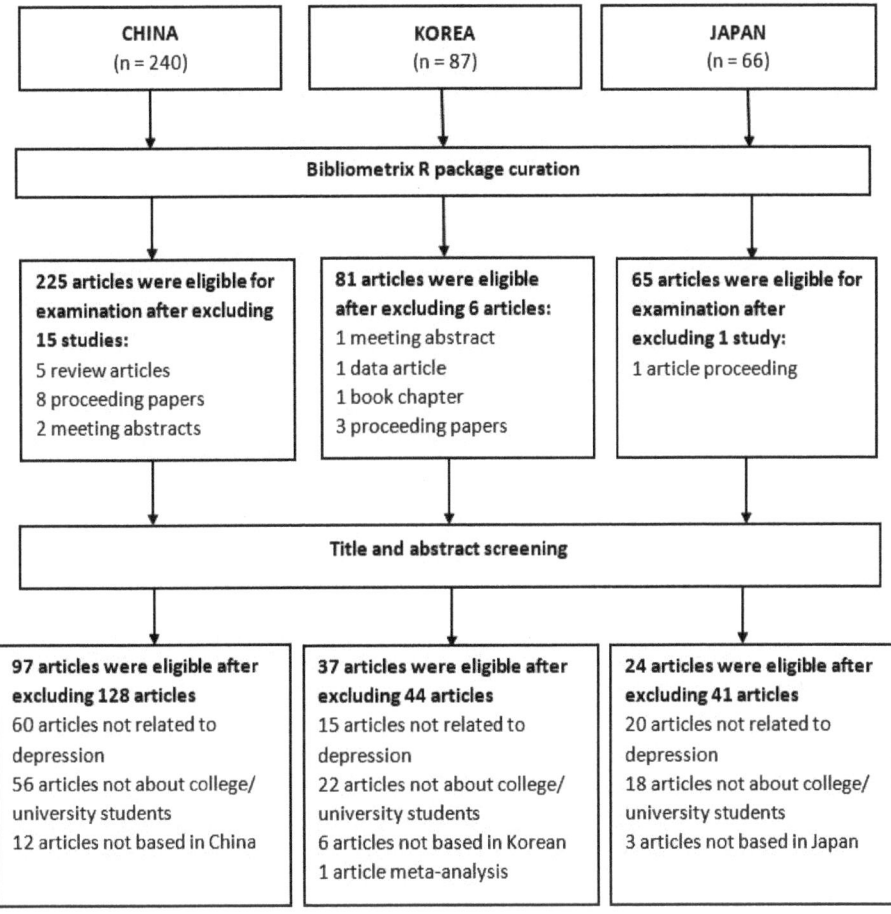

Figure 1. The flow chart for excluding ineligible articles.

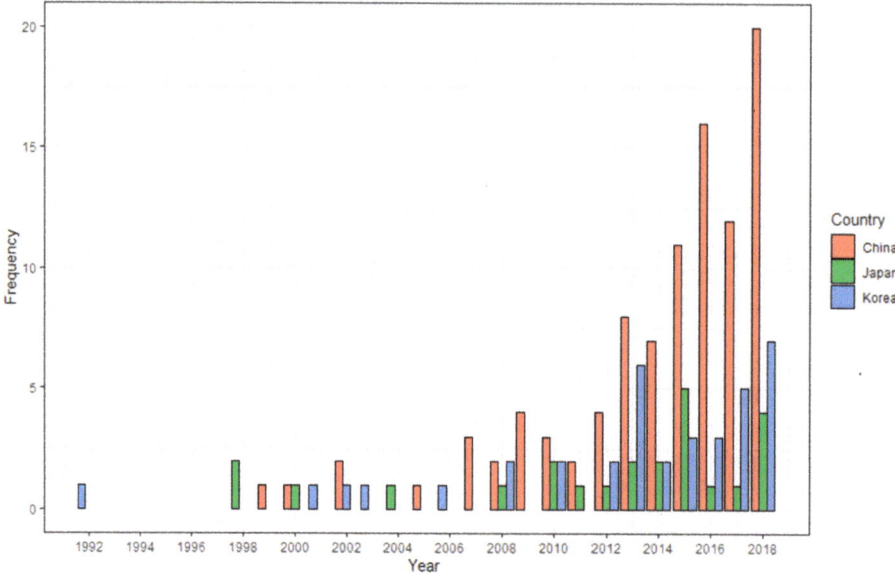

Figure 2. The number of publications from 1992 to 2018.

3.2.2. Research Targets

Figure 3 displays the types of universities, target groups, and sub-group that were studied in China, Korea, and Japan. Common universities were places in which studies regarding depressive disorder among students were most frequently implemented in China (80%), Korea (84%), and Japan (96%). Among the three countries, China had the most diverse research locations. Studies implemented in technical or medical universities in China accounted for 20% of all publications. In contrast, studies in Japan merely focused on students in common universities. Only one study was conducted in medical universities [37].

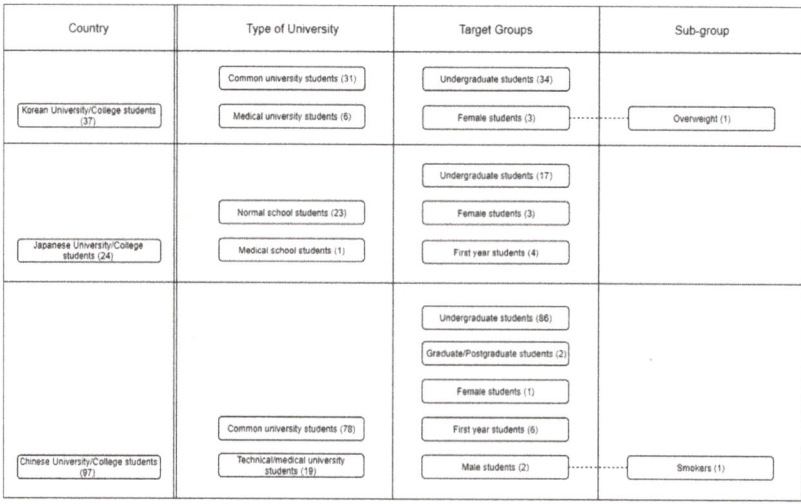

Figure 3. Types of university and target groups.

For the variety of target groups, China was also outstanding compared to its counterparts with five target groups and a sub-group, which was male smokers [38]. The target groups of studies in Japan were more diverse than those in Korea with three different target groups. Although there were only two target groups that were studied in Korea, researchers delved into the character of female students [39].

3.3. Scientific Collaboration Patterns

Until 2018, China obtained the highest percentage of internationally collaborated publications with 44% of its total publications about depressive disorder among university students, while Korea and Japan came after with 32% and 21%, respectively (see Figure 4). Collaboration among domestic researchers was still the most dominant pattern in Japan (50%), Korea (49%), and China (47%). Different from China, in which other types of collaborations besides domestic and international collaborations were limited, Japan acquired a relatively high percentage of papers published solo by a domestic researcher (17%) and a group of purely foreign researchers (13%).

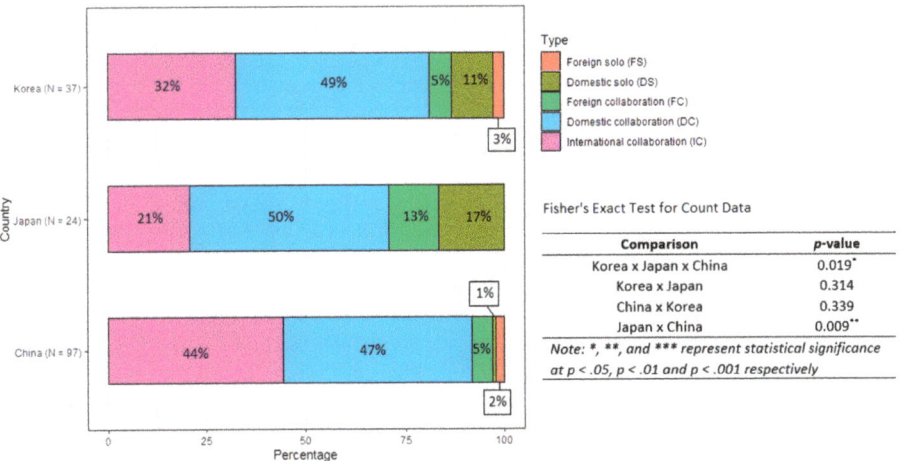

Figure 4. The proportion of collaboration types.

The Fisher exact's test was employed to examine the difference in the proportion of collaboration types among Korea, Japan, and China. The collaboration proportion among Korea, Japan, and China is statistically significantly different at $p < 0.05$. The differences in collaboration type proportion of China–Korea and Korea–Japan were found to be statistically insignificant, while the difference between China and Japan was found to be statistically significant at $p < 0.01$

Figure 5 displays the number of international collaborations in China, Korea, and Japan from 2000 to 2018. As presented, Japan and China were the first countries obtaining papers coauthored internationally in researching depressive disorder among university students. The first article in Korea appeared three years later in 2003. China experienced a substantial hike in the number of international collaborations, and the number peaked in 2016 and 2018 with nine international collaborations. On the contrary, Japan was comparatively not keen on coauthoring internationally, with only five times collaborating with foreign researchers. The number of international collaborations in Korea was rare before 2013, but it became more regular during 2013 and 2017. In 2018, the number of internationally collaborated articles surged with four papers published.

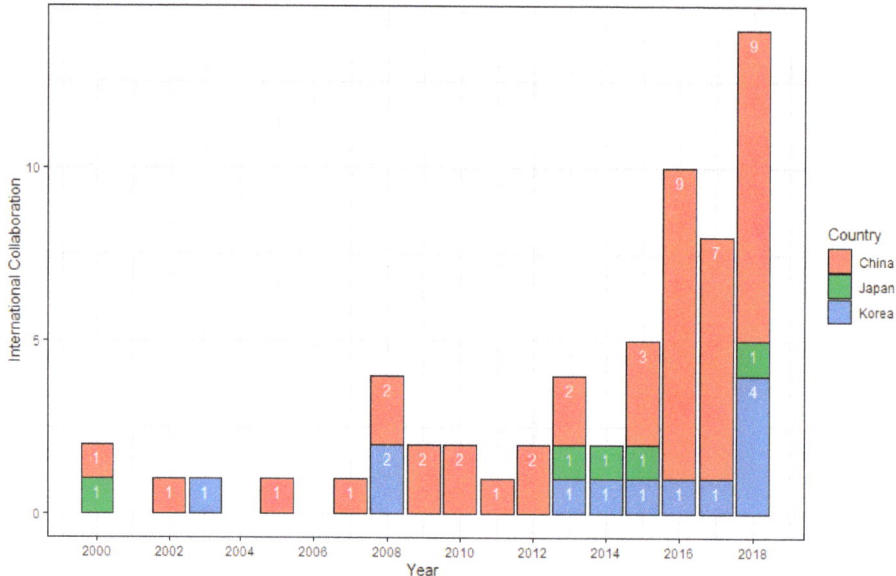

Figure 5. The number of internationally collaborated articles from 2006 to 2018.

The USA was the most frequently collaborated partner of China, Korea, and Japan. In three countries, Korea was the most frequent country to collaborate with the USA with 75% (9/12) of total international collaborations. China and Japan's collaborations with the USA accounted for roughly 63% (27/43) and 60% (3/5) of total internationally collaborated papers. In terms of the variety of partners, China had a broader collaborating network across Asia and Europe than Korea and Japan (see Table A1).

3.4. Funding situation

Research funding in China was relatively more generous and consistent than its counterparts. China had the first funded project in 2007 [40], while Japan and Korea had their first funded projects one year later [34] (see Figure 6). It is noteworthy that the study of Saint Arnault and Kim [41] was the first funded study in Korea and Japan concurrently, and their funding was provided by a foreign government. During the 2007-2018 period, the number of funded projects in China grew significantly and peaked in 2018 at 16 publications. In contrast, after the first funded project in 2008, only five studies in Japan regarding depressive disorder among university students were funded. For Korea, even though funding for research started simultaneously with Japan, the funding was given more frequently than Japan. Only in three years (2009, 2011, and 2014), no funding was granted.

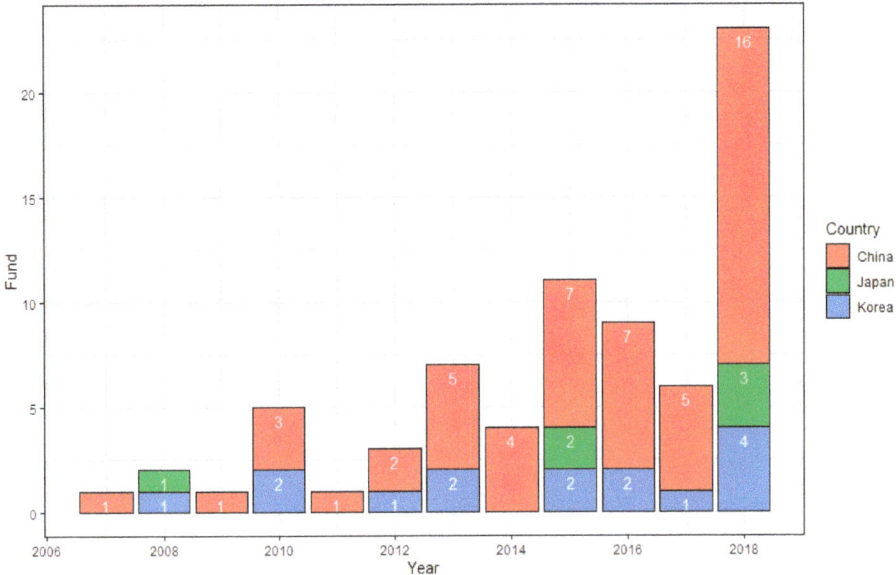

Figure 6. The number of funded projects from 2006 to 2018.

In China, most of the funding was given by the central government (32%) and local government (28%). The third-largest funding contributor was academic institutes with 26% (see Figure 7). The local and central governments played important roles in funding provision in China, but in Japan and Korea, only the central government's funds were provided. In Korea, academic institutes (44%) contributed more substantially than governmental agencies (37%) in funding provided to studies related to depressive disorder among university students, 11% of total mentions of funding sources derived from non-profit organizations. In Japan, a major funding source was still governmental organizations (34%), but the role of academic institutes was less significant than the other two counterparts (8%). Studies related to depressive disorder among university students in Japan was considerably dependent on funding from social sources (33%) and foreign sources (25%). It is noted that a study can receive funding from two or more sources, so the share of governmental sources in Japan was fairly low, although the central government had funded four out of six studies in Japan.

Table 2 shows the Fisher's exact test result regarding the difference in the percentage of funds provided and the percentage of government funds provided among Korea, Japan, and China. The results suggest a statistically significant difference between the proportion of funds provided in China and Japan. Interestingly, even though the proportion of funds provided is not different between China and Korea, their proportion of government funds provided is statistically significantly different. In general, the funding proportion and government funding proportion among Korea, Japan, and China were statistically significantly different.

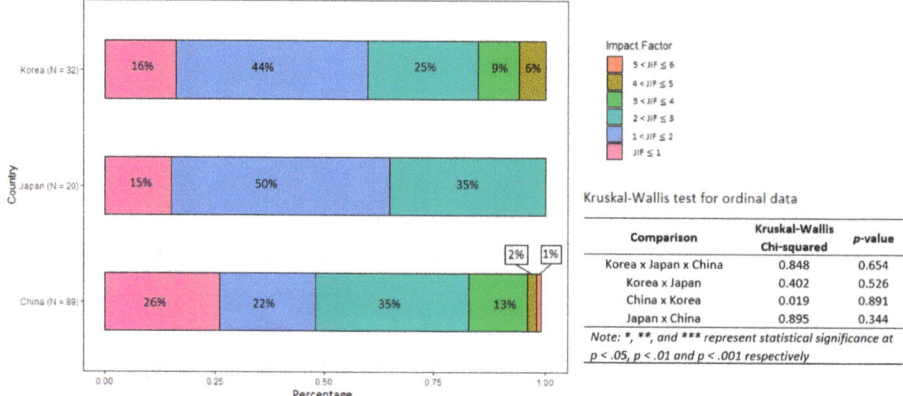

Figure 7. The proportions of studies according to Journal Impact Factor (JIF) levels among Korea, Japan, and China.

Table 2. Fisher's exact test on funding provision.

Comparison	*p*-Value (Funding Provision)	*p*-Value (Government Funding Provision)
Korea × Japan × China	0.031 *	0.011 *
Korea × Japan	0.260	1
China × Korea	0.408	0.018 *
Japan × China	0.045 *	0.076

Note: *, **, and *** represent statistical significance at $p < 0.05$, $p < 0.01$ and $p < 0.001$ respectively. Funding Provision: Receiving fund >< not receiving fund Government Funding Provision: Receiving fund from the government >< not receiving fund from the government.

3.5. Scientific Impact—Number of Citations

To avoid bias from the year of publication that (1) older publications tend to have a higher number of citations and (2) the Journal Impact Factor since the publication time might have changed significantly until 2018, only articles within the last ten years, between 2008 and 2018, were included in this section.

3.5.1. A Brief Overview

Articles related to depressive disorder among university students in China, Korea, and Japan received a relatively small number of citations. From 2008 to 2018, there were merely two articles acquiring citations equal to or greater than 50 in Korea and China, whereas Japan obtained no article (see Table 3). In China, the highest number of times an article was cited was 125 [42], which was double the highest citation an article received in Korea with 63 citations [43] and six times higher than Japan's with 24 citations [44]. Nevertheless, the relative citation indexes of funded and internationally collaborated articles in China were lowest with 0.72 and 0.82, respectively. In the case of Japan, the relative citation index of internationally collaborated papers highlighted the impact of studies with an international corporation. Still, funded articles were less impactful than non-funded articles. The impact of internationally collaborated or funded articles was generally similar to articles without international corporations or funding.

Table 3. Citation during the period 2008–2018.

	Korea	Japan	China
The highest number of citations	63	24	125
Number of highly cited articles (>=50)	2	0	2
Average citation—International collaboration	12.45	9	9.23
Average citation—No international collaboration	12.15	6.81	11.3
Relative citation index [1]	**1.03**	**1.32**	**0.82**
Average citation—Funding	11.93	6.67	9.12
Average citation—No funding	12.56	7.5	12.61
Relative citation index [2]	**0.95**	**0.89**	**0.72**

Relative citation index [1] is defined as the ratio of the average citation of papers that had international collaborations over that of paper having no international collaboration. Relative citation index [2] is defined as the ratio of the average citation of papers that received funding over that of paper having no funding.

The average citations of studies in Korea were relatively higher than those in China and Japan across categories. In contrast, despite a greater relative citation index than China and even Korea in terms of international collaboration, Japan had the lowest average number of citations in all categories.

3.5.2. Journal Impact Factor

We utilized the Journal Impact Factor (JIF) for measuring the quality of scientific research. To identify the JIF of the journal in which a study was published, we referred to the Journal Citation Report (JCR) in 2017, which was used to qualify journals in the WoS database during the time that the data in the current study were retrieved.

Figure 8 illustrates the percentage of studies published in journals with different JIF levels and the results of the Kruskal–Wallis test among Korea, Japan, and China. In Japan, half of the articles were published in journals with $1 < JIF \leq 2$, and there was no article published in a journal with JIF > 3. Korea obtained 40% of articles published in journals with JIF > 2. 51% of studies published in journals with JIF > 2 made China significantly surpass the other two countries in terms of scientific quality. However, it is notable that China also accounted for a larger percentage of studies published in journals with JIF ≤ 1 than the other two countries. Despite some differences between Korea, Japan, and China, the Kruskal–Wallis test produced statistically insignificant results in all cases: Korea vs. Japan vs. China, China vs. Japan, Japan vs. Korea, and Korea vs. China.

Funded studies in Japan presented the most transparent improvement in scientific quality. No funded studies were published in journals with JIF ≤ 1 (see Table 4). The difference between funded and non-funded studies was also confirmed by a Kruskal–Wallis test (chi-sqr = 3.963 and $p < 0.05$). Korea's funded studies seemed to be published in higher impact factor journals than non-funded studies, 26% of funded studies were published in journals with JIF > 3, while that percentage of non-funded studies was only 6%. Nonetheless, the results provided by Kruskal–Wallis was not statistically significant. As for China, the difference in scientific quality between funded and non-funded articles was ambiguous and statistically insignificant. As for the international collaboration, none of the three countries expressed a clear and statistically significant difference, which hints at the ineffectiveness of the current international collaboration practices of three countries in raising scientific quality (see Table 5).

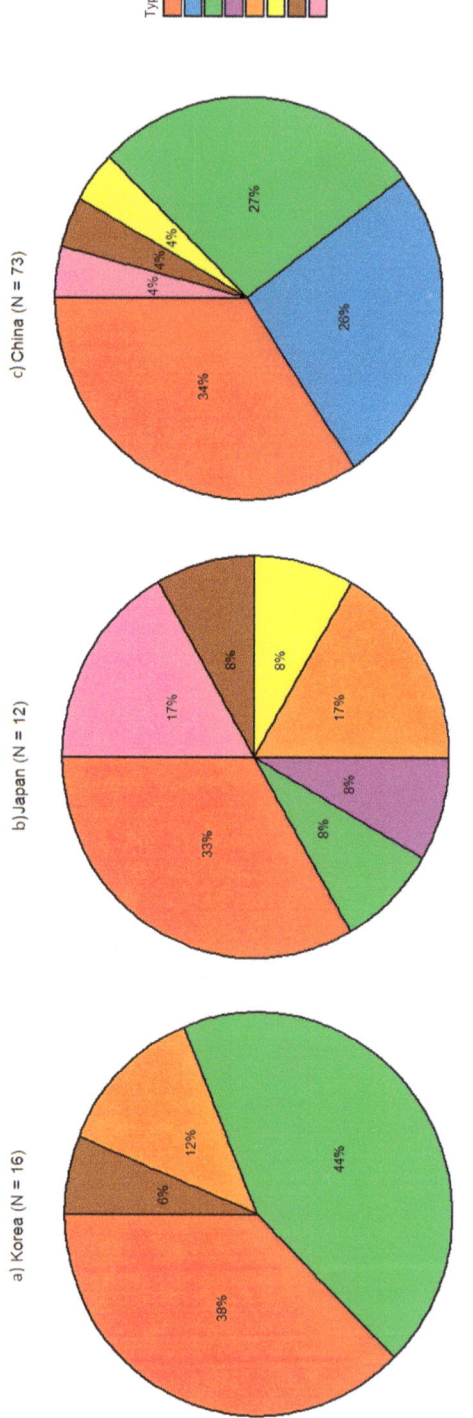

Figure 8. The proportions of funding sources based on the total mentioned sources in (**a**) Korea, (**b**) Japan, and (**c**) China.

Table 4. Percentage of JIF levels by funding provision.

	Korea		Japan		China	
	Yes (N = 15)	No (N = 17)	Yes (N = 6)	No (N = 9)	Yes (N = 51)	No (N = 38)
JIF ≤ 1	20%	12%	0%	33%	25%	26%
1 < JIF ≤ 2	27%	59%	33%	33%	20%	26%
2 < JIF ≤ 3	27%	24%	67%	33%	37%	32%
3 < JIF ≤ 4	13%	6%	0%	0%	14%	13%
4 < JIF ≤ 5	13%	0%	0%	0%	2%	3%
5 < JIF ≤ 6	0%	0%	0%	0%	2%	0%
Kruskal–Wallis Chi-squared	1.117		3.963		0.241	
p-value	0.291		0.047		0.623	

Table 5. Percentage of JIF levels by international collaboration.

	Korea		Japan		China	
	Yes (N = 11)	No (N = 21)	Yes (N = 4)	No (N = 16)	Yes (N = 39)	No (N = 50)
JIF ≤ 1	9%	19%	0%	19%	23%	28%
1 < JIF ≤ 2	55%	38%	75%	44%	28%	18%
2 < JIF ≤ 3	27%	24%	25%	38%	23%	44%
3 < JIF ≤ 4	9%	10%	0%	0%	18%	10%
4 < JIF ≤ 5	0%	10%	0%	0%	5%	0%
5 < JIF ≤ 6	0%	0%	0%	0%	3%	0%
Kruskal–Wallis Chi-squared	0.028		0.003		0.472	
p-value	0.867		0.959		0.492	

3.6. Poisson Regression Analysis

To assess the effectiveness of international collaboration, funding provision, and the number of co-authors on raising the scientific impact of the research articles during 2008-2018, we regressed three independent variables "*InterCollab*", "*Funding*", and "*Author*" against the dependent variable "*ToCitation*" without control variable "*Year*" (model 1) and with control variable "*Year*" (model 2). Before conducting the regression analysis, we also employed the correlation analysis and found that there was no multicollinearity among independent variables (see Tables A2–A4). The regressed results are shown in Table 6. In Korea, the association between "*InterCollab*" and "*ToCitation*" is not statistically significant, while "*ToCitation*" is statistically positively associated with "*Author*" and statistically negatively associated with "*Funding*". These results hint at the ineffectiveness, or even worse, of international collaboration and funding provision in raising the scientific impact measured by the total citation.

In Japan, the first model suggests the negative associations of "*ToCitation*" with "*InterCollab*" and "*Funding*", even though the associations are not statistically significant. Nonetheless, when "*Year*" is controlled, the associations become positive, although they are still not statistically significant. One point worth mentioning here is the positive impact of the number of co-authors on the scientific impact of the article. Both estimations from the two models show "*InterCollab*" and "*Funding*" are not effective in increasing scientific citations, but "*Author*" is.

Table 6. Poisson regression estimates with "ToCitation" as dependent variable.

Dependent variable "ToCitation"	Korea				Japan				China			
	Model (1)		Model (2)		Model (1)		Model (2)		Model (1)		Model (2)	
	β	z value	β	z value	β	z value	β	z value	β	z value	β	z value
"InterCollab"	0.079	0.743	−0.001	−0.017	−0.003	−0.015	0.273	1.158	−0.322	−4.720***	−0.516	−7.408***
"Funding"	−0.045	−0.424	−0.203	−1.843	−0.230	−1.182	0.016	0.089	−0.397	−5.970***	−0.004	−0.070
"Author"	0.038	2.096*	0.060	3.422***	0.094	2.150*	0.122	2.723**	0.053	4.794***	0.023	1.661
"Year"			−0.173	−10.399***			−0.209	−6.877***			−0.291	−25.564***
Constant	2.307	21.888***	352.281	10.470***	1.599	7.883***	422.706	6.907***	2.399	30.989***	588.688	25.678***
AIC	730.5		623.4		179.5		133.0		1820.7		1127.7	

Note: *, **, *** represents statistically significance at $p < 0.05$, $p < 0.01$ and $p < 0.001$ respectively; Model (1): Year the article was published is not controlled; Model (2): Year the article was not published is controlled.

Table 7. Poisson regression estimates with "JIF.Lev" as the dependent variable.

Dependent variable "JIF.Lev"	Korea				Japan				China			
	Model (1)		Model (2)		Model (1)		Model (2)		Model (1)		Model (2)	
	β	z value	β	z value	β	z value	β	z value	β	z value	β	z value
"InterCollab"	−0.052	−0.219	−0.004	−0.180	0.017	0.041	0.025	0.057	0.088	0.646	0.086	0.637
"Funding"	0.142	0.609	0.124	0.525	0.276	0.837	0.299	0.893	0.031	0.226	0.045	0.329
"Author"	0.037	0.975	0.040	1.039	0.010	0.131	0.013	0.171	0.041	1.774	0.039	1.668
"Year"			−0.028	−0.751			−0.017	−0.321			−0.018	−0.765
Constant	0.690	2.979**	58.034	0.447	0.647	1.881*	34.987	0.327	0.611	3.483***	37.889	0.777
AIC	107.74		109.18		64.712		66.61		293.4		294.83	

Note: *, **, *** represents statistically significance at $p < 0.05$, $p < 0.01$ and $p < 0.001$ respectively. Model (1): Year the article was published is not controlled. Model (2): Year the article was not published is controlled.

The effectiveness of *"InterCollab"* and *"Funding"* in China is not an improvement compared to the other two countries, rather even worse. The first model indicates statistically significant negative associations of *"ToCitation"* with *"InterCollab"* and *"Funding"* at $p < 0.01$. Even though in the second model, the association between *"ToCitation"* and *"Funding"* turns to be statistically insignificant, the coefficient is still negative. Similar to the other two countries, *"Author"* also possesses a positive association with *"ToCiation"*.

As for the regression against the dependent variable *"JIF.Lev"*, no statistically significant association was found across three countries (see Table 7). These regression results indicated that neither *"Funding"*, *"InterCollab"*, nor *"Author"* affected the scientific quality measured by the levels of JIF.

4. Discussion

4.1. Publication Trend

The current study found that there was a sharp increase in the number of articles regarding depressive disorder among university students in Korea during 2008 and 2018, but the growth rate was not stable. The rising number of publications might result from the development of community health service programs in 2007, in which juveniles are the targeted subjects [45]. Our results also showed that the research targets of depressive disorder studies in Korea are not diverse, and no studies on special student groups (e.g., international students, first-year students, post-graduate students, etc.) had been conducted besides few studies on female students. Given the fact that the prevalence and risk factors of depressive disorder were different among types of students [21,22,26], paying more focus on various groups of students is suggested as a way to enhance the effectiveness of depression treatment and prevention services in higher education.

For Japan, findings show that the number of studies regarding depressive disorder among university students in Japan is scarce. There were only 24 articles published until 2018, which was only equal to one-fifth of the total number of publications in China. After 2010, Japan witnessed a positive growing signal in the number of articles. The positive signal might emerge as a consequence of the Mental Health Policy Framing Conference in conjunction with the Ministry of Health, Labor, and Welfare in 2010. The conference accomplished with committees' recommendations to improve health care for children-adolescents and depression [46]. Despite some positive changes, the number of publications in Japan was still inadequate to cope with a relatively high prevalence of depression and suicide rates. This might be because of the shortage of the number of researchers in the mental health of children and adolescents. Only 0.025% of psychiatrists in Japan is certified to treat children and adolescents [47,48]. Besides the inadequate publication number in Japan, the lack of diversity in research targets is also a primary concern that requires more attention from the scientific policy-makers, given the increasing demand of international workforces in Japan [49–52].

In China, we found that even though the first publication emerged in 1999, relatively later than the other two countries, the number of studies related to depressive disorder among university students started to increase more substantially and consistently than Korea and Japan in 2007. With only eight publications by 2007, the number of publications in China had emerged significantly by more than 12 folds to 97 publications by 2018. Not only the publication outcome is improved dramatically, but the diversity in the research topic is also commendable Such impressive changes might be the outcome of the '686 Project' launched in China in 2004. The project's aims are to improve the capacity of the community in mental health prevention, treatment, and management [53,54]. Additionally, endeavors in policy reform of the Chinese government, e.g., Healthy China 2020, Healthy China 2030, National Mental Health Law 2013, etc., should not be excluded.

Overall, some positive changes in terms of publication outcomes are witnessed with the most outstanding performance from China. Such improvements are more or less influenced by the orientation of policymaking in Korea, Japan, and China. Given the acute mental problems adolescents currently suffer from in Japan and Korea, more scientific researches are needed.

4.2. Scientific Collaboration Patterns

The results from Fisher's Exact test show that there is a statistically significant difference in terms of collaboration construction among Korea, Japan, and China. The difference is most significant between China and Japan. However, except for China, the collaboration network in Korea and Japan is narrow and monotonous. Moreover, while the current international collaboration in Korea and Japan is ineffective in raising scientific impact measured by the number of total citations and quality measured by the JIF level, the association between international collaboration and scientific impact in China was statistically significantly negative (see Tables 6 and 7).

In Korea, we found that the three most common patterns of collaboration are collaborating domestically (49%), collaborating internationally (32%), and research conducted alone by a researcher affiliated with a Korean institute (11%). Thanks to the stable number of international cooperations since 2013, the proportion of international collaboration in Korea has become relatively higher than that in Japan, but still lower than in China. A tight scientific cooperation relationship between Korea and the USA, which contributes up to 75% of the total number of mentioned international collaborations, can help boost the number of collaborated projects quickly due to existing collaborating network, but adversely, it can hinder the exchange of diverse knowledge with other scientific communities. Furthermore, the international collaborations during 2008–2018 were also found to be ineffective in increasing the scientific impact of the study. Hence, diversifying the international collaboration network and pre-evaluating the effectiveness of international collaboration is necessary to improve the quality of the research, knowledge exchange, and expand the scientific collaboration network [55–57].

International collaboration is an effective way to increase scientific productivity. However, we found that the international collaboration rate in Japan was relatively low, with only 21%. Most of the studies related to depressive disorder among university students were accomplished by a domestic researcher (17%) and a group of domestic researchers (50%). Another 13% of publications were conducted by a group of foreign researchers. This suggests foreign scientists are willing to learn about the depressive disorder among Japanese university students.

Interestingly, among the top highly-cited papers in Japan, 3 out of 10 papers were written by a group of foreign researchers. Moreover, despite statistical insignificance, the results of Poisson regression analysis hint at the positive influence of international collaboration on scientific impact measured by the total citations. Based on these findings, we recommend policymakers and academic institutes in Japan to promote international collaboration for raising scientific productivity and exchanging knowledge in depressive disorder among Japanese university students [55–57].

In China, we found a considerable contribution from international collaborations in the collaboration pattern with 44%, which is much higher than the other two countries. Also, health promotion is even integrated into the economic and political initiatives of China. In response to the proposition of the Belt and Road Initiative in 2013, China also formed the Health Sub-Alliance of the University Alliance of the Silk Road (UASR-HAS) in 2015 to encourage international collaboration in health-related research and education [58]. Our results of the international collaboration were in line with the time the UASR-HAS was established. Specifically, the international collaborations after 2015 in China accounted for almost 60% (25/43) of the total international collaborations. Nevertheless, the adverse impact of international collaboration on scientific influence was seen. These results might point out the advantages (increase in scientific output) as well as disadvantages (low scientific impact) of integration issues, both political and economic, in scientific collaboration.

Therefore, besides the implementation of international collaboration promotion policies, we recommend governments, especially the Chinese government, initiate an evaluation system for internationally collaborated research to increase scientific impact and public trust [59–61]. Further research regarding the effect of integrating political-economic issues into scientific collaboration on the research quality should be conducted.

4.3. Funding Provision

According to our data, starting in 2008, the amount of funding granted to topics related to depressive disorder among university students in Korea has been relatively steady. Funding was provided every year, with the exception of 2009, 2011, and 2014. This result might also be the evidence of Korea's endeavors in promoting community health service programs for adolescents and response to the Mental Health Action Plan: 2013–2020 of WHO [62]. The plan urges nations to increase funding into community-based services and integrate mental health into general health care settings. The study's result also highlighted the greater contribution of academic institutes (44%) than the central government (37%) in funding provision. Despite the expansion of investment into mental health research and development of central government in Korea, there was a huge disproportion in directing the investment, with only 10% of the budget [63] is spent on studies of mental health policies, services, and humanities and social sciences issues, etc., while another 90% was spent on basic research, therapy, and diagnosis studies. As the depressive level and healthcare usage are significantly affected by multiple social-cultural-economic aspects [25,64–71], such disproportionate distribution of investment might result in insufficient depression prevention and treatment among particular populations, such as university students. Re-allocation of the investment is, therefore, essential to protect the mental health of the young generation.

Despite funding provision being an effective way to increase scientific productivity and attract international collaboration in the Korean case, Japan didn't converge to the same path. Findings revealed that the funding granted for studies of depressive disorder among university students in Japan was quite finite. During the time between 2007 and 2018, only six studies were funded. The central government provided funds to four of those studies (2 in 2015 and 2 in 2018). In 2013, "the previous Healthcare Policy" was approved by the Japanese cabinet for better allocating the medical R&D budget [72]. The budget allocation for studies related to depressive disorder among university students was seemingly not enough to create impactful improvement in depression prevention and treatment services in higher education [73]. Given that funded articles were found to have higher scientific quality than those not funded, and mental health treatment services in Japan are mainly centered on institutional settings, more investment in community- and school-based services, especially scientific activities, are recommended [60,61,74,75].

Efforts to reform mental health care in China are also reflected in its investment in mental health research. Our findings reveal that since 2009, the number of studies related to depressive disorder among university students had been funded more consistently, especially the number of funds granted per year after 2013, accounting for approximately 85% of total funds given, were leveraged compared to the previous period. This is aligned with the implementation of the health care reform in 2009 and the National Mental Health Law in 2013 [76,77]. The law's purposes are to encourage and support scientific research in mental health as well as improve and maintain the psychological well-being of students.

As for the association between the funding provision and scientific impact, China possessed a negative correlation, while Korea and Japan obtained no significant correlation. The negative association between China's funding provision and the scientific impact can be due to the misallocation of research funds, since the decisions for funding may be influenced by extraneous factors, such as social networks or political patronage, besides scientific merits [78]. In addition, no association across countries between funding provision and scientific quality measured by JIF levels was statistically significant. Therefore, along with policies promoting financial support in studies regarding depressive disorder among university students, a proper evaluation system for funded research in three countries, especially China, is also necessary to enhance the scientific influence of the research output and public trust [59–61]. In China, the evaluation system should be focused on government-funded research, while in Korea, funds from institutes need more careful and rigorous evaluation. Additionally, in all three cases, the number of co-authors is positively associated with scientific impact. Given the scientific development regarding depressive disorder among university students in Korea, Japan, and

China is at the initial stage, team-based research should be promoted to improve the outcome's quality and quantity.

4.4. Limitations

The current study has several limitations. First, the total number of citations cannot completely represent the scientific impact, as it may include self-citations, which tends to overstate the real impact of the study. Second, even though we found the ineffectiveness of the current funding provision and international collaboration in raising scientific impact and scientific quality, we could not specify what types of funding and international collaboration are ineffective. Third, employing only the WoS database and including only research articles provide several scientific production biases. For example, a number of Japanese researchers tend to publish in Japanese journals indexed in the CiNii database, and in terms of social sciences research, Japanese researchers prefer to publish in the form of a book than an article. Forth, to some theoretical extent, the total number of citations and the impact factor level can be used to measure scientific impact and scientific quality, but due to the lack of pragmatic data on real-life impacts, such as social responses and treatment effectiveness, the result of this study should only be considered as a point of reference for policymaking. More conclusive findings will emerge in a more comprehensive study.

5. Conclusions

The current scientometric study aims to describe the scientific research situation of depressive disorder among university students and evaluate the effectiveness of international collaboration and funding provision on enhancing scientific impact in Korea, Japan, and China, based on data from the WoS database. Findings reveal that: The research outputs in Korea and Japan are relatively low, and they also lack international collaborations, funding provisions, and diversity in research targets. This result is aligned with the findings from the bibliometric study of Larivière and Grant that Korea and Japan have lower scientific production than the world average [14]. Meanwhile, China's research outputs, number of international collaborations, funding provisions outstand its counterparts.

To some extent, the international collaboration and funding provision in Japan and Korea remain ineffective in raising scientific impact and scientific quality, while the situation is worse in China (the negative associations of the total citations with international collaboration and funding provision).

As the younger generations will be the main contributors to sustainable development in the future, keeping them physically and mentally healthy is like protecting the "root" of sustainable development. Thus, we recommend policymakers in Japan and Korea to promote scientific research regarding mental health among university students through international collaborations, funding provisions, and resource reallocation. It is also necessary to implement an adequate evaluation system for internationally collaborated and funded scientific output, especially in China.

Author Contributions: Conceptualization, M.-H.N. and Q.-Y.T.N.; methodology, M.-H.N. and V.-P.L.; software, M.-H.N.; validation, Q.-H.V., M.-T.H. (Manh-Toan Ho) and M.-T.H. (Manh-Tung Ho); formal analysis, M.-H.N., Q.-Y.T.N., and M.-C.N.; investigation, M.-T.H. (Manh-Toan Ho), M.-C.N. and T.-T.V.; resources, M.-T.H. (Manh-Tung Ho), Q.-Y.T.N. and T.-T.L.; data curation, M.-H.N., M.-T.H. (Manh-Tung Ho) and Q.-Y.T.N.; writing—original draft preparation, M.-H.N., Q.-Y.T.N., M.-T.H. (Manh-Toan Ho), and T.-T.L.; writing—review and editing, M.-H.N., M.-T.H. (Manh-Tung Ho), T.-T.V., and M.-T.H. (Manh-Toan Ho); visualization, V.-P.L., M.H.N and Q.-Y.T.N.; supervision, Q.-H.V.; project administration, Q.-H.V.; funding acquisition, Q.-H.V. All authors have read and agreed to the published version of the manuscript.

Funding: This research received no external funding.

Conflicts of Interest: The authors declare no conflict of interest.

Appendix A

Table A1. Total mentions of international collaborations by collaborated countries.

Countries	Korea	Japan	China
Singapore	1	1	4
China	1	1	
Taiwan	1	1	1
Korea		1	1
Japan	1		4
UK	1		3
US	9	3	27
Australia	1	1	8
France		1	
Canada			4
Germany			1
Norway			1
New Zealand			1
Malaysia		1	
Total mentions	15	10	55

Table A2. Correlation analysis—Korea.

Korea	"ToCitation"	"JIF.Lev"	"Author"	"InterCollab"	"Fund"	"Year"
"ToCitation"	1					
"JIF.Lev"	0.479	1				
"Author"	0.074	0.314	1			
"InterCollab"	0.025	−0.071	−0.016	1		
"Fund"	0.003	0.234	0.254	−0.020	1	
"Year"	−0.384	−0.194	0.080	0.032	−0.070	1

Table A3. Correlation analysis—Japan.

Japan	"ToCitation"	"JIF.Lev"	"Author"	"InterCollab"	"Fund"	"Year"
"ToCitation"	1					
"JIF.Lev"	0.230	1				
"Author"	0.222	0.189	1			
"InterCollab"	0.136	0.036	0.481	1		
"Fund"	−0.059	0.450	0.233	−0.054	1	
"Year"	−0.612	−0.025	0.183	0.131	0.247	1

Table A4. Correlation analysis—China.

China	"ToCitation"	"JIF.Lev"	"Author"	"InterCollab"	"Fund"	"Year"
"ToCitation"	1					
"JIF.Lev"	0.137	1				
"Author"	0.068	0.272	1			
"InterCollab"	−0.076	0.110	0.078	1		
"Fund"	−0.099	0.058	0.137	−0.061	1	
"Year"	−0.575	−0.128	−0.095	−0.014	0.146	1

References

1. The United Nations Youth and the SDGs. Available online: https://www.un.org/sustainabledevelopment/youth/ (accessed on 15 December 2019).
2. UNCTAD Youth Prioritized as Sustainable Development Innovators. Available online: https://unctad.org/en/pages/newsdetails.aspx?OriginalVersionID=2009 (accessed on 15 December 2019).

3. Ibrahim, A.K.; Kelly, S.J.; Adams, C.E.; Glazebrook, C. A systematic review of studies of depression prevalence in university students. *J. Psychiatr. Res.* **2013**, *47*, 391–400. [CrossRef] [PubMed]
4. Vu, H.T.T.; Nguyen, T.X.; Nguyen, H.T.T.; Le, T.A.; Nguyen, T.N.; Nguyen, A.T.; Nguyen, T.T.H.; Nguyen, H.L.; Nguyen, C.T.; Tran, B.X.; et al. Depressive symptoms among elderly diabetic patients in Vietnam. *DMSO* **2018**, *11*, 659–665. [CrossRef] [PubMed]
5. Vu, T.; Le, T.; Dang, A.; Nguyen, L.; Nguyen, B.; Tran, B.; Latkin, C.; Ho, C.; Ho, R. Socioeconomic vulnerability to depressive symptoms in patients with chronic hepatitis B. *Int. J. Environ. Res. Public Health* **2019**, *16*, 255. [CrossRef]
6. Simon, G.E.; Coleman, K.J.; Rossom, R.C.; Beck, A.; Oliver, M.; Johnson, E.; Whiteside, U.; Operskalski, B.; Penfold, R.B.; Shortreed, S.M.; et al. Risk of suicide attempt and suicide death following completion of the patient health questionnaire depression module in community practice. *J. Clin. Psychiatry* **2016**, *77*, 221–227. [CrossRef]
7. Pan, Y.-J.; Juang, K.-D.; Lu, S.-R.; Chen, S.-P.; Wang, Y.-F.; Fuh, J.-L.; Wang, S.-J. Longitudinal risk factors for suicidal thoughts in depressed and non-depressed young adolescents. *Aust. N. Z. J. Psychiatry* **2017**, *51*, 930–937. [CrossRef]
8. Miller, A.B.; Eisenlohr-Moul, T.; Giletta, M.; Hastings, P.D.; Rudolph, K.D.; Nock, M.K.; Prinstein, M.J. A within-person approach to risk for suicidal ideation and suicidal behavior: Examining the roles of depression, stress, and abuse exposure. *J. Consult. Clin. Psychol.* **2017**, *85*, 712–722. [CrossRef] [PubMed]
9. Jenkins, R. Global mental health and sustainable development 2018. *BJPsych Int.* **2019**, *16*, 34–37. [CrossRef] [PubMed]
10. Tran, B.X.; Ha, G.H.; Vu, G.T.; Nguyen, L.H.; Latkin, C.A.; Nathan, K.; McIntyre, R.S.; Ho, C.S.; Tam, W.W.; Ho, R.C. Indices of change, expectations, and popularity of biological treatments for major depressive disorder between 1988 and 2017: A scientometric analysis. *Int. J. Environ. Res. Public Health* **2019**, *16*, 2255. [CrossRef]
11. Tran, B.X.; McIntyre, R.S.; Latkin, C.A.; Phan, H.T.; Vu, G.T.; Nguyen, H.L.T.; Gwee, K.K.; Ho, C.S.H.; Ho, R.C.M. The current research landscape on the artificial intelligence application in the management of depressive disorders: A bibliometric analysis. *Int. J. Environ. Res. Public Health* **2019**, *16*, 2150. [CrossRef]
12. Wang, X.-Q.; Peng, M.-S.; Weng, L.-M.; Zheng, Y.-L.; Zhang, Z.-J.; Chen, P.-J. Bibliometric study of the comorbidity of pain and depression research. *Neural Plast.* **2019**, *2019*, 1657498. [CrossRef]
13. Nature Index. The Top 10 Countries for Scientific Research in 2018. Available online: https://www.natureindex.com/news-blog/top-ten-countries-research-science-twenty-nineteen (accessed on 15 December 2019).
14. Larivière, V.; Grant, J. Bibliometric analysis of mental health research: 1980–2008. *Rand Health Q.* **2017**, *6*, 12. [PubMed]
15. OECD Suicide Rates. Available online: https://data.oecd.org/healthstat/suicide-rates.htm (accessed on 15 December 2019).
16. Kyodo School Issues are No. 1 Reason behind Youth Suicides in 2018, Japanese Government White Paper. Available online: https://www.japantimes.co.jp/news/2019/07/16/national/social-issues/school-matters-no-1-issue-behind-youth-suicides-2018-japanese-government-white-paper-finds/#.Xfj61mQzZEY (accessed on 18 December 2019).
17. Kwak, C.W.; Ickovics, J.R. Adolescent suicide in South Korea: Risk factors and proposed multi-dimensional solution. *Asian J. Psychiatry* **2019**, *43*, 150–153. [CrossRef] [PubMed]
18. WHO Suicide Rate Estimates, Crude Estimates by Country. Available online: http://apps.who.int/gho/data/view.main.MHSUICIDEv?lang=en (accessed on 15 December 2019).
19. Nguyen, T.V.; Ho-Le, T.P.; Le, U.V. International collaboration in scientific research in Vietnam: An analysis of patterns and impact. *Scientometrics* **2017**, *110*, 1035–1051. [CrossRef]
20. National Institute of Mental Health Depression. Available online: https://www.nimh.nih.gov/health/topics/depression/index.shtml (accessed on 20 January 2020).
21. Nguyen, M.-H.; Serik, M.; Vuong, T.-T.; Ho, M.-T. Internationalization and its discontents: Help-seeking behaviors of students in a multicultural environment regarding acculturative stress and depression. *Sustainability* **2019**, *11*, 1865. [CrossRef]
22. Ogunsanya, M.E.; Bamgbade, B.A.; Thach, A.V.; Sudhapalli, P.; Rascati, K.L. Determinants of health-related quality of life in international graduate students. *Curr. Pharm. Teach. Learn.* **2018**, *10*, 413–422. [CrossRef]

23. Cao, C.; Meng, Q.; Shang, L. How can Chinese international students' host-national contact contribute to social connectedness, social support and reduced prejudice in the mainstream society? Testing a moderated mediation model. *Int. J. Intercult. Relat.* **2018**, *63*, 43–52. [CrossRef]
24. Constantine, M.G.; Okazaki, S.; Utsey, S.O. Self-concealment, social self-efficacy, acculturative stress, and depression in African, Asian, and Latin American international college students. *Am. J. Orthopsychiatry* **2004**, *74*, 230–241. [CrossRef]
25. Nguyen, M.; Le, T.; Meirmanov, S. Depression, acculturative stress, and social connectedness among international university students in Japan: A statistical investigation. *Sustainability* **2019**, *11*, 878. [CrossRef]
26. Nguyen, M.-H.; Ho, M.-T.; Nguyen, Q.-Y.T.; Vuong, Q.-H. A dataset of students' mental health and help-seeking behaviors in a multicultural environment. *Data* **2019**, *4*, 124. [CrossRef]
27. Aria, M.; Cuccurullo, C. Bibliometrix: An R-tool for comprehensive science mapping analysis. *J. Informetr.* **2017**, *11*, 959–975. [CrossRef]
28. Kim, H.-Y. Statistical notes for clinical researchers: Chi-squared test and Fisher's exact test. *Restor. Dent. Endod.* **2017**, *42*, 152. [CrossRef] [PubMed]
29. McDonald, J.H. *Handbook of Biological Statistics*, 3rd ed.; Sparky House Publishing: Baltimore, MD, USA, 2014.
30. Coxe, S.; West, S.G.; Aiken, L.S. The analysis of count data: A gentle introduction to Poisson regression and its alternatives. *J. Personal. Assess.* **2009**, *91*, 121–136. [CrossRef] [PubMed]
31. Hutchinson, M.K.; Holtman, M.C. Analysis of count data using Poisson regression. *Res. Nurs. Health* **2005**, *28*, 408–418. [CrossRef] [PubMed]
32. Crittenden, K.S.; Fugita, S.S.; Bae, H.; Lamug, C.B.; Un, C. A cross-cultural study of self-report depressive symptoms among college students. *J. Cross-Cult. Psychol.* **1992**, *23*, 163–178. [CrossRef]
33. Kim, O. Sex differences in social support, loneliness, and depression among Korean college students. *Psychol. Rep.* **2001**, *88*, 521–526. [CrossRef]
34. Anderson, C.A. Attributional style, depression, and loneliness: A cross-cultural comparison of American and Chinese students. *Personal. Soc. Psychol. Bull.* **1999**, *25*, 482–499. [CrossRef]
35. Sakamoto, S. The effects of self-focus on negative mood among depressed and nondepressed Japanese students. *J. Soc. Psychol.* **1998**, *138*, 514–523. [CrossRef]
36. Sakamoto, S.; Kambara, M. A longitudinal study of the relationship between attributional style, life events, and depression in Japanese undergraduates. *J. Soc. Psychol.* **1998**, *138*, 229–240. [CrossRef]
37. Takayama, Y.; Miura, E.; Miura, K.; Ono, S.; Ohkubo, C. Condition of depressive symptoms among Japanese dental students. *Odontology* **2011**, *99*, 179–187. [CrossRef]
38. Cai, L.; Xu, F.; Cheng, Q.; Zhan, J.; Xie, T.; Ye, Y.; Xiong, S.; McCarthy, K.; He, Q. Social smoking and mental health among Chinese male college students. *Am. J. Health Promot.* **2017**, *31*, 226–231. [CrossRef]
39. Kim, Y.-R.; Hwang, B.I.; Lee, G.Y.; Kim, K.H.; Kim, M.; Kim, K.K.; Treasure, J. Determinants of binge eating disorder among normal weight and overweight female college students in Korea. *Eat. Weight Disord. Stud. Anorex. Bulim. Obes.* **2018**, *23*, 849–860. [CrossRef] [PubMed]
40. Liu, C.; Xie, B.; Chou, C.-P.; Koprowski, C.; Zhou, D.; Palmer, P.; Sun, P.; Guo, Q.; Duan, L.; Sun, X.; et al. Perceived stress, depression and food consumption frequency in the college students of China seven cities. *Physiol. Behav.* **2007**, *92*, 748–754. [CrossRef] [PubMed]
41. Saint Arnault, D.; Kim, O. Is there an Asian idiom of distress? *Arch. Psychiatr. Nurs.* **2008**, *22*, 27–38. [CrossRef] [PubMed]
42. Ni, X.; Yan, H.; Chen, S.; Liu, Z. Factors influencing internet addiction in a sample of freshmen university students in China. *Cyberpsychol. Behav.* **2009**, *12*, 327–330. [CrossRef] [PubMed]
43. Song, Y.; Lindquist, R. Effects of mindfulness-based stress reduction on depression, anxiety, stress and mindfulness in Korean nursing students. *Nurse Educ. Today* **2015**, *35*, 86–90. [CrossRef] [PubMed]
44. Igarashi, H.; Hasui, C.; Uji, M.; Shono, M.; Nagata, T.; Kitamura, T. Effects of child abuse history on borderline personality traits, negative life events, and depression: A study among a university student population in Japan. *Psychiatry Res.* **2010**, *180*, 120–125. [CrossRef] [PubMed]
45. Heo, Y.-C.; Kahng, S.K.; Kim, S. Mental health system at the community level in Korea: Development, recent reforms and challenges. *Int. J. Ment. Health Syst.* **2019**, *13*, 9. [CrossRef]
46. Setoya, Y. Overview of the Japanese mental health system. *Int. J. Ment. Health* **2012**, *41*, 3–18. [CrossRef]
47. Sakano, M.; Snowden, N. Paving the way for the future of child and adolescent mental health in Japan. *Lond. J. Prim. Care* **2018**, *10*, 123–125. [CrossRef]

48. The Japanese Society for Child and Adolescent Psychiatry Certified Physician. Available online: http://child-adolesc.jp/nintei/ninteii/ (accessed on 15 December 2019).
49. Vuong, Q.H.; Napier, N.K. Acculturation and global mindsponge: An emerging market perspective. *Int. J. Intercult. Relat.* **2015**, *49*, 354–367. [CrossRef]
50. Pekerti, A.A.; Vuong, Q.H.; Napier, N.K. Double edge experiences of expatriate acculturation: Navigating through personal multiculturalism. *J. Glob. Mobil.* **2017**, *5*, 225–250. [CrossRef]
51. Nagata, K. Firms Go Abroad by Hiring Foreign Students Here. Available online: https://www.japantimes.co.jp/news/2013/02/26/reference/firms-go-abroad-by-hiring-foreign-students-here/#.XjHF2mgzZPY (accessed on 15 December 2019).
52. JIJI Japanese Government Bolsters Support for Foreign Students Seeking Jobs. Available online: https://www.japantimes.co.jp/news/2019/12/20/national/japan-ups-support-for-foreign-student-job-seekers/#.XjHF2mgzZPY (accessed on 15 December 2019).
53. Ma, H. Integration of hospital and community services-the 686 Project-is a crucial component in the reform of China's mental health services. *Shanghai Arch. Psychiatry* **2012**, *24*, 172–174. [PubMed]
54. Xiang, Y.-T.; Ng, C.H.; Yu, X.; Wang, G. Rethinking progress and challenges of mental health care in China. *World Psychiatry* **2018**, *17*, 231–232. [CrossRef] [PubMed]
55. Freshwater, D.; Sherwood, G.; Drury, V. International research collaboration: Issues, benefits and challenges of the global network. *J. Res. Nurs.* **2006**, *11*, 295–303. [CrossRef]
56. Vuong, Q.-H.; Napier, N.K.; Ho, T.M.; Nguyen, V.H.; Vuong, T.-T.; Pham, H.H.; Nguyen, H.K.T. Effects of work environment and collaboration on research productivity in Vietnamese social sciences: Evidence from 2008 to 2017 Scopus data. *Stud. High. Educ.* **2019**, *44*, 2132–2147. [CrossRef]
57. Widmer, R.J.; Widmer, J.M.; Lerman, A. International collaboration: Promises and challenges. *Rambam Maimonides Med. J.* **2015**, *6*, e0012. [CrossRef]
58. Wang, Y.; Sun, X.; Wang, L.; Zhou, Z.; Fang, Y.; Zhou, L.; Cai, H.; Qi, X.; Han, T.; Zhuang, G.; et al. International collaboration to promote global health: The 2017 Belt and Road Initiative Global Health International Congress & 2017 Chinese Preventive Medicine Association—Chinese Society on Global Health Annual Meeting. *Glob. Health J.* **2017**, *1*, 34–43.
59. Zhou, W.; Yu, Y.; Zhao, X.; Xiao, S.; Chen, L. Evaluating China's mental health policy on local-level promotion and implementation: A case study of Liuyang Municipality. *BMC Public Health* **2019**, *19*, 24. [CrossRef]
60. Vuong, Q.-H. Breaking barriers in publishing demands a proactive attitude. *Nat. Hum. Behav.* **2019**, *3*, 1034. [CrossRef]
61. Vuong, Q.-H. The (ir) rational consideration of the cost of science in transition economies. *Nat. Hum. Behav.* **2018**, *2*, 5. [CrossRef]
62. World Health Organization. *Mental Health Action Plan 2013–2020*; World Health Organization: Geneva, Switzerland, 2013.
63. Roh, S.; Lee, S.-U.; Soh, M.; Ryu, V.; Kim, H.; Jang, J.W.; Lim, H.Y.; Jeon, M.; Park, J.-I.; Choi, S.; et al. Mental health services and R&D in South Korea. *Int. J. Ment. Health Syst.* **2016**, *10*, 45. [PubMed]
64. Abdel Wahed, W.Y.; Hassan, S.K. Prevalence and associated factors of stress, anxiety, and depression among medical Fayoum University students. *Alex. J. Med.* **2017**, *53*, 77–84. [CrossRef]
65. Pham, T.; Bui, L.; Nguyen, A.; Nguyen, B.; Tran, P.; Vu, P.; Dang, L. The prevalence of depression and associated risk factors among medical students: An untold story in Vietnam. *PLoS ONE* **2019**, *14*, e0221432. [CrossRef] [PubMed]
66. Tennant, C. Life events, stress, and depression: A review of recent findings. *Aust. N. Z. J. Psychiatry* **2002**, *36*, 173–182. [CrossRef]
67. Vuong, Q.H. Be rich or don't be sick: Estimating Vietnamese patients' risk of falling into destitution. *SpringerPlus* **2015**, *4*, 529. [CrossRef]
68. Vuong, Q.-H.; Ho, T.-M.; Nguyen, H.-K.; Vuong, T.-T. Healthcare consumers' sensitivity to costs: A reflection on behavioural economics from an emerging market. *Palgrave Commun.* **2018**, *4*, 1–10. [CrossRef]
69. Vuong, Q.-H.; Vuong, T.-T.; Ho, T.; Nguyen, H. Psychological and socio-economic factors affecting social sustainability through impacts on perceived health care quality and public health: The case of Vietnam. *Sustainability* **2017**, *9*, 1456. [CrossRef]

70. Vuong, Q.-H.; Nghiem, K.-C.; La, V.-P.; Vuong, T.-T.; Nguyen, H.-K.; Ho, M.-T.; Tran, K.; Khuat, T.-H.; Ho, M.-T. Sex differences and psychological factors associated with general health examinations participation: Results from a Vietnamese cross-section dataset. *Sustainability* **2019**, *11*, 514. [CrossRef]
71. Vuong, Q.H. Data on Vietnamese patients' behavior in using information sources, perceived data sufficiency and (non) optimal choice of health care provider. *Data Brief* **2016**, *7*, 1687–1695. [CrossRef]
72. Japanese Cabinet. *The Healthcare Policy*; Japanese Cabinet: Tokyo, Japan, 2014.
73. Kasai, K.; Ando, S.; Kanehara, A.; Kumakura, Y.; Kondo, S.; Fukuda, M.; Kawakami, N.; Higuchi, T. Strengthening community mental health services in Japan. *Lancet Psychiatry* **2017**, *4*, 268–270. [CrossRef]
74. Kanata, T. Japanese mental health care in historical context: Why did Japan become a country with so many psychiatric care beds? *Soc. Work* **2016**, *52*, 471–489. [CrossRef]
75. OECD. *OECD Health Overview: Health Policy in Japan*; OECD: Paris, France, 2017.
76. Chen, H.; Phillips, M.; Cheng, H.; Chen, Q.; Chen, X.; Fralick, D.; Zhang, Y.; Liu, M.; Huang, J.; Bueber, M. Mental health law of the People's Republic of China (English translation with annotations): Translated and annotated version of China's new mental health law. *Shanghai Arch. Psychiatry* **2012**, *24*, 305–321.
77. Shao, Y.; Wang, J.; Xie, B. The first mental health law of China. *Asian J. Psychiatry* **2015**, *13*, 72–74. [CrossRef]
78. Xie, Y.; Zhang, C.; Lai, Q. China's rise as a major contributor to science and technology. *Proc. Natl. Acad. Sci. USA* **2014**, *111*, 9437–9442. [CrossRef]

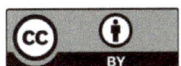

© 2020 by the authors. Licensee MDPI, Basel, Switzerland. This article is an open access article distributed under the terms and conditions of the Creative Commons Attribution (CC BY) license (http://creativecommons.org/licenses/by/4.0/).

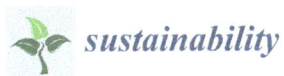

Article

Dietary Health-Related Risk Factors for Women in the Polish and Croatian Population Based on the Nutritional Behaviors of Junior Health Professionals

Dominika Głąbska [1,*], Valentina Rahelić [2], Dominika Guzek [3], Kamila Jaworska [1], Sandra Bival [2], Zlatko Giljević [4,5] and Eva Pavić [2]

1. Department of Dietetics, Faculty of Human Nutrition and Consumer Sciences, Warsaw University of Life Sciences (WULS-SGGW), 159c Nowoursynowska Str., 02-776 Warsaw, Poland; kamila_jaworska@onet.eu
2. Department of Nutrition and Dietetics, University Hospital Centre Zagreb, 12 Kišpatićeva Str., 10-000 Zagreb, Croatia; valentina.rahelic@kbc-zagreb.hr (V.R.); sandra.bival@kbc-zagreb.hr (S.B.); eva.pavic@kbc-zagreb.hr (E.P.)
3. Department of Organization and Consumption Economics, Faculty of Human Nutrition and Consumer Sciences, Warsaw University of Life Sciences (WULS-SGGW), 159c Nowoursynowska Str., 02-776 Warsaw, Poland; dominika_guzek@sggw.pl
4. Department of Internal Medicine, University Hospital Centre, 12 Kišpatićeva Str., 10-000 Zagreb, Croatia; zlatko.giljevic@kbc-zagreb.hr
5. School of Medicine, Department of Internal Medicine, University of Zagreb, 3 Šalata Str., 10-000 Zagreb, Croatia
* Correspondence: dominika_glabska@sggw.pl; Tel.: +48-22-59-371-26

Received: 4 August 2019; Accepted: 13 September 2019; Published: 17 September 2019

Abstract: In Poland and Croatia, similarly as for a number of European countries, anemia and osteoporosis are common diet-related diseases in women, while for both the proper nutritional behaviors and preventive education are crucial. However, for the proper nutritional education there are some barriers, including those associated with an educator, his own nutritional behaviors and beliefs. The aim of the study was to assess the dietary health risk factors for women in the Polish and Croatian population based on the nutritional behaviors of junior health professionals. The study was conducted in Polish (n = 70) and Croatian (n = 80) female students of the faculties associated with public health at the universities in capital cities. Their diets were assessed based on 3-day dietary records. Nutritional value and consumption of food products, as well as the dietary risk factors for anemia and osteoporosis, were compared. While assessing the risk factors for anemia, in the Polish group, the higher intake of iron and folate, as well as vitamin B_{12} per 1000 kcal, was observed; and for folate, the higher frequency of inadequate intake was stated for Croatian women. While assessing the risk factors for osteoporosis, in the Polish group, compared with the Croatian, the higher intake of calcium per 1000 kcal was observed, but for vitamin D, there were no differences. Differences of the intake between the Polish and the Croatian group of junior health professionals may result in various dietary health risks for women. Based on the assessment of dietary intake, for anemia, compared to Polish women, a higher risk may be indicated for Croatian women, but for osteoporosis, similar risks may be indicated for Polish and Croatian women. Therefore, for public health, adequate nutritional education of junior health professionals is necessary.

Keywords: diet; nutrition; intake; public health; health professionals; dietary risk

1. Introduction

According to the World Health Organization (WHO), a number of women die because of noncommunicable diseases before they reach the age of 70—it was estimated that there were 4.7 million of such deaths in 2012 [1]. Women also generally suffer due to decreased quality of life and well-being—this indicates that there is a need to work toward improving the health and well-being of women and girls, beyond maternal and child care [2].

A number of noncommunicable diseases are diet-related; hence, nutritional education is crucial to prevent these diseases. However, it has been observed that it is not enough for nutritional educators to have the proper qualifications, including the right knowledge and skills, to affect change—the educators' own beliefs may influence health education [3]. The nutritional educators' own nutritional behaviors and beliefs may influence the information that is presented to patients and may interfere with the process of imparting knowledge [4]. At the same time, nutritional educators should follow diet recommendations; previous studies have shown that if educators had excessive body mass, it negatively affected the perception of their credibility, level of trust, and inclination of the patient to follow their advice [5].

Providing dietary recommendations is a serious problem as, generally, physicians do not even engage in nutritional counseling [6], while the other nutritional educators often do not have adequate knowledge and skills [7–9]; sometimes, even dietitians do not have it [10–12]. Although some studies indicate that dietitians follow their own advice of maintaining a well-balanced diet [13], others conclude that the nutritional behaviors of dietitians generally are not in agreement with their own recommendations; both dietitians and other nutritional educators consume inadequate amounts of fruits and vegetables [14–16] and fish [14,17]—they also consume sweets [17] and fast food meals [16] too often. This data corresponds to the excessive body mass commonly reported for physicians [18], nurses [19], educators [20], and also for dietitians [21]. Moreover, malnutrition has also been reported in dietitians [15] and the lower body mass is often related with symptoms of orthorexia nervosa [22]. The improper nutritional behaviors of health professionals are associated with a diet that is characterized by inadequate intake of fiber [23,24], calcium [23,25], iron [19,23], potassium [23], vitamin A [19], vitamin D [23], riboflavin [19], folate [19,23], and vitamin B_{12} [19].

Taking all this information into account, two major problems can be highlighted. These problems are related with educators providing misleading information to their patients based on their own beliefs, which results in the patients maintaining an unhealthy diet; in other cases, patients do not follow the nutritional educators' recommendations because of loss of trust and confidence in them. Consequently, it may be assumed that proper nutritional behaviors of nutritional educators may be crucial for effective education; if the educators do not follow proper nutritional behavior, they may directly generate health-related dietary risk factors for patients.

Anemia [26] and osteoporosis [27] are the diet-related diseases typical for women. The two conditions may be associated, and when they occur at the same time, they cause even more serious reduction of the quality of life in the affected individuals [28].

The frequency of decreased blood hemoglobin concentration (< 120 g/L), interpreted as the occurrence of anemia according to the WHO [29] definition, is high even for the developed regions of the world, especially for women [30]. According to WHO estimations, the prevalence of anemia in nonpregnant women aged 15–49 is 22.5% (ranging from 16.4 to 30.1%) in the European region, being 23% in Poland and 24% in Croatia; for pregnant women, the frequency is even higher [31]. The primary diet-related reasons for anemia are deficiencies of iron [32], folate [33], and vitamin B_{12} [34], although WHO indicated iron deficiency as the most prominent contributor [35].

The frequency of osteoporosis, according to the statistics of the International Osteoporosis Foundation (IOF) [36], for European countries is also high, as for women aged over 50 (the group especially prone to osteoporosis), its occurrence is 21–24%, contributing to an estimated lifetime risk of hip fracture of 22.8%. In this age group, the frequency of osteoporosis in Poland is also estimated at about 20%, contributing to hip fractures in 3% of the female population [37]. As was observed by Cvijetić et al. [38], for Croatia, there are no detailed osteoporosis statistics; but it is estimated that 39% of individuals aged over 60 have osteoporosis, with 95% of them being women [39]. At the same time, based on the data for Zagreb (the capital city of Croatia), the frequency of vertebral fractures for women in the group aged over 50 was estimated as 9.7% [40]. As calcium intake is directly associated with bone mass, it is the primary diet-related influencing factor [41]; however, vitamin D is also a factor that contributes to better calcium absorption and bone mineralization, and thus bone mineral density [42].

In this study, our aim was to assess the dietary health risk factors for women in the Polish and Croatian population based on the nutritional behaviors of junior health professionals. Taking into account the comprehensive quality of diet, we planned to assess not only the daily intake, but also the proportions of macronutrients (the share of energy contribution), as well as the nutrient density of diet [43] (expressed as daily intake recalculated per 1000 kcal). Moreover, we also included the assessment of food products intake and food products intake recalculated per 1000 kcal. In order to include issues related to the environmental effects of food production, we decided to assess, under food products intake, animal-derived products separately; under the intake of protein, we decided to assess animal and plant protein separately. Western populations generally have too high total protein intake [44]; it has also been observed that environmental impact reduction is proportional to the animal products share reduction [45]. This study was planned to be conducted by assessing the dietary risk factors for anemia and osteoporosis, which are the most common diet-related diseases for women and may influence the social sustainability level in populations.

2. Materials and Methods

2.1. Ethical Statement

The study was conducted according to the guidelines of the Declaration of Helsinki. It was approved by the Bioethical Commission of the National Food and Nutrition Institute in Warsaw (No. 0701/2015). All the participants provided their informed consent to participate in the study.

2.2. Studied Group

The study was conducted among two groups of junior health professionals who were students of faculties associated with public health at universities located in capital cities. It was decided to recruit students that in the future should be characterized by a general nutritional knowledge only, and not specialists in dietetics or medicine. Hence, students of dietary and medical courses were not included; only those who planned to become general nutritional specialists conducting group nutritional education in and outside of hospitals were recruited. For Poland, it was the Warsaw University of Life Sciences (WULS-SGGW) in Warsaw, whereas for Croatia it was the University of Applied Health Sciences (Zdravstveno Veleučilište u Zagrebu—ZVU) in Zagreb.

The students were invited to participate in the study in the semester when they had their dietitian classes to assess nutritional behaviors of students characterized by a similar level of nutritional knowledge. The inclusion criteria were as follows:

- female;
- aged 19–25;
- living in the capital city or around it;
- student of faculty associated with health science and promotion; and
- providing written informed consent to participate.

The exclusion criteria were as follows:

- being pregnant or breastfeeding;
- any chronic diet-related disease diagnosed;
- currently trying to lose weight; and
- following any special diet.

In the indicated universities, based on the indicated inclusion and exclusion criteria, two independent groups of participants were recruited: 70 young women in the Polish group and 80 young women in the Croatian group.

2.3. Assessment of the Diet

The assessment of the diet was based on a 3-day dietary record, according to widely applicable rules [46]. The dietary assessment was conducted by respondents during three random and nonconsecutive days, which were commanded to be typical and two of them were to be weekdays and one weekend day. The study's participants had a structured form to be completed with the information about consumed meals: the place where they were consumed, consumption time, and detailed description (products included, applied culinary and cooking techniques, serving size). The serving size was to be indicated either in grams (if they possessed a kitchen scale or consumed packed products with such information on the packaging) or in a descriptive manner (as a standard household measures). The respondents were instructed about the need to note all the products and all the beverages in a scrupulous manner. Moreover, they were informed about the need to not change their typical dietary habits because of keeping the dietary record.

Both groups of respondents were given identical forms (in their native language, either Polish or Croatian) and identical instructions to conduct the 3-day dietary record. The instructions were translated into Polish/Croatian by native Polish/Croatian speakers who were dietitians to obtain an accurate description of necessary issues, including some examples as to how to keep the dietary record.

Subsequently, to obtain a comparable analysis of the diet, independent from the applied databases, the same tables of nutritional value of food products and dishes were applied for both groups. The Polish tables were selected; therefore, the dietary records obtained for the Croatian group were translated to Polish, as in the previously conducted own study [47]. The translation was independently conducted in two stages: two English-speaking Croatian dietitians translated them from Croatian to English (while describing the specific dishes and providing the photographs of typical Croatian products and information about recipes, if needed), and afterwards two English-speaking Polish dietitians independently translated Croatian dietary records from English to Polish (verifying all the doubts with Croatian dietitians, if needed). The applied procedure resulted in obtaining both Polish and Croatian dietary records translated into Polish to be analyzed using the same database (the Polish one).

The Polish 3-day dietary records and the Croatian ones, translated into Polish (in a 2-step process via English), were afterwards analyzed in four ways as follows:

- The typical nutritional value of the diet, which was assessed for the energy value of the diet and the following nutrients: total protein, animal protein, plant protein, protein as a share of energy value, fat, saturated fatty acids, monounsaturated fatty acids, polyunsaturated fatty acids, cholesterol, fat as a share of energy value, total carbohydrates, sucrose, lactose, starch, fiber, carbohydrate as a share of energy value (macronutrients), sodium, potassium, calcium, phosphorus, iron, magnesium, zinc, copper, manganese, iodine (minerals), thiamine, riboflavin, niacin, vitamin B_6, folate, vitamin B_{12}, vitamin A, vitamin E, vitamin C, vitamin D (vitamins). The nutritional value was assessed for a mean daily intake and was calculated using the tables of nutritional value of food products and dishes by the Polish National Food and Nutrition Institute in Warsaw [48] and the Polish dietitian software Energia 4.1.;
- The typical nutritional value of the diet recalculated per 1000 kcal of the diet, which was assessed for the nutrients, independently recalculated to enable reliable comparison;
- The typical consumption of food products, which was assessed for the following groups: milk and dairy beverages, cottage cheese, hard cheese, eggs, meat, cold cuts, fish and fish products, butter, sour cream (animal-derived products), vegetables, legumes, fruits, potatoes, bread, other cereal products, oil, margarine, nuts, mushrooms, sugar, jam and honey, chocolate sweets, cakes and cookies, alcoholic beverages, sweetened beverages (other food products). The consumed dishes

were deconstructed into food products, and they were then divided into listed groups, which are commonly applied for assessing the intake of food products [49];
- The typical consumption of food products recalculated per 1000 kcal of the diet, which was assessed for the food product groups, independently recalculated to enable reliable comparison.

While assessing sodium intake, the salt added to dishes was not calculated, but only that naturally present in food products or in processed food products. This is because, in general, dietary intake assessment is not a recommended method to analyze sodium intake; the 24-hour urine collection is the 'gold standard' for this assessment [50] and is commonly applied [51]. Moreover, dietary intake assessment methods usually do not capture the amount of sodium obtained from salt added to dishes consumed [52]. This is because, in western countries, excessive sodium intake is common; in practice, the risk of inadequate intake does not exist [53].

Subsequently, the groups were compared for the obtained nutritional value and the intake of food products. Moreover, the dietary health risk factors were specified for each population, and the most common ones for young women's diet-related health risks were selected and the related nutrients were analyzed as follows: anemia (iron, folate, and vitamin B_{12}) [54] and osteoporosis (calcium and vitamin D) [55]. Vitamin D was included in the analysis in spite of the fact that it is mainly generated in skin after sunshine exposure [56]. However, inadequate exposure that is commonly stated results in need for at least adequate dietary intake [57]. Combined inadequate sunshine exposure and inadequate intake result in vitamin D deficiency [58] that is observed both for Poland [59] and Croatia [60].

The intakes of indicated nutrients in groups were compared with the recommended intake values, as specified by National Institutes of Health [61], while the Estimated Average Requirement (EAR) values were selected as a reference to estimate the prevalence of inadequate intake [62]. We applied the following reference values: calcium (800 mg), iron (8.1 mg), folate (320 µg), vitamin B_{12} (2 µg), and vitamin D (10 µg) [61].

2.4. Statistical Analysis

The distribution was verified using the Shapiro-Wilk test. Afterwards, the t-Student test (for parametric distributions) and the U Mann-Whitney test (for nonparametric distributions) were applied for comparison of the typical intakes. At the same time, the chi^2 test was applied for comparison of the prevalence of inadequate intake.

The statistical analysis was conducted for the accepted level of significance of $p \leq 0.05$ and while using Statistica, version 8.0 (Statsoft Inc., Tulsa, OK, USA).

3. Results

Comparison of energy value and macronutrients intake in groups of junior health professionals from Poland and Croatia is presented in Table 1. In the analyzed group, Polish women, while compared with Croatian ones, were characterized by a higher protein ($p = 0.0001$), but lower carbohydrates share in energy value of the diet ($p = 0.0068$). At the same time, they were characterized by lower intake of sucrose ($p = 0.0109$) and starch ($p = 0.0098$), but higher intake of fiber ($p = 0.0002$).

Comparison of macronutrients intake per 1000 kcal in groups of junior health professionals from Poland and Croatia is presented in Table 2. In the analyzed group, Polish women, while compared with Croatian ones, were characterized by a higher total protein ($p = 0.0001$), animal protein ($p = 0.0190$), plant protein ($p = 0.0270$), polyunsaturated fatty acids ($p = 0.0071$), lactose ($p = 0.0205$) and fiber intake ($p < 0.0001$). At the same time, they were characterized by lower intake of sucrose ($p = 0.0098$) and starch ($p = 0.0015$).

Table 1. Comparison of energy value and macronutrients intake in groups of junior health professionals from Poland and Croatia.

	Polish Group		Croatian Group		p **
	Mean ± SD	Median (Range)	Mean ± SD	Median (Range)	
Energy value (kcal)	1492.3 ± 420.7	1415.4 * (756.8–2870.0)	1569.0 ± 561.0	1466.0 * (718.3–3743.9)	0.4115
Total protein (g)	79.5 ± 24.6	80.5 * (19.6–178.3)	73.7 ± 24.8	69.9 * (34.2–157.2)	0.0700
Animal protein (g)	53.5 ± 22.4	51.7 (0.2–124.1)	50.3 ± 20.5	49.1 (9.8–103.2)	0.3465
Plant protein (g)	26.0 ± 11.8	23.4 * (7.1–65.7)	23.4 ± 9.1	22.2 * (7.1–60.5)	0.4741
Protein (% EV)	22.0 ± 5.0	22.0 (5–33)	13.0 ± 5.0	12.0 * (5–26)	0.0001
Total fat (g)	56.1 ± 20.9	52.9 (21.3–116.1)	58.0 ± 25.8	52.5 * (19.7–143.6)	0.8595
Saturated fatty acids (g)	18.7 ± 9.1	17.1 * (4.0–45.9)	21.2 ± 10.0	19.4 * (6.8–45.9)	0.0851
Monounsaturated fatty acids (g)	22.4 ± 10.2	21.3 * (4.8–58.6)	23.2 ± 11.6	21.5 * (6.7–64.6)	0.8168
Polyunsaturated fatty acids (g)	10.6 ± 5.9	8.9 * (2.3–30.5)	8.9 ± 4.9	8.1 * (2.3–26.0)	0.0773
Cholesterol (mg)	316.9 ± 240.1	230.0 * (28.0–878.5)	266.6 ± 138.0	227.4 * (26.9–609.1)	0.8832
Fat (% of EV)	34.0 ± 8.0	34.0 (15–50)	33.0 ± 8.0	33.0 (14–56)	0.5963
Total carbohydrates (g)	190.2 ± 65.3	180.8 * (81.5–386.9)	204.7 ± 81.7	193.3 * (52.2–501.4)	0.1449
Sucrose (g)	27.1 ± 20.3	21.7 * (5.1–118.7)	34.2 ± 32.9	28.5 * (1.7–207.6)	0.0109
Lactose (g)	13.2 ± 7.5	12.34 (0.0–37.0)	11.7 ± 6.7	10.7 * (0.0–32.8)	0.1589
Starch (g)	92.1 ± 48.7	82.1 * (13.6–224.6)	107.6 ± 41.6	102.9 * (30.2–217.0)	0.0098
Fiber (g)	25.2 ± 10.4	25.8 * (7.7–52.1)	19.2 ± 11.4	18.2 * (7.2–79.1)	0.0002
Carbohydrate (% EV)	44.0 ± 10.0	44.0 (35–67)	47.0 ± 9.0	47.0 * (16–71)	0.0068

EV—Energy Value; * nonparametric distribution (verified using the Shapiro-Wilk test; $p < 0.05$); ** compared using the t-Student test (for parametric distributions) or the U Mann-Whitney test (for nonparametric distributions).

Table 2. Comparison of macronutrients intake per 1000 kcal in groups of junior health professionals from Poland and Croatia.

	Polish Group		Croatian Group		p **
	Mean ± SD	Median (Range)	Mean ± SD	Median (Range)	
Total protein (g)	54.3 ± 12.7	55.5 (12.5–83.2)	47.9 ± 10.7	46.8 * (29.7–79.3)	0.0001
Animal protein (g)	36.9 ± 14.4	36.2 (0.2–67.4)	32.7 ± 11.7	29.9 (13.5–65.5)	0.0190
Plant protein (g)	17.4 ± 6.2	16.7 * (5.1–39.8)	15.2 ± 4.5	14.5 (6.4–35.9)	0.0270
Total fat (g)	37.4 ± 8.7	37.3 (17.1–55.8)	36.6 ± 8.6	36.8 * (15.1–62.1)	0.3842
Saturated fatty acids (g)	12.3 ± 4.3	11.78 (2.5–23.9)	13.4 ± 4.2	12.9 * (5.8–24.4)	0.1338
Monounsaturated fatty acids (g)	15.0 ± 5.3	14.4 (5.3–26.9)	14.6 ± 4.4	14.4 * (4.4–29.8)	0.6539
Polyunsaturated fatty acids (g)	7.1 ± 3.2	6.4 * (1.5–13.9)	5.6 ± 2.2	5.3 * (2.0–14.1)	0.0071
Cholesterol (mg)	216.5 ± 165.1	163.1 * (25.2–597.8)	171.8 ± 78.8	162.5 * (37.4–419.0)	0.8773
Total carbohydrates (g)	127.6 ± 25.0	125.8 (71.5–186.0)	130.5 ± 23.0	132.9 * (46.9–198.4)	0.2237
Sucrose (g)	18.1 ± 12.0	14.9 * (4.3–75.5)	20.9 ± 10.2	18.6 * (65.8–1.5)	0.0098
Lactose (g)	9.4 ± 5.9	8.8 * (0.0–37.6)	7.5 ± 3.8	7.6 * (0.0–23.4)	0.0205
Starch (g)	60.4 ± 24.6	60.2 * (15.7–128.2)	69.1 ± 16.9	72.5 * (27.1–109.8)	0.0015
Fiber (g)	17.3 ± 7.1	16.6 * (5.6–40.7)	12.5 ± 4.4	11.9 * (6.2–27.4)	<0.0001

* Nonparametric distribution (verified using the Shapiro-Wilk test; $p < 0.05$); ** compared using the t-Student test (for parametric distributions) or the U Mann-Whitney test (for nonparametric distributions).

Comparison of minerals intake in groups of junior health professionals from Poland and Croatia is presented in Table 3. In the analyzed group, Polish women, while compared with Croatian ones, were characterized by a higher potassium ($p = 0.0059$), phosphorus ($p = 0.0002$), iron ($p = 0.0062$), magnesium ($p < 0.0001$), zinc ($p = 0.0086$), copper ($p = 0.0001$), manganese ($p = 0.0166$), and iodine intake ($p = 0.0001$).

Comparison of minerals intake per 1000 kcal in groups of junior health professionals from Poland and Croatia is presented in Table 4. In the analyzed group, Polish women, while compared with Croatian ones, were characterized by a higher potassium ($p = 0.0007$), calcium ($p = 0.0111$), phosphorus ($p < 0.0001$), iron ($p < 0.0001$), magnesium ($p < 0.0001$), zinc ($p < 0.0001$), copper ($p < 0.0001$), manganese ($p = 0.0015$), and iodine intake ($p < 0.0001$).

Comparison of vitamins intake in groups of junior health professionals from Poland and Croatia is presented in Table 5. In the analyzed group, Polish women, while compared with Croatian ones, were characterized by a higher riboflavin ($p = 0.0063$), vitamin B_6 ($p = 0.0040$), folate ($p = 0.0027$), vitamin A ($p = 0.0008$), and vitamin E intake ($p = 0.0119$). At the same time, they were characterized by lower intake of niacin ($p = 0.0043$).

Table 3. Comparison of minerals intake in groups of junior health professionals from Poland and Croatia.

	Polish Group		Croatian Group		p **
	Mean ± SD	Median (Range)	Mean ± SD	Median (Range)	
Sodium (mg)	1229.6 ± 662.5	1087.0 * (289.9–3179.8)	1342.5 ± 723.1	1218.9 * (125.7–3589.7)	0.3883
Potassium (mg)	3242.4 ± 1003.1	3239.8 * (1215.9–5279.2)	2812.1 ± 979.3	2602.2 (1327.2–7484.2)	0.0059
Calcium (mg)	751.7 ± 294.8	746.8 (194.2–1640.2)	700.1 ± 315.7	647.3 * (168.5–1469.0)	0.2324
Phosphorus (mg)	1480.9 ± 419.6	1473.6 (575.9–3010.1)	1257.2 ± 422.5	1163.2 * (588.3–3273.0)	0.0002
Iron (mg)	12.1 ± 5.2	10.9 * (4.3–25.0)	10.1 ± 4.1	9.2 * (4.7–31.1)	0.0062
Magnesium (mg)	360.1 ± 128.9	347.0 * (154.1–738.3)	280.8 ± 134.0	260.2 * (129.4–958.6)	<0.0001
Zinc (mg)	10.3 ± 3.6	9.7 * (3.7–22.0)	8.9 ± 3.2	8.4 * (4.2–21.3)	0.0086
Copper (mg)	1.4 ± 0.6	1.2 * (0.5–3.4)	1.0 ± 0.4	1.0 * (0.5–2.7)	0.0001
Manganese (mg)	4.7 ± 1.9	4.3 * (1.5–10.3)	4.0 ± 2.4	3.8 * (0.8–15.5)	0.0166
Iodine (mg)	71.4 ± 62.2	47.6 * (3.4–302.2)	41.4 ± 32.1	31.6 * (6.3–193.6)	0.0001

* Nonparametric distribution (verified using the Shapiro-Wilk test; $p < 0.05$); ** compared using the t-Student test (for parametric distributions) or the U Mann-Whitney test (for nonparametric distributions).

Table 4. Comparison of minerals intake per 1000 kcal in groups of junior health professionals from Poland and Croatia.

	Polish Group		Croatian Group		p **
	Mean ± SD	Median (Range)	Mean ± SD	Median (Range)	
Sodium (mg)	823.4 ± 370.4	745.5 * (238.1–1810.1)	834.9 ± 299.3	819.3 (175.0–1483.1)	0.6110
Potassium (mg)	2241.4 ± 701.1	3229.8 * (1220.2–3960.3)	1850.0 ± 514.3	1815.3 * (928.2–3314.3)	0.0007
Calcium (mg)	525.5 ± 209.5	503.8 (123.5–1161.6)	440.3 ± 133.5	437.3 (151.3–743.2)	0.0111
Phosphorus (mg)	1016.4 ± 236.5	1007.0 (366.3–1676.0)	811.2 ± 148.2	802.5 * (569.4–1312.3)	<0.0001
Iron (mg)	8.4 ± 3.7	7.4 * (2.9–26.1)	6.451.6	6.1 * (4.2–12.0)	< 0.0001
Magnesium (mg)	249.5 ± 92.6	224.4 * (111.1–653.0)	182.3 ± 48.6	176.7 * (106.9–332.2)	<0.0001
Zinc (mg)	7.0 ± 1.9	6.9 (2.4–12.0)	5.7 ± 1.2	5.7 * (3.6–12.0)	<0.0001
Copper (mg)	1.0 ± 0.4	0.9 * (0.4–2.0)	0.7 ± 0.2	0.7 * (0.4–1.3)	<0.0001
Manganese (mg)	3.2 ± 1.3	3.0 * (1.1–7.3)	2.6 ± 1.0	2.5 (0.8–5.4)	0.0015
Iodine (mg)	49.2 ± 2.9	36.2 * (2.4–218.2)	27.9 ± 25.0	19.2 * (3.0–126.0)	<0.0001

* Nonparametric distribution (verified using the Shapiro-Wilk test; $p < 0.05$); ** compared using the t-Student test (for parametric distributions) or the U Mann-Whitney test (for nonparametric distributions).

Table 5. Comparison of vitamins intake in groups of junior health professionals from Poland and Croatia.

	Polish Group		Croatian Group		p **
	Mean ± SD	Median (Range)	Mean ± SD	Median (Range)	
Thiamine (mg)	1.1 ± 0.4	1.1 * (0.4–2.9)	1.2 ± 0.5	1.12 * (0.5–3.0)	0.8212
Riboflavin (mg)	1.8 ± 0.6	1.8 (0.4–3.2)	1.6 ± 0.6	1.5 * (0.7–3.4)	0.0063
Niacin (mg)	14.9 ± 6.5	13.9 * (4.2–38.6)	17.82 ± 8.2	16.8 * (5.0–50.1)	0.0043
Vitamin B_6 (mg)	2.2 ± 0.7	2.0 (0.6–4.1)	1.9 ± 0.8	1.7 * (0.9–5.4)	0.0040
Folate (ug)	380.7 ± 157.9	370.9 (124.0–776.6)	310.6 ± 137.9	284.0 * (143.7–891.8)	0.0027
Vitamin B_{12} (ug)	4.2 ± 2.4	3.8 * (0.0–10.3)	3.6 ± 2.1	3.1 * (0.6–11.9)	0.0712
Vitamin A (ug)	1700.9 ± 1599.9	1126.7 * (176.6–9278.2)	939.1 ± 691.8	792.2 * (225.4–3473.4)	0.0008
Vitamin E (mg)	11.9 ± 6.6	10.6 (2.3–35.7)	9.3 ± 4.9	8.4 * (2.6–26.8)	0.0119
Vitamin C (mg)	156.2 ± 114.3	126.5 * (6.2–490.5)	130.7 ± 93.5	101.6 * (18.4–229.9)	0.2915
Vitamin D (ug)	3.1 ± 4.0	1.8 * (0.0–26.2)	2.4 ± 2.2	1.9 * (0.1–12.4)	0.6814

* Nonparametric distribution (verified using the Shapiro-Wilk test; $p < 0.05$); ** compared using the t-Student test (for parametric distributions) or the U Mann-Whitney test (for nonparametric distributions).

Comparison of vitamins intake per 1000 kcal in groups of junior health professionals from Poland and Croatia is presented in Table 6. In the analyzed group, Polish women, while compared with Croatian ones, were characterized by a higher riboflavin ($p < 0.0001$), vitamin B_6 ($p = 0.0011$), folate ($p = 0.0006$), vitamin B_{12} ($p = 0.0074$), vitamin A ($p = 0.0004$), and vitamin E intake ($p = 0.0015$). At the same time, they were characterized by lower intake of niacin ($p = 0.0176$).

Comparison of animal-derived products intake in groups of junior health professionals from Poland and Croatia is presented in Table 7. In the analyzed group, Polish women, while compared with Croatian ones, were characterized by a higher cottage cheese ($p = 0.0062$), but lower cold cuts intake ($p = 0.0023$).

Comparison of animal-derived products intake per 1000 kcal in groups of junior health professionals from Poland and Croatia is presented in Table 8. In the analyzed group, Polish women, while compared with Croatian ones, were characterized by a higher cottage cheese ($p = 0.0084$), but lower cold cuts intake ($p = 0.0035$).

Table 6. Comparison of vitamins intake per 1000 kcal in groups of junior health professionals from Poland and Croatia.

	Polish Group		Croatian Group		p **
	Mean ± SD	Median (Range)	Mean ± SD	Median (Range)	
Thiamine (mg)	0.8 ± 0.2	0.8 (0.3–1.7)	0.8 ± 0.2	0.8 (0.4–1.3)	0.7920
Riboflavin (mg)	1.3 ± 0.4	1.2 (0.3–2.1)	1.0 ± 0.2	1.0 * (0.6–1.6)	<0.0001
Niacin (mg)	10.2 ± 4.0	9.4 (4.5–20.9)	11.7 ± 4.3	11.3 * (4.1–23.2)	0.0176
Vitamin B$_6$ (mg)	1.5 ± 0.6	1.5 * (0.7–3.0)	1.3 ± 0.4	1.2 * (0.6–2.5)	0.0011
Folate (ug)	268.8 ± 133.3	235.5 * (83.1–808.0)	204.8 ± 73.8	187.1 * (105.3–497.8)	0.0006
Vitamin B$_{12}$ (ug)	2.9 ± 1.6	2.6 * (0.0–7.5)	2.4 ± 1.4	1.9 * (0.8–8.6)	0.0074
Vitamin A (ug)	1212.9 ± 1191.6	724.3 * (121.1–6699.8)	200.3 ± 77.4	196.4 * (16.3–424.3)	0.0004
Vitamin E (mg)	8.1 ± 3.9	7.8 (1.4–17.2)	6.0 ± 2.4	5.4 * (2.7–13.0)	0.0015
Vitamin C (mg)	156.2 ± 114.3	126.5 * (6.2–490.5)	88.2 ± 60.7	69.4 * (8.1–352.0)	0.1836
Vitamin D (ug)	2.1 ± 2.8	1.3 * (0.0–17.5)	1.6 ± 1.3	1.2 * (0.3–7.3)	0.7204

* Nonparametric distribution (verified using the Shapiro-Wilk test; $p < 0.05$); ** compared using the t-Student test (for parametric distributions) or the U Mann-Whitney test (for nonparametric distributions).

Table 7. Comparison of animal-derived products intake in groups of junior health professionals from Poland and Croatia.

	Polish Group		Croatian Group		p **
	Mean ± SD	Median (Range)	Mean ± SD	Median (Range)	
Milk, dairy beverages (g)	202.2 ± 138.6	200.0 * (0–550)	201.0 ± 130.2	168.5 * (0–550)	0.8966
Cottage cheese (g)	63.5 ± 89.4	33.0 * (0–500)	20.0 ± 30.0	0.0 * (0–134)	0.0062
Hard cheese (g)	9.6 ± 15.8	0.0 * (0–55)	12.5 ± 20.1	3.0 * (0–106)	0.1786
Eggs (g)	46.8 ± 60.5	0.0 * (0–200)	26.6 ± 30.2	17.0 * (0–110)	0.4137
Meat (g)	79.4 ± 70.2	100.0 * (0–300)	99.0 ± 53.2	98.5 * (0–224)	0.0952
Cold cuts (g)	7.6 ± 18.5	0.0 * (0–90)	19.8 ± 31.8	1.0 * (0–134)	0.0023
Fish and fish products (g)	39.4 ± 60.5	0.0 * (0–233)	29.5 ± 40.8	13.0 * (0–167)	0.6745
Butter (g)	3.3 ± 7.1	0.0 * (0–30)	0.9 ± 2.1	0.0 * (0–10)	0.5429
Sour cream (g)	2.6 ± 9.9	0.0 * (0–60)	2.9 ± 11.4	0.0 * (0–60)	0.8212

* Nonparametric distribution (verified using the Shapiro-Wilk test; $p < 0.05$); ** compared using the t-Student test (for parametric distributions) or the U Mann-Whitney test (for nonparametric distributions).

Table 8. Comparison of animal-derived products intake per 1000 kcal in groups of junior health professionals from Poland and Croatia.

	Polish Group		Croatian Group		p **
	Mean ± SD	Median (Range)	Mean ± SD	Median (Range)	
Milk, dairy beverages (g)	147.3 ± 117.2	138.8 * (0–636.6)	132.3 ± 87.6	115.5 * (0–414.8)	0.5682
Cottage cheese (g)	45.5 ± 64.8	22.9 * (0–320.9)	15.0 ± 25.9	0.0 * (0–144.7)	0.0084
Hard cheese (g)	7.0 ± 12.0	0.0 * (0–52.9)	7.5 ± 11.1	2.0 * (0–60.4)	0.2208
Eggs (g)	32.8 ± 42.9	0.0 * (0–142.1)	17.7 ± 21.3	11.6 * (0–107.5)	0.4300
Meat (g)	54.8 ± 47.1	60.3 * (0–162.4)	65.6 ± 24.1	60.1 (0–144.4)	0.1162
Cold cuts (g)	5.3 ± 12.4	0.0 * (0–51.4)	12.5 ± 22.3	0.6 * (0–119.4)	0.0035
Fish and fish products (g)	26.3 ± 40.4	0.0 * (0–168.3)	21.0 ± 28.9	8.9 * (0–104.6)	0.6071
Butter (g)	2.2 ± 4.2	0.0 * (0–18.1)	0.6 ± 1.5	0.0 * (0–9.8)	0.5355
Sour cream (g)	2.2 ± 8.3	0.0 * (0–48.5)	1.8 ± 6.7	0.0 * (0–35.2)	0.8080

* Nonparametric distribution (verified using the Shapiro-Wilk test; $p < 0.05$); ** compared using the t-Student test (for parametric distributions) or the U Mann-Whitney test (for nonparametric distributions).

Comparison of other products intake in groups of junior health professionals from Poland and Croatia is presented in Table 9. In the analyzed group, Polish women, while compared with Croatian ones, were characterized by a higher vegetables ($p = 0.0049$), oil ($p = 0.0238$), nuts ($p = 0.0455$), and jam/honey intake (p = 0.0471). At the same time, they were characterized by lower intake of potatoes (p < 0.0001), chocolate sweets (p = 0.0042), and cakes/cookies (p = 0.0006).

Comparison of other products intake per 1000 kcal in groups of junior health professionals from Poland and Croatia is presented in Table 10. In the analyzed group, Polish women, while compared with Croatian ones, were characterized by a higher vegetables (p = 0.0035), oil (p = 0.0114), nuts (p = 0.0419), and jam/honey intake (p = 0.0425). At the same time, they were characterized by lower intake of potatoes (p < 0.0001), chocolate sweets (p = 0.0041), and cakes/cookies (p = 0.0044).

Table 9. Comparison of other products intake in groups of junior health professionals from Poland and Croatia.

	Polish Group		Croatian Group		p **
	Mean ± SD	Median (Range)	Mean ± SD	Median (Range)	
Vegetables (g)	305.2 ± 230.9	275 * (0–1000)	205.7 ± 151.7	160.0 * (13–810)	0.0049
Legumes (g)	17.5 ± 69.7	0.0 * (0–550)	6.9 ± 24.8	0.0 * (0–200)	0.6952
Fruits (g)	183.8 ± 119.6	152 * (0–540)	193.7 ± 145.3	167.0 * (0–800)	0.9970
Potatoes (g)	31.3 ± 69.1	0.0 * (0–267)	65.9 ± 67.5	50.0 * (0–333)	<0.0001
Bread (g)	69.9 ± 63.6	62.0 * (0–210)	72.8 ± 48.4	65.0 * (0–183)	0.3873
Other cereal products (g)	79.7 ± 57.6	66.0 * (0–270)	87.4 ± 77.8	65.5 * (0–390)	0.9474
Oil (g)	11.1 ± 10.5	10.0 * (0–55)	8.1 ± 11.3	4.5 * (0–63)	0.0238
Margarine (g)	0.0	0.0 * (0–0)	0.1 ± 0.5	0.0 * (0–3)	0.6938
Nuts (g)	14.8 ± 21.0	0.5 * (0–65)	6.7 ± 11.4	0.0 * (0–64)	0.0455
Mushrooms (g)	1.7 ± 10.2	0.0 * (0–70)	1.8 ± 7.3	0.0 * (0–34)	0.7360
Sugar (g)	0.7 ± 3.4	0.0 * (0–20)	0.6 ± 1.7	0.0 * (0–10)	0.5122
Jam and honey (g)	2.8 ± 9.3	0.0 * (0–50)	2.4 ± 5.0	0.0 * (0–32)	0.0471
Chocolate sweets (g)	10.8 ± 29.6	0.0 * (0–133)	11.7 ± 15.6	1.5 * (0–58)	0.0042
Cakes and cookies (g)	18.5 ± 45.3	0.0 * (0–250)	34.1 ± 44.8	20 * (0–234)	0.0006
Alcoholic beverages (g)	4.3 ± 20.7	0.0 * (0–120)	10.7 ± 45.3	0.0 * (0–33)	0.5517
Sweetened beverages (g)	10.3 ± 63.2	0.0 * (0–470)	40.3 ± 143.8	0.0 * (0–1167)	0.0589

* Nonparametric distribution (verified using the Shapiro-Wilk test; p < 0.05); ** compared using the t-Student test (for parametric distributions) or the U Mann-Whitney test (for nonparametric distributions).

Table 10. Comparison of other products intake per 1000 kcal in groups of junior health professionals from Poland and Croatia.

	Polish Group		Croatian Group		p **
	Mean ± SD	Median (Range)	Mean ± SD	Median (Range)	
Vegetables (g)	215.7 ± 168.2	198.3 * (0–839.0)	144.8 ± 119.3	109.1 * (8.4–622.3)	0.0035
Legumes (g)	11.2 ± 45.4	0.0 * (0–361.8)	5.4 ± 18.4	0.0 * (0–144.4)	0.7360
Fruits (g)	133.7 ± 102.2	116.1 * (0–604.9)	128.8 ± 97.7	107.8 * (0–482.9)	0.6203
Potatoes (g)	20.2 ± 43.0	0.0 * (0–165.4)	45.6 ± 49.2	34.4 * (0–217.0)	<0.0001
Bread (g)	45.0 ± 40.2	39.8 * (0–158.6)	46.6 ± 30.0	43.1 * (0–131.0)	0.4278
Other cereal products (g)	53.6 ± 36.3	45.5 * (0–206.4)	54.1 ± 39.6	45.6 * (0–187.6)	0.8124
Oil (g)	7.5 ± 7.0	7.1 * (0–36.8)	4.8 ± 5.8	3.2 * (0–20.8)	0.0114
Margarine (g)	0.0	0.0 * (0–0)	0.1 ± 0.4	0.0 * (0–2.7)	0.6938
Nuts (g)	9.2 ± 12.1	0.5 * (0–44.8)	4.6 ± 8.4	0.0 * (0–45.9)	0.0419
Mushrooms (g)	1.1 ± 6.5	0.0 * (0–40.8)	1.4 ± 5.5	0.0 * (0–26.9)	0.7360
Sugar (g)	0.5 ± 2.1	0.0 * (0–11.4)	0.3 ± 0.9	0.0 * (0–4.4)	0.5231
Jam and honey (g)	1.7 ± 5.4	0.0 * (0–31.8)	1.7 ± 3.6	0.0 * (0–21.5)	0.0425
Chocolate sweets (g)	6.5 ± 17.6	0.0 * (0–82.3)	8.2 ± 11.6	0.9 * (0–53.6)	0.0041
Cakes and cookies (g)	10.8 ± 25.3	0.0 * (0–141.8)	21.2 ± 25.1	15.1 * (0–132.5)	0.0004
Alcoholic beverages (g)	1.9 ± 9.3	0.0 * (0–52.7)	5.9 ± 24.7	0.0 * (0–184.2)	0.5530
Sweetened beverages (g)	6.7 ± 40.9	0.0 * (0–298.9)	18.1 ± 47.2	0.0 * (0–311.7)	0.0599

* Nonparametric distribution (verified using the Shapiro-Wilk test; p < 0.05); ** compared using the t-Student test (for parametric distributions) or the U Mann-Whitney test (for nonparametric distributions).

Comparison of the estimated prevalence of inadequate intake of chosen nutrients, while compared with the reference values [61], in groups of junior health professionals from Poland and Croatia is presented in Table 11. In the analyzed group, for folate (p = 0.0023), in the Polish group there is a lower risk of inadequate intake, while compared with the Croatian one.

Table 11. Comparison of the estimated prevalence of inadequate intake of chosen nutrients, while compared with the reference values [61], in groups of junior health professionals from Poland and Croatia.

Nutrient *	Polish Group		Croatian Group		p **
	Respondents with Inadequate Intake—n (%)	Respondents with Adequate Intake—n (%)	Respondents with Inadequate Intake—n (%)	Respondents with Adequate Intake—n (%)	
Calcium	42 (60%)	28 (40%)	51 (64%)	29 (36%)	0.7616
Iron	15 (21%)	55 (79%)	18 (22%)	52 (78%)	0.6901
Folate	28 (40%)	42 (60%)	53 (67%)	27 (33%)	0.0023
Vitamin B_{12}	9 (13%)	61 (87%)	13 (16%)	67 (84%)	0.7226
Vitamin D	66 (94%)	4 (6%)	79 (99%)	1 (1%)	0.2876

* The following reference values were applied: calcium (800 mg), iron (8.1 mg), folate (320 µg), vitamin B_{12} (2 µg), vitamin D (10 µg), [61]; ** compared using the chi^2 test.

4. Discussion

While comparing the nutritional value of the diets and the intake of products between groups of junior health professionals from Poland and Croatia, a number of differences cropped up. While comparing the estimated prevalence of inadequate dietary intake of chosen nutrients, such differences were stated only for folate; however, in both groups, a number of respondents were characterized by an inadequate dietary intake of other nutrients. It should be mentioned that such a situation results from following an improperly balanced diet [63]. As shown by the Food and Agriculture Organization of the United Nations (FAO) [64], in a properly balanced diet that is based on nutritional recommendations, a healthy individual can easily obtain the recommended intake of a majority of nutrients. Consequently, an inadequate intake of specific nutrients may be treated as an indicator of an improperly balanced diet. FAO [65] further emphasizes that a healthy diet associated with an adequate intake of nutrients may be obtained from various combinations of food products.

4.1. Potential Influence of Health Professional Dietary Habits on Their Patients

While analyzing the nutritional value of the diets of junior health professionals, it must be above all emphasized that they will educate the Polish and Croatian populations about recommended nutritional behaviors in the future. Consequently, their nutritional inadequacies may generate nutritional inadequacies for a number of individuals and may contribute to dietary health risk factors. This is based on the association between personal dietary habits and attitudes toward preventive counseling, which was observed in a group of physicians and medical students [66]. Furthermore, their own improper dietary behaviors may generate a lack of confidence in the ability to counsel patients regarding lifestyle that is commonly observed [67].

Some patients perceive their dietitian as a role model and focus on both the presented recommendations and the body size or shape; therefore, a number of dietitians are aware that they should also follow the same dietary recommendations that they present to their patients [68]. Furthermore, these educators who include information about they themselves following recommended dietary habits are perceived by patients to be not only healthier, but also more believable and motivating than others [69]. Similarly, the review by Lobelo and Quevedo [70] reported that healthcare providers who are physically active are more likely to provide physical counseling for their patients compared to others. Furthermore, they stated that healthcare providers can play an important role by becoming early adopters of physical activity and diet behaviors and, in turn, become role models for their patients and communities [71].

As the presented study was planned to assess the dietary intake of female junior health professionals, their diets were also analyzed from the point of view of future female patients and the diet-related diseases common in this group were analyzed.

4.2. Dietary Risk Factors for Anemia

According to the WHO [72], anemia, in industrialized countries, is diagnosed for one in ten women and for one in four pregnant women. However, the systematic analysis of population-representative data by Stevens et al. [73] indicated, based on hemoglobin concentration, a higher frequency of 29% in nonpregnant women and 38% in pregnant ones. This problem may lead to significant health-related consequences such as increased mortality [74].

In the presented study, a higher intake of iron and folate was observed in the Polish group compared to the Croatian group. Also, such an observation was noted in case of intake of vitamin B_{12} per 1000 kcal. A higher iron and vitamin B_{12} intake for Polish women was observed despite a higher intake of cold cuts (which are within their sources) in Croatian women. However, the frequency of inadequate intake was rather high for both countries. Moreover, a higher frequency of inadequate intake for folate was stated more commonly for Croatian women than Polish ones, that may have resulted from the lower vegetable intake in Croatian women. The observations correspond with the results of other studies indicating inadequate intake of iron, for Polish [75] and Croatian young women [76], as well as of folate, for Polish [77] and Croatian young women [76].

Based on the assessment of intake adequacy, the risk of anemia for young women in both countries is quite high. Furthermore, for Croatia, it may be even higher than that for Poland despite a higher intake of cold cuts. Although the intake of traditional meat products is high in Croatia, corresponding to high intake of cold cuts reported in this study, it mainly results in high fat intake [78]; however, it may not influence iron intake significantly.

4.3. Dietary Risk Factors for Osteoporosis

Osteoporosis is another disease that is commonly more observed in women than men because it is estimated that one in two women, but only one in three men, will experience osteoporotic fractures [79]. However, the prevention of osteoporosis is especially important because progressive bone mass loss is observed after the age of 30 [80], contributing to the high risk for osteoporosis [81].

In the presented study, a higher intake of calcium per 1000 kcal was observed in the Polish group compared to the Croatian group. This may have been associated with a higher cottage cheese intake in Polish women. However, a very low intake was observed for vitamin D in both groups; therefore, for both countries, the frequency of inadequate intake was high. The observations correspond with inadequate intake of calcium, observed for Polish [82] and Croatian young women [83]; however, some studies reported higher intake of calcium in Croatia [84]. Furthermore, the inadequate intake of vitamin D is commonly stated for both Polish [85] and Croatian [86] young women [47].

Based on the conducted assessment of the adequacy of intake, it must be stated that the risk of osteoporosis for young women in both countries is high and comparable, resulting primarily from the inadequate intake of vitamin D. Moreover, as the vitamin D status both in Poland [59] and Croatia [60] is commonly not adequate, due to insufficient sunshine exposure, it must be emphasized that the inadequate vitamin D intake probably is not compensated by the endogenous synthesis. Taking it into account, even if the inadequate intake of calcium is not so common, the risk of osteoporosis must be stated.

Taking into account, that it is stated, that health professionals commonly do not have proper healthy lifestyle behaviors that impact chronic diseases, they are often not prepared properly for preventive counseling with their patients, and do not present dietary recommendation to their patients [86], so the necessary actions should be taken to obtain a properly balanced diet following. It may be stated, that adequate nutritional education is needed, in order to improve their nutritional behaviors, embolden them to educate their patients, and increase the number of patients being counseled.

Although the present study provided new insight for identifying potential dietary health risks for women in Poland and Croatia, some limitations must be noted. For further studies, it would be valuable to conduct similar assessments in groups consisting of other nutritional knowledge providers (including physicians); male educators should also be analyzed. It should be emphasized that, both in

Poland and Croatia, nutritional faculties are not present only in capital cities, so including specialists from other regions would allow us to gain a broader perspective.

5. Conclusions

A number of differences in the nutrients and food products intake between the Polish and the Croatian group of junior health professionals may result in various dietary health risks for women in these countries. For anemia, compared to Polish women, a higher risk may be indicated for Croatian women because of lower iron, folate, and vitamin B_{12} intake, and more common inadequate intake of folate. For osteoporosis, similar risks may be indicated for Polish and Croatian women because of very low vitamin D intake in both countries. Therefore, adequate nutritional education of junior health professionals is necessary.

Author Contributions: Conceptualization, D.G. (Dominika Głąbska), V.R., D.G. (Dominika Guzek); methodology, D.G. (Dominika Głąbska); formal analysis, D.G. (Dominika Głąbska), V.R., D.G. (Dominika Guzek), K.J.; investigation, V.R., K.J., S.B., E.P.; data curation, D.G. (Dominika Głąbska), V.R., D.G. (Dominika Guzek), K.J., S.B., Z.G., E.P.; writing—original draft preparation, D.G. (Dominika Głąbska), V.R., D.G. (Dominika Guzek), K.J., S.B., Z.G., E.P.; writing—review and editing, D.G. (Dominika Głąbska), V.R., D.G. (Dominika Guzek), K.J., S.B., Z.G., E.P.; project administration, D.G. (Dominika Głąbska), V.R.

Funding: The research was financed by the Polish Ministry of Science and Higher Education with funds from the Faculty of Human Nutrition and Consumer Sciences, Warsaw University of Life Sciences (WULS), for scientific research.

Conflicts of Interest: The authors declare no conflict of interest.

References

1. World Health Organization (WHO). Ten Top Issues for Women's Health. Available online: https://www.who.int/life-course/news/commentaries/2015-intl-womens-day/en/ (accessed on 29 August 2019).
2. World Health Organization (WHO). Strategy on women's health and well-being in the WHO European Region. In Proceedings of the Regional Committee for Europe, 66th Session Copenhagen, Copenhagen, Denmark, 12–15 September 2016.
3. Jonas, K.; Crutzen, R.; Krumeich, A.; Roman, N.; van den Borne, B.; Reddy, P. Healthcare workers' beliefs, motivations and behaviours affecting adequate provision of sexual and reproductive healthcare services to adolescents in Cape Town, South Africa: A qualitative study. *BMC Health Serv. Res.* **2018**, *18*, 109. [CrossRef] [PubMed]
4. Cao, R.; Stone, T.E.; Petrini, M.A.; Turale, S. Nurses' perceptions of health beliefs and impact on teaching and practice: A Q-sort study. *Int. Nurs. Rev.* **2018**, *65*, 131–144. [CrossRef] [PubMed]
5. Puhl, R.M.; Gold, J.A.; Luedicke, J.; DePierre, J.A. The effect of physicians' body weight on patient attitudes: Implications for physician selection, trust and adherence to medical advice. *Int. J. Obes.* **2013**, *37*, 1415–1421. [CrossRef] [PubMed]
6. Adamski, M.; Gibson, S.; Leech, M.; Truby, H. Are doctors nutritionists? What is the role of doctors in providing nutrition advice? *Nutr. Bull.* **2018**, *43*, 147–152. [CrossRef]
7. Ahmed, A.; Jabbar, A.; Zuberi, L.; Islam, M.; Shamim, K. Diabetes related knowledge among residents and nurses: A multicenter study in Karachi, Pakistan. *BMC Endocr. Disord.* **2012**, *12*, 18. [CrossRef] [PubMed]
8. Findlow, L.A.; McDowell, J.R.S. Determining registered nurses' knowledge of diabetes mellitus. *J. Diabetes Nurs.* **2002**, *6*, 170–175.
9. Irazusta, A.; Gil, S.; Ruiz, F.; Gondra, J.; Jauregi, A.; Irazusta, J.; Gil, J. Exercise, physical fitness, and dietary habits of first-year female nursing students. *Biol. Res. Nurs.* **2006**, *7*, 175–186. [CrossRef] [PubMed]
10. Albuquerque, A.G.; Pontes, C.M.; Osorio, M.M. Knowledge of educators and dieticians on food and nutrition education in the school environment. *Rev. Nutr.* **2013**, *26*, 291–300. [CrossRef]
11. Schaefer, J.T.; Zullo, M.D. US Registered Dietitian Nutritionists' Knowledge and Attitudes of Intuitive Eating and Use of Various Weight Management Practices. *J. Acad. Nutr. Diet.* **2017**, *117*, 1419–1428. [CrossRef]
12. Winham, D.M.; Hutchins, A.M.; Thompson, S.V.; Dougherty, M.K. Arizona Registered Dietitians Show Gaps in Knowledge of Bean Health Benefits. *Nutrients* **2018**, *10*, 52. [CrossRef]

13. Fredericks, S.C.; Hamilton, C. Dietary Intakes of Registered Dietitians. *J. Amer. Diet. Ass.* **1996**, *96*, 25. [CrossRef]
14. Kowalze, K.; Turyk, Z.; Drywień, M. Nutrition of students from dietetics profile education in the Siedlce University of Natural Sciences and Humanities compared with students from other academic centres. *Rocz. Panstw. Zakl. Hig.* **2016**, *67*, 51–58.
15. Mealha, V.; Ferreira, C.; Guerra, I.; Ravasco, P. Students of dietetics & nutrition; a high risk group for eating disorders? *Nutr. Hosp.* **2013**, *28*, 1558–1566. [CrossRef] [PubMed]
16. Almajwal, A.M. Stress, shift duty, and eating behavior among nurses in Central Saudi Arabia. *Saudi Med. J.* **2016**, *37*, 191–198. [CrossRef] [PubMed]
17. Głąbska, D.; Włodarek, D. Analysis of the declared nutritional behaviours in a group of diabetology nurses educating patients about diabetes diet therapy. *Rocz. Panstw. Zakl. Hig.* **2015**, *66*, 345–351. [PubMed]
18. Bleich, S.N.; Bennett, W.L.; Gudzune, K.A.; Cooper, L.A. Impact of physician BMI on obesity care and beliefs. *Obesity* **2012**, *20*, 999–1005. [CrossRef] [PubMed]
19. Gupta, S. Dietary Practices and Nutritional Profile of Female Nurses from Government Hospitals in Delhi, India. *Iran. J. Nurs. Midwifery Res.* **2017**, *22*, 348–353. [CrossRef] [PubMed]
20. Miller, S.K.; Alpert, P.T.; Cross, C.L. Overweight and obesity in nurses, advanced practice nurses, and nurse educators. *J. Am. Acad. Nurse Pract.* **2008**, *20*, 259–265. [CrossRef]
21. Tremelling, K.; Sandon, L.; Vega, G.L.; McAdams, C.J. Orthorexia Nervosa and Eating Disorder Symptoms in Registered Dietitian Nutritionists in the United States. *J. Acad. Nutr. Diet.* **2017**, *117*, 1612–1617. [CrossRef]
22. Asil, E.; Sürücüoğlu, M.S. Orthorexia Nervosa in Turkish Dietitians. *Ecol. Food Nutr.* **2015**, *54*, 303–313. [CrossRef]
23. Przeor, M.; Goluch-Koniuszy, Z. Ocena stanu odżywienia oraz sposobu żywienia pielęgniarek będących w okresie okołomenopauzalnym pracujących w systemie zmianowym. [Evaluation of nutrition and diet of nurses during perimenopause while working in a shift system]. *Prob. Hig. Epidemiol.* **2013**, *94*, 797–801. (In Polish)
24. Stefańska, E.; Ostrowska, L.; Radziejewska, I.; Kardasz, M. Sposób żywienia studentów Uniwersytetu Medycznego w Białymstoku w zależności od miejsca zamieszkania w trakcie studiów. [Mode of nutrition in students of the Medical University of Bialystok according to their place of residence during the study period]. *Prob. Hig. Epidemiol.* **2010**, *91*, 585–590. (In Polish)
25. Kubiak, J.; Różańska, D.; Regulska-Ilow, B.; Kawicka, A.; Salomon, A.; Konikowska, K. Ocena jakości diet studentek dietetyki na podstawie wskaźnika DQI (Diet Quality Index). [Assessment of the quality of the dietetics students diets based on the diet quality index (DQI)]. *Bromat. Chem. Toksykol.* **2015**, *3*, 429–432. (In Polish)
26. Warner, M.J.; Kamran, M.T. Anemia, Iron Deficiency. Available online: https://www.ncbi.nlm.nih.gov/books/NBK448065/ (accessed on 29 August 2019).
27. Alswat, K.A. Gender Disparities in Osteoporosis. *J. Clin. Med. Res.* **2017**, *9*, 382–387. [CrossRef]
28. Toxqui, L.; Vaquero, M.P. Chronic iron deficiency as an emerging risk factor for osteoporosis: A hypothesis. *Nutrients* **2015**, *7*, 2324–2344. [CrossRef]
29. World Health Organization (WHO). Haemoglobin Concentrations for the Diagnosis of Anaemia and Assessment of Severity. Available online: https://www.who.int/vmnis/indicators/haemoglobin.pdf (accessed on 29 August 2019).
30. World Health Organization (WHO). Focusing on Anaemia—Towards an Integrated Approach for Effective Anaemia Control. Available online: https://www.who.int/nutrition/publications/micronutrients/WHOandUNICEF_statement_anaemia/en (accessed on 29 August 2019).
31. World Health Organization (WHO). *The Global Prevalence of Anaemia in 2011*; World Health Organization: Geneva, Switzerland, 2015.
32. DeLoughery, T.G. Iron Deficiency Anemia. *Med. Clin. N. Am.* **2017**, *101*, 319–332. [CrossRef]
33. O'Malley, E.G.; Cawley, S.; Kennedy, R.A.K.; Reynolds, C.M.E.; Molloy, A.; Turner, M.J. Maternal anaemia and folate intake in early pregnancy. *J. Public Health* **2018**, *40*, 296–302. [CrossRef]
34. Green, R. Vitamin B12 deficiency from the perspective of a practicing hematologist. *Blood* **2017**, *129*, 2603–2611. [CrossRef]

35. World Health Organization, Centers for Disease Control and Prevention. Assessing the Iron Status of Populations. Available online: https://www.who.int/nutrition/publications/micronutrients/anaemia_iron_deficiency/9789241596107/en/ (accessed on 4 August 2019).
36. International Osteoporosis Foundation (IOF). Facts and Statistics. Available online: https://www.iofbonehealth.org/facts-statistics (accessed on 29 August 2019).
37. Svedbom, A.; Hernlund, E.; Ivergård, M.; Compston, J.; Cooper, C.; Stenmark, J.; McCloskey, E.V.; Jönsson, B.; Kanis, J.A.; EU Review Panel of IOF. Osteoporosis in the European Union: A compendium of country-specific reports. *Arch. Osteoporos.* **2013**, *8*, 137. [CrossRef]
38. Cvijetić Avdagić, S.; Grazio, S.; Kaštelan, D.; Koršić, M. Epidemiologija osteoporoze. *Arhiv. za higijenu rada i toksikologiju* **2007**, *58*, 13–18. [CrossRef]
39. Giljević, Z. Znaaj problema osteoporoze u Hrvatskoj. In Proceedings of the Svjetski Dan Osteoporoze, Zagreb, Croatia, 20–22 October 2005; Sveučilište u Zagrebu: Zagreb, Croatia, 2005.
40. Grazio, S.; Korsić, M.; Jajić, I. Prevalence of vertebral fractures in an urban population in Croatia aged fifty and older. *Wien. Klin. Wochenschr.* **2005**, *117*, 42–47. [CrossRef]
41. Tai, V.; Leung, W.; Grey, A.; Reid, I.R.; Bolland, M.J. Calcium intake and bone mineral density: Systematic review and meta-analysis. *BMJ* **2015**, *351*, 4183. [CrossRef]
42. Laird, E.; Ward, M.; McSorley, E.; Strain, J.J.; Wallace, J. Vitamin D and bone health: Potential mechanisms. *Nutrients* **2010**, *2*, 693–724. [CrossRef]
43. Drewnowski, A.; Dwyer, J.; King, J.C.; Weaver, C.M. A proposed nutrient density score that includes food groups and nutrients to better align with dietary guidance. *Nutr. Rev.* **2019**, *77*, 404–416. [CrossRef]
44. Metges, C.C.; Barth, C.A. Metabolic consequences of a high dietary-protein intake in adulthood: Assessment of the available evidence. *J. Nutr.* **2000**, *130*, 886–889. [CrossRef]
45. Springmann, M.; Wiebe, K.; Mason-D'Croz, D.; Sulser, T.B.; Rayner, M.; Scarborough, P. Health and nutritional aspects of sustainable diet strategies and their association with environmental impacts: A global modelling analysis with country-level detail. *Lancet Planet. Health* **2018**, *2*, 451–461. [CrossRef]
46. Głąbska, D.; Guzek, D.; Ślązak, J.; Włodarek, D. Assessing the Validity and Reproducibility of an Iron Dietary Intake Questionnaire Conducted in a Group of Young Polish Women. *Nutrients* **2017**, *9*, 199. [CrossRef]
47. Głąbska, D.; Uroić, V.; Guzek, D.; Pavić, E.; Bival, S.; Jaworska, K.; Giljević, Z.; Lange, E. The Possibility of Applying the Vitamin D Brief Food Frequency Questionnaire as a Tool for a Country with No Vitamin D Data in Food Composition Tables. *Nutrients* **2018**, *10*, 1278. [CrossRef]
48. Kunachowicz, H.; Nadolna, J.; Przygoda, B.; Iwanow, K. (Eds.) *Food Composition Tables*; PZWL: Warsaw, Poland, 2005. (In Polish)
49. Głąbska, D.; Jusinska, M. Analysis of the choice of food products and the energy value of diets of female middle- and long-distance runners depending on the self-assessment of their nutritional habits. *Rocz. Panstw. Zakl. Hig.* **2018**, *69*, 155–163.
50. Committee on the Consequences of Sodium Reduction in Populations; Food and Nutrition Board; Board on Population Health and Public Health Practice; Institute of Medicine; Strom, B.L.; Yaktine, A.L.; Oria, M. (Eds.) *Sodium Intake in Populations: Assessment of Evidence*; National Academies Press: Washington, DC, USA, 2013. Available online: https://www.ncbi.nlm.nih.gov/books/NBK201516/ (accessed on 5 September 2019).
51. Chen, S.L.; Dahl, C.; Meyer, H.E.; Madar, A.A. Estimation of Salt Intake Assessed by 24-Hour Urinary Sodium Excretion among Somali Adults in Oslo, Norway. *Nutrients* **2018**, *10*, 900. [CrossRef]
52. Cogswell, M.E.; Maalouf, J.; Elliott, P.; Loria, C.M.; Patel, S.; Bowman, B.A. Use of Urine Biomarkers to Assess Sodium Intake: Challenges and Opportunities. *Annu. Rev. Nutr.* **2015**, *35*, 349–387. [CrossRef]
53. Vega-Vega, O.; Fonseca-Correa, J.I.; Mendoza-De la Garza, A.; Rincón-Pedrero, R.; Espinosa-Cuevas, A.; Baeza-Arias, Y.; Dary, O.; Herrero-Bervera, B.; Nieves-Anaya, I.; Correa-Rotter, R. Contemporary Dietary Intake: Too Much Sodium, Not Enough Potassium, yet Sufficient Iodine: The SALMEX Cohort Results. *Nutrients* **2018**, *10*, 816. [CrossRef]
54. Johnson-Wimbley, T.D.; Graham, D.Y. Diagnosis and management of iron deficiency anemia in the 21st century. *Therap. Adv. Gastroenterol.* **2011**, *4*, 177–184. [CrossRef]
55. Sunyecz, J.A. The use of calcium and vitamin D in the management of osteoporosis. *Ther. Clin. Risk Manag.* **2008**, *4*, 827–836. [CrossRef]
56. European Food Safety Authority (EFSA). Scientific opinion on the tolerable upper intake level of vitamin D. *EFSA J.* **2012**, *10*, 2813.

57. Van Schoor, N.M.; Lips, P. Worldwide vitamin D status. *Best Pract. Res. Clin. Endocrinol. Metab.* **2011**, *25*, 671–680. [CrossRef]
58. Cashman, K.D.; Dowling, K.G.; Škrabáková, Z.; Gonzalez-Gross, M.; Valtueña, J.; De Henauw, S.; Moreno, L.; Damsgaard, C.T.; Michaelsen, K.F.; Mølgaard, C.; et al. Vitamin D deficiency in Europe: Pandemic? *Am. J. Clin. Nutr.* **2016**, *103*, 1033–1044. [CrossRef]
59. Płudowski, P.; Ducki, C.; Konstantynowicz, J.; Jaworski, M. Vitamin D status in Poland. *Pol. Arch. Med. Wewn.* **2016**, *126*, 530–539. [CrossRef]
60. Colić Barić, I.; Keser, I.; Bituh, M.; Rumbak, I.; Rumora Samarin, I.; Beljan, K.; Gežin, L.; Lazinica, G. *Vitamin D Status and Prevalence of Inadequacy in Croatian Population*; Book of Abstracts of 4th International Congress of Nutritionists: Zadar, Hrvatska, 2016; p. 97.
61. Nutrient Recommendations: Dietary Reference Intakes (DRI). Available online: https://ods.od.nih.gov/Health_Information/Dietary_Reference_Intakes.aspx (accessed on 4 August 2019).
62. Institute of Medicine. *Dietary Reference Intakes: Applications in Dietary Assessment*; The National Academies Press: Washington, DC, USA, 2000. Available online: https://www.nap.edu/catalog/9956/dietary-reference-intakes-applications-in-dietary-assessment (accessed on 4 August 2019). [CrossRef]
63. Shao, A.; Drewnowski, A.; Willcox, D.C.; Krämer, L.; Lausted, C.; Eggersdorfer, M.; Mathers, J.; Bell, J.D.; Randolph, R.K.; Witkamp, R.; et al. Optimal nutrition and the ever-changing dietary landscape: A conference report. *Eur. J. Nutr.* **2017**, *56*, 1–21. [CrossRef]
64. Food and Agriculture Organization of the United Nations (FAO). Food-Based Dietary Guidelines. Available online: http://www.fao.org/nutrition/education/food-dietary-guidelines/en/ (accessed on 29 August 2019).
65. Food and Agriculture Organization of the United Nations (FAO). Food-Based Approaches to Meeting Vitamin and Mineral Needs. Available online: http://www.fao.org/3/y2809e/y2809e08.htm (accessed on 29 August 2019).
66. Duperly, J.; Lobelo, F.; Segura, C.; Sarmiento, F.; Herrera, D.; Sarmiento, O.L.; Frank, E. The association between Colombian medical students' healthy personal habits and a positive attitude toward preventive counseling: Cross-sectional analyses. *BMC Public Health* **2009**, *9*, 218. [CrossRef]
67. Howe, M.; Leidel, A.; Krishnan, S.M.; Weber, A.; Rubenfire, M.; Jackson, E.A. Patient-related diet and exercise counseling: Do providers' own lifestyle habits matter? *Prev. Cardiol.* **2010**, *13*, 180–185. [CrossRef]
68. Cant, R.P. Communication competence within dietetics: dietitians' and clients' views about the unspoken dialogue—the impact of personal presentation. *J. Hum. Nutr. Diet.* **2009**, *22*, 504–510. [CrossRef]
69. Frank, E.; Breyan, J.; Elon, L. Physician disclosure of healthy personal behaviors improves credibility and ability to motivate. *Arch. Fam. Med.* **2000**, *9*, 287–290. [CrossRef]
70. Lobelo, F.; de Quevedo, I.G. The Evidence in Support of Physicians and Health Care Providers as Physical Activity Role Models. *Am. J. Lifestyle Med.* **2016**, *10*, 36–52. [CrossRef]
71. Lobelo, F.; de Quevedo, I.G. Weighing in on residents' body mass index: A teachable moment for physicians and patients alike? *J. Grad. Med. Educ.* **2013**, *5*, 521–523. [CrossRef]
72. World Health Organization (WHO). *Iron Deficiency Anaemia Assessment, Prevention and Control a Guide for Programme Managers*; World Health Organization: Geneva, Switzerland, 2001.
73. Stevens, G.A.; Finucane, M.M.; De-Regil, L.M.; Paciorek, C.J.; Flaxman, S.R.; Branca, F.; Peña-Rosas, J.P.; Bhutta, Z.A.; Ezzati, M.; Nutrition Impact Model Study Group (Anaemia). Global, regional, and national trends in haemoglobin concentration and prevalence of total and severe anaemia in children and pregnant and non-pregnant women for 1995-2011: A systematic analysis of population-representative data. *Lancet Glob. Health* **2013**, *1*, 16–25. [CrossRef]
74. Khaskheli, M.N.; Baloch, S.; Sheeba, A.; Baloch, S.; Khaskheli, F.K. Iron deficiency anaemia is still a major killer of pregnant women. *Pak. J. Med. Sci.* **2016**, *32*, 630–634. [CrossRef]
75. Skolmowska, D.; Głąbska, D. Analysis of Heme and Non-Heme Iron Intake and Iron Dietary Sources in Adolescent Menstruating Females in a National Polish Sample. *Nutrients* **2019**, *11*, 1049. [CrossRef]
76. Satalic, Z.; Baric, I.C.; Keser, I. Diet quality in Croatian university students: Energy, macronutrient and micronutrient intakes according to gender. *Int. J. Food Sci. Nutr.* **2007**, *58*, 398–410. [CrossRef]
77. Głąbska, D.; Książek, A.; Guzek, D. Development and Validation of the Brief Folate-Specific Food Frequency Questionnaire for Young Women's Diet Assessment. *Int. J. Environ. Res. Public Health* **2017**, *14*, 1574. [CrossRef]

78. Lešić, T.; Krešić, G.; Koprivnjak, O.; Kovečević, D.; Gross-Bošković, A.; Sokolić, D.; Jurković, M.; Pleadin, J. Estimation of dietary fat intake via the consumption of traditional meat products. *Croat. J. Food Technol. Biotechnol. Nutr.* **2016**, *11*, 138–144.
79. Ross, P.D. Osteoporosis. Frequency, consequences, and risk factors. *Arch. Intern. Med.* **1996**, *156*, 1399–1411. [CrossRef]
80. Benjamin, R.M. Bone health: Preventing osteoporosis. *J. Am. Diet. Assoc.* **2010**, *110*, 498. [CrossRef]
81. Osterhoff, G.; Morgan, E.F.; Shefelbine, S.J.; Karim, L.; McNamara, L.M.; Augat, P. Bone mechanical properties and changes with osteoporosis. *Injury* **2016**, *2*, 11–20. [CrossRef]
82. Lewiński, A.; Skowrońska-Jóźwiak, E. Calcium and vitamin D supply in Polish population—facts and myths. *Ann. Agric. Environ. Med.* **2014**, *21*, 455–456.
83. Mandić-Puljek, M.; Mandić, M.L.; Perl, A.; Kenjerić, D. Calcium intake, food sources and seasonal variations in eastern Croatia. *Coll. Antropol.* **2005**, *29*, 503–507.
84. Douglas, C.C.; Rumbak, I.; Barić, I.C.; Kovačina, M.; Piasek, M.; Ilich, J.Z. Are new generations of female college-student populations meeting calcium requirements: Comparison of American and Croatian female students. *Nutrients* **2010**, *2*, 599–610. [CrossRef]
85. Wyka, J.; Żechałko-Czajkowska, A. Vitamins and minerals in diets of first year female students of the Wrocław university of environmental and life sciences. *Pol. J. Food Nutr. Sci.* **2008**, *58*, 131–137.
86. Hidalgo, K.D.; Mielke, G.I.; Parra, D.C.; Lobelo, F.; Simões, E.J.; Gomes, G.O.; Florindo, A.A.; Bracco, M.; Moura, L.; Brownson, R.C.; et al. Health promoting practices and personal lifestyle behaviors of Brazilian health professionals. *BMC Public Health* **2016**, *16*, 1114. [CrossRef]

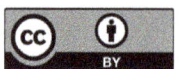

© 2019 by the authors. Licensee MDPI, Basel, Switzerland. This article is an open access article distributed under the terms and conditions of the Creative Commons Attribution (CC BY) license (http://creativecommons.org/licenses/by/4.0/).

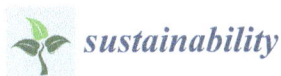

Article

Research on the Efficiency of Local Government Health Expenditure in China and Its Spatial Spillover Effect

Mengying Wang and Chunhai Tao *

School of Statistics, Jiangxi University of Finance and Economics, No. 169, East Shuanggang Road, Nanchang 330013, China; wangmengying@stu.jxufe.cn
* Correspondence: taochunhai@jxufe.edu.cn; Tel.: + 86-0791-8381-6995

Received: 6 March 2019; Accepted: 22 April 2019; Published: 26 April 2019

Abstract: The efficiency of the local government health expenditure (GHE) in China determines the level of public health services. However, the local government does not pay much attention to that efficiency, though the scale of local GHE is increasing. In this paper, first, we use the data envelopment analysis (DEA) method to measure the static overall efficiency of the local government health expenditure (GHE) in each region of China from 2007 to 2016. Then, based on the spatial statistical theory, global and local spatial Moran's I value is utilized to investigate its spatial correlation and spatial agglomeration phenomenon. Finally, the spatial spillover effect (SSE) of the static overall efficiency of local GHE in each region is measured by constructing a spatial Durbin model (SDM). It is demonstrated that there are significant differences in the efficiency of the local GHE between different regions of China. In addition, it is shown that Moran's I value of the static overall efficiency of the local GHE from 2007 to 2016 is positive. It passed the test of the 5% significance level, indicating that there is a positive spatial correlation between the efficiency of the local GHE and a spatial spillover effect. On the other hand, the decomposition of the SDM reveals that the proportion of GHE to financial expenditure, gross domestic product (GDP) per capita, and population density have a positive effect on the efficiency of the local GHE. Hence, their growth will improve the GHE efficiency in the local region and neighboring regions. In contrast, the proportion of urban population, illiteracy, and fiscal decentralization have a negative effect. Thus, their growth will decrease the GHE efficiency in the local region and neighboring regions. The results are discussed and suggestions are given based on the analysis in this paper. The main contribution of this work is to consider the spatial spillover effect in terms with realistic meaning. The results obtained can be used as a reference for optimizing the structure and improving the efficiency of government health inputs. It breaks the government's GDP-only theory-based assessment system and helps to improve it by assessing the GHE efficiency.

Keywords: government health expenditure (GHE) efficiency; data envelopment analysis (DEA) method; Moran's I value; spatial spillover effect (SSE); spatial Durbin model (SDM)

1. Introduction

For a long time, China has been committed to building an efficient and sustainable social public health system (SPHS). Relevant policies are proposed by the government to improve efficiency and sustainability. Lots of science founding are established to make a substantial contribution to the improvement of public health. In addition, we know that the efficiency of government health expenditure (GHE) and healthcare sustainability can affect each other. However, the current Chinese medical and health services cannot meet the new requirements, that is, the people's growing demand for healthcare, the high quality of health services, and the wide coverage of the medical insurance.

It is also very difficult to achieve the goal of an equal and sustainable healthcare service. Thus, it is important to study the GHE efficiency.

Nowadays, it is difficult and expensive to see a doctor in China, which is an outstanding social issue, and the relationship between doctors and patients is becoming terrible. In this context, the scale and efficiency of the government's social public health services supply have received much attention in all sectors of our society and they also constitute a hot research topic. On the one hand, it is an important perspective for local governments in exploring the causes of the imbalance in the national wealth and livelihood. On the other hand, local governments' insufficient input in social public health services or high-input-low-output (HILO) will also affect its supply efficiency. At present, many scholars have empirically analyzed that local governments have a policy bias toward ignoring public service expenditures in the process of fiscal expenditure [1,2]. However, there is little researche on the HILO problem. With the constraint of the relative lack of public service input in China [3], we need to determine how to improve the efficiency of local government's public service supply, in order to improve the output effect with an equal input, since this plays a decisive role in improving the efficiency of the Chinese public service. In particular, with the increase of local government social public health service input, a slight change in supply efficiency will have a great influence on the achievement of the set goals [4].

In view of this, this paper intends to use the mainstream methods of health economic supply theory and empirical research to analyze the input and output of the government's social public health service. Then, we measure the government's health expenditure efficiency in different regions of China, based on the spatial correlated test and spatial panel measurement model. According to the results of the empirical analysis, some suggestions are proposed to help design the government's new health input mechanism, which can accelerate the construction of a healthy China, improve the national health policy, and deepen the reform of the medical and health system.

2. Literature Review

Since the data envelopment analysis (DEA) method was proposed by Farrell in 1957 [5], and developed by Charnes, Cooper, and Rhodes (CCR) in 1978 [6], the quantitative evaluation theory and empirical research methods of local government social public health service supply efficiency have made great progress in the past 30 years. For example, Afonso and Fernandes (2006) used the DEA two-step analysis method to study the efficiency and influencing factors of local GHEs in Europe and Portugal [7]. Hadad et al. (2013) used the DEA estimation model to estimate the efficiency of the healthcare system and found that, in the Organization for Economic Co-operation and Development (OECD) countries, the number of stable healthcare systems is higher [8]. On the other hand, many Chinese scholars have also conducted some related research. Han and Miao (2010) used the DEA-Tobit two-stage analysis framework to measure the efficiency and influencing factors of GHEs in various provinces or cities in China [9]. Luo (2012) used the DEA-Bootstrap two-stage analysis framework to measure the efficiency of Chinese local fiscal expenditures and their influencing factors [10]. Guan et al. (2014) used the DEA four-stage analysis framework to measure the efficiency of the social public healthcare input in 30 provinces in China and the results show that the provincial social public health expenditure has an annual efficiency loss of 29.5% [11]. Jin and Song (2012) used the DEA and Malmquist productivity index to analyze the differences in government health expenditure efficiency among different regions in China [12]. Thus, in terms of evaluation methods, DEA solves the difficulty by integrating the efficiency of different project units and multiple-input-multiple-output (MIMO), so that it is easy to compare the efficiency values of different projects.

There is no typical academic and practical method to simply measure the supply efficiency of the government public health service. The most important thing to do is explore how to improve the efficiency of government health expenditure. It is found from the existing literature that scholars mainly pay attention to the evaluation of social public health expenditure efficiency, ignoring the research on the efficiency of regional public health expenditure. However, the level of economic and social development among different regions is obviously different. We need to consider the regional disparities in the calculation of the expenditure efficiency of different regions. In 2009, as a Chinese policy goal, the improvement of the utilization of health resources in the new healthcare reform was clearly proposed. Nowadays, with the increasing convenience of social transportation, the sharing of health resources among different regions is more convenient and the spatial nature of medical and health services is more obvious. This makes it more practical to study the efficiency of healthcare utilization and we can propose some policy suggestions to improve government supply efficiency based on this study.

Some scholars have studied the spatiality of government health expenditures and most studies show that the allocation of health resources in China is spatial. Wang et al. (2015) pointed out that the efficiency of health resources is a multi-dimensional and comprehensive problem closely related to factors, such as the economy, population, and regional development [13]. At the same time, the combination of traditional statistical methods and spatial statistical methods can better reveal the advantages and disadvantages of the health field, with a spatial distribution [13]. Han et al. (2016) believed that the total allocation of health resources in Chinese provinces or cities is basically consistent with the economic development of the regions [14]. Gu (2014) pointed out that when we study the allocation of health support areas, we should not only investigate the characteristics and needs of local areas, but also consider the influence of neighboring areas [15].

On the one hand, many scholars have conducted research on the output indicators in studying the efficiency of GHE. Retzlaff-Roberts (2004) [16] and Hadad et al. (2013) [8] selected life expectancy and infant mortality (survival) as output indicators. Liu et al. (2014) [17] selected the number of health institutions, health personnel and beds as intermediate output indicators. The number of outpatients and inpatients, emergency mortality, and observation room mortality were considered as final output indicators. Xiao al. (2014) [18] selected maternal mortality and infant mortality as output indicators.

On the other hand, scholars have conducted a lot of research on the factors affecting the efficiency of GHE. Most research starts from the economic, social, and political factors. For example, Tu (2012) pointed out that the factors that have a great impact on hospital efficiency include the fiscal decentralization, proportion of GHE, urbanization level, density of medical institutions, and medical technology level. Among them, only the fiscal decentralization, proportion of GHE, and medical technology level were considered to be the major factors affecting the efficiency of primary healthcare institutions [19]. Li and Wang (2015) conducted a study on the efficiency of local GHEs. The results showed that there were obvious regional differences in the efficiency of local GHEs during the sample period. The main factors affecting efficiency include the fiscal decentralization, household registration system, healthcare reform, urbanization level, economic development level, population density, and education level [20].

Among the existing research, many scholars have conducted fruitful research on the efficiency of GHE. Relevant research has a strong reference effect in the improvement of the supply efficiency of local governments' public health services in China. However, the characteristics of social public health services make it difficult to measure local governments' supply. Thus, it has not yet formed a comprehensive, consistent, and general evaluation system, methods, indicators, and research conclusions. In addition, the existing literature has the following limitations:

First, the discussion on the efficiency of GHE in the existing literature is relatively simple, if the low efficiency, caused by the uneven allocation of health resources, is not considered.

Secondly, due to the difficulty associated with accurately evaluating government health inputs and outputs, most scholars choose life expectancy and child mortality as output variables in studying the efficiency of GHE. However, health resources, such as the number of institutional beds and technicians, are the most direct outputs of GHE.

Finally, the spillover effect of health resource utilization efficiency has not been considered in the existing literature in studying the efficiency of GHE. Therefore, due to the special nature of public health services, there are still no comprehensive, consistent, general evaluation systems, methods, indicators, and research conclusions, though many scholars have conducted a lot of research on the efficiency of GHE.

3. Methods and Materials

3.1. Study Settings and Potential Data Sources

The research object of this paper was 31 provinces, municipalities directly under the central government and autonomous regions in China. The relevant indicator data of each region from 2007 to 2016 were obtained from the China Statistical Yearbook [21], China Health Statistical Yearbook [22] and China Financial Yearbook [23]. The geographical distance between provincial capitals and cities in different regions was drawn from Wikipedia.

3.2. Variable Selection

3.2.1. Input Variable Selection

In this paper, the local GHE in 31 provinces (municipalities, autonomous regions) of China were selected as the sole input variable. Considering the comparability of the economy and data, Hong Kong, Macao, and Taiwan were not included in the calculation.

Figure 1 shows the local GHE in China from 2007 to 2016. From Figure 1, it can be seen that the local GHE in China had a rapid growth trend, from 199.58 billion Chinese yuan in 2007 to 1306.76 billion Chinese yuan in 2016, with a 650% increase. Among them, the largest absolute growth was in 2014, up 188.34 billion Chinese yuan from 2013. While the local government has increased health expenditure year by year, the problems in China, including it being difficult and expensive to see a doctor, are still serious. In addition, we often need to consider the spatial correlation when there is spatial distribution in the economic subjects, however, the traditional econometric models often neglect spatial correlation because of the irrelevance in the regional data. Spatial econometrics, as a branch of econometrics, incorporates the spatial weight matrix into the regression model, which is widely used in regional science, urban economics, geoeconomics, and development economics. Spatial econometrics studies how to deal with spatial heterogeneity (spatial structure) and spatial correlation (spatial interaction) in regression models. This paper will measure the efficiency of the local GHE and its spatial spillover effect. The selection of output and influencing factor variables are given as follows.

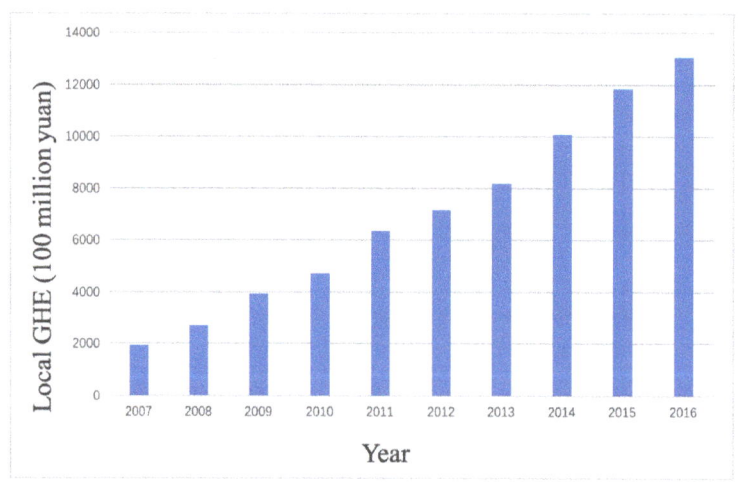

Figure 1. Chinese local government health expenditures from 2007 to 2016.

3.2.2. Output and Influencing Factor Variables Selection

The basic goal of GHE is to achieve the optimal supply of public health services under the condition of limited health resources in order to obtain the maximum health output. From this point of view, we can divide the target of GHE into an intermediate target and a final target (see Figure 2).

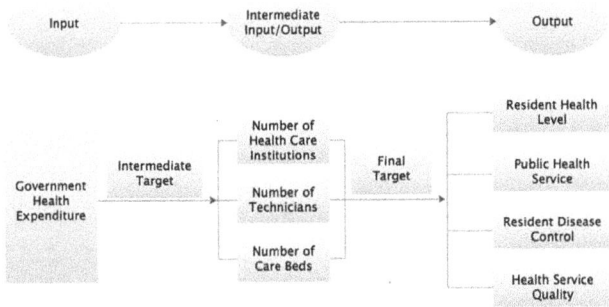

Figure 2. Government health expenditure (GHE) target.

Therefore, according to the final goal of the local GHE, this paper chooses the following seven indicators to show the inputs and outputs of local governments in the field of health services: (1) Severe malnutrition rate among children under five years old and the mortality rate, reflecting the health level of residents; (2) the number of outpatient visits and the medical expenses per capita of outpatients and inpatients, reflecting public health services; (3) infectious disease incidence rate of Class A and B statutory reports and infectious disease mortality rate, reflecting the residents' diseases control; and (4) hospital bed utilization rate, reflecting the quality of healthcare services. The output of local government public health services from 2007 to 2016 is shown in Table 1.

Table 1. Outputs of government-invested public health service from 2007 to 2016.

Indicator Name	Maximum	Minimum	Mean	Standard Deviation
Outpatient consultation (100 million)	2.56	0.53	1.88	0.75
Infectious disease incidence rate of Class A and B statutory reports (%)	302.00	232.13	262.89	25.37
Outpatient and inpatient medical expenses per capita (Chinese yuan)	5077.44	9141.66	7225.28	1388.96
Bed use rate (%)	76.52	89.00	85.03	3.50
Severe malnutrition rate among children under 5 years old (%)	1.33	2.06	1.56	0.26
Population mortality rate (%)	5.83	6.07	5.95	0.09
Infectious disease mortality rate (%)	0.89	1.26	1.11	0.12

Based on the existing research results, this paper will consider the urban and rural, cultural, economic, and demographic factors, which may have an important impact on the spatial spillover effect of the local GHE efficiency. Therefore, the proportion of urban population, illiteracy rate, the GHE accounting for the proportion of fiscal expenditure, gross domestic product (GDP) per capita, fiscal decentralization, and population density are selected as explanatory variables, which are shown in detail in Table 2.

Table 2. Selection of influencing factors of spatial measurement model.

Indicator (Unit)	Calculation Method
Proportion of urban population (%)	Regional urban population/region permanent resident population * 100%
Illiteracy rate (%)	Number of illiterates over 15 years old/total population over 15 years old * 100%
Proportion of government health expenditure to financial expenditure (%)	Local government health expenditure/local fiscal expenditure * 100%
GDP per capita (Chinese yuan/person)	Gross regional product/regional resident population
Fiscal decentralization (%)	Local finance general budget expenditure/important fiscal expenditure * 100%
Population density (person/km^2)	Regional permanent population/region total area

3.3. Method

3.3.1. DEA Method

The DEA method, occasionally called frontier analysis, was developed by Charnes, Cooper, and Rhodes (CCR) in 1978 [6]. DEA models are classified into the model of Banker, Charnes, and Cooper (BCC) [24] and the CCR model. The BCC model is an output-oriented model and the CCR model is an input-oriented model. This paper chooses the output-oriented BCC model to study the efficiency of the local GHE. The specific model is shown as follows.

Assuming that the DEA model has J decision-making units (DMUs), $DMU_j (j = 1, 2, \cdots, J)$, each DMU has M input items, $X_j = (x_{1j}, x_{2j}, x_{3j}, \cdots x_{Mj})$, and N output items, $Y_j = (y_{1j}, y_{2j}, y_{3j}, \cdots y_{Nj})$. Thus, the overall efficiency of j_0-th DMU can be obtained from the following linear programming.

$$\max \ \eta_{j_0} = \frac{\sum_{n=1}^{N} \alpha_n y_{nj_0}}{\sum_{m=1}^{M} \beta_m x_{mj_0}}$$

$$s.t. \begin{cases} \frac{\sum_{n=1}^{N} \alpha_n y_{nj}}{\sum_{m=1}^{M} \beta_m x_{mj}} \leq 1 & (j = 1, 2, \cdots, J) \\ \alpha_n \geq 0 & (n = 1, 2, \cdots, M), \beta_m \geq 0 (m = 1, 2, \cdots, M) \end{cases} \quad (1)$$

where η_{j_0} is the desired overall efficiency and α_n and β_m are the weights for the outputs and inputs, respectively.

The purpose of this paper is to study the input of local governments in the field of public health services and to maximize the output of medical and health services with a certain amount of scale of health resources. Thus, this paper chooses the BCC model to calculate the efficiency of the local GHE in China. Furthermore, with the increasing convenience of social transportation and the more convenient sharing of health resources among different regions, the spatial spillover effect of public health services in different regions will be more obvious. In view of this, we continue to explore the temporal and spatial correlation and evolution trend of the local GHE efficiency in order to obtain a deeper understanding of the efficiency of the local GHE in China, which has great significance for optimizing the results of financial expenditure and improving the GHE efficiency.

3.3.2. Spatial Econometric Model Method

(1) Morland Index

The First Law of Geography asserts that everything is related and the closer the things are, the higher the degree of correlation will be [25]. We record the geospatial data of n regions as $\{x_i, x_j\}_{i=1, j=1}^{n}$, where i and j represent region i and region j, respectively. The distance between region i and region j is recorded as w_{ij}, which can be defined as a spatial weight matrix as follows.

$$W = \begin{pmatrix} w_{11} & \cdots & w_{1n} \\ \vdots & \vdots & \vdots \\ w_{n1} & \cdots & w_{nn} \end{pmatrix}, \quad (2)$$

where the elements on the principal diagonal are equal to 0, i.e., $w_{11} = \cdots = w_{nn} = 0$ (the distance of the same region is expressed as 0). It should be noted that the commonly used spatial weight matrix is the spatial adjacent weight matrix, which can be expressed as follows:

$$w_{ij} = \begin{cases} 1, & \text{regions } i \text{ and } j \text{ are neighbors} \\ 0, & \text{regions } i \text{ and } j \text{ are not neighbors} \end{cases}. \quad (3)$$

As we know, the spatial measurement method can be used when there is spatial correlation among the data. If there is no spatial correlation, the general measurement method is used. "Spatial autocorrelation" means that regions have similar values of variables to other similar regions. Spatial autocorrelation can be divided into positive spatial correlation and negative spatial correlation. The most widely used method to measure spatial correlation is the Moran index, which is given as follows.

$$I = \frac{\sum_{i=1}^{n}\sum_{j=1}^{n} w_{ij}(x_i - \bar{x})(x_j - \bar{x})}{s^2 \sum_{i=1}^{n}\sum_{j=1}^{n} w_{ij}}, \tag{4}$$

where $s^2 = \frac{\sum_{i=1}^{n}(x_i - \bar{x})^2}{n}$ is the sample variance and $\sum_{i=1}^{n}\sum_{j=1}^{n} w_{ij}$ is the sum of all spatial weight matrixes.

The value range of the Moran index is [−1,1]. If the Moran index I is greater than 0, there is a positive spatial correlation among different regions. If I is less than 0, there is a negative spatial correlation. If I is close to 0, the correlation among different regions is weak. The Moran index can be decomposed into the global Moran index and the local Moran index. The global Moran index represents the overall correlation, while the local Moran index decomposes the Moran index of each region in a certain year, which indicates a clustering phenomenon in this region. The Moran index can be regarded as the correlation coefficient between the observed value and its spatial lag.

The global Moran index is decomposed to obtain the Moran index value of each sample individual. The spatial dependence of each sample individual and its adjacent individual can be judged by plotting the value of each sample individual and its spatial adjacent individual as a scatter plot. Generally, four quadrants are obtained using scatter plots of the local Moran index. Each quadrant corresponds to a spatial structure, representing a set of special relationships between the value of individual variables and the mean value of adjacent individual variables, and each sample individual is grouped into a quadrant. Specifically, the value of individual variables in the first quadrant is high (H) and that of adjacent individuals is also high (H) and is expressed as HH, which is a common spatial expression pattern of a high-high cluster. The value of individual variables in the third quadrant is low (L), and the value of variables in adjacent individuals is low (L) and expressed by LL, which is a typical low-low cluster. The number of individuals in the second quadrant and the fourth quadrant is relatively small, where the value of individual variables is low, with high-value neighboring individual variables, and the value of individual variables is high, with low-value neighboring individual variables; this can be expressed by the LH and HL clusters, respectively. Furthermore, positive spatial correlation refers to the high-high or low-low cluster, while negative spatial correlation refers to the high-low or low-high cluster. There is no spatial correlation among the HL or LH cluster regions with random distribution. In this way, we can find the identity of the population and economic clusters in China by identifying the Chinese provinces using the HH and LL characteristics and the local Moran index.

(2) Spatial Econometric Model

➢ Model Selection

First, the spatial autoregressive model of the panel should be examined. The specific formula is as follows.

$$y_{it} = \rho w'_i y_i + x'_{it}\beta + \mu_i + \varepsilon_{it}, (i = 1, \cdots, n; t = 1, \cdots, T), \tag{5}$$

where w'_i is the i-th row of the spatial weight matrix W, $w'_i y_i = \sum_{j=1}^{n} w_{ij} y_{jt}$, w_{ij} is the (i, j)-th element of the spatial weight matrix W, and μ_i is the individual effect of region i. If μ_i is related to x_{it}, it is a fixed effects model; otherwise, it is a random effects model. The usual Hausman test can be used to determine whether a fixed-effect or a random-effect model should be used and it is shown as follows.

$$\begin{cases} y_{it} = \tau y_{i,t-1} + \rho \omega_i' y_t + x_{it}\beta + d_i' X_t \delta + u_i + \gamma_t + \varepsilon_{it} \\ \varepsilon_{it} = \lambda m_i' \varepsilon_t + v_{it} \end{cases} \quad (6)$$

where $y_{i,t-1}$ is the first-order lag of the interpreted variable y_{it}, $d_i' X_t \delta$ is the spatial lag of the explanatory variable, d_i^i is the i-th row of the corresponding spatial weight matrix D, γ_t is the time effect, and m_i' is the i-th row of the disturbance item space weight matrix M. The following items explain how to distinguish the spatial autoregressive models [26].

(a) If $\lambda = 0$, it is a Spatial Durbin Model (SDM);
(b) If $\lambda = 0$ and $\delta = 0$, it is a Spatial Autoregression Model (SAR);
(c) If $\tau = 0$ and $\delta = 0$, it is a Spatial Autocorrelation Model (SAC);
(d) If $\tau = \rho = 0$ and $\delta = 0$, it is a Spatial Error Model (SEM).

➤ Decomposition Mechanism of the Special Spillover Effect

The spatial Durbin model can decompose the explanatory variable-spillover effect using the partial differential method proposed by LeSage and Pace in 2009 [27], considering the total, direct, and indirect effects. Among them, the direct effect is the influence on the local region caused by the explanatory variables, while the indirect effect is the influence on the result of the explanatory variables in the neighboring regions. The specific calculation method is given as follows.

$$Y = (I_n - \ell W)^{-1} \alpha l_n + (I_n - \ell W)^{-1}(X_t \beta + W X_t \theta) \alpha l_n + (I_n - \ell W)^{-1} \varepsilon, \quad (7)$$

which can be rewritten as

$$Y = \sum_{r=1}^{k} S_r(W) x_r + V(W) l_n \alpha + V(W) \varepsilon, \quad (8)$$

where we have $S_r(W) = V(W)(I_n \beta_r + W \theta_r)$, $V(W) = (I_n - \ell W)^{-1}$ and I_n is an n-order identity matrix. In addition, the above equation can be converted into a matrix form, shown as

$$\begin{bmatrix} y_1 \\ y_2 \\ \vdots \\ y_n \end{bmatrix} = \sum_{r=1}^{k} \begin{bmatrix} S_r(W)_{11} & S_r(W)_{12} & \cdots & S_r(W)_{1n} \\ S_r(W)_{21} & S_r(W)_{22} & \cdots & S_r(W)_{2n} \\ \vdots & \vdots & \ddots & \vdots \\ S_r(W)_{n1} & S_r(W)_{n1} & \cdots & S_r(W)_{nn} \end{bmatrix} \begin{bmatrix} x_{1r} \\ x_{2r} \\ \vdots \\ x_{nr} \end{bmatrix} + V(W) l_n \alpha + V(W) \varepsilon, \quad (9)$$

Thus, the total, direct, and indirect effects are obtained as

$$\overline{M}(r)_{\text{ATI}} = n^{-1} I_n S_r(W)_{I_n}, \quad (10)$$

$$\overline{M}(r)_{\text{ADI}} = n^{-1} \text{trace} S_r(W), \quad (11)$$

$$\overline{M}(r)_{\text{AII}} = n^{-1} \{ I_n S_r(W)_{I_n} - \text{trace} S_r(W) \}. \quad (12)$$

4. Results

4.1. Efficiency Analysis of Local Government Health Expenditure

In this paper, we used the output-oriented BCC model and Deap 2.1 software to process the input and output data in order to obtain the efficiency of the local GHE from 2007 to 2016. The results are shown in Figure 3.

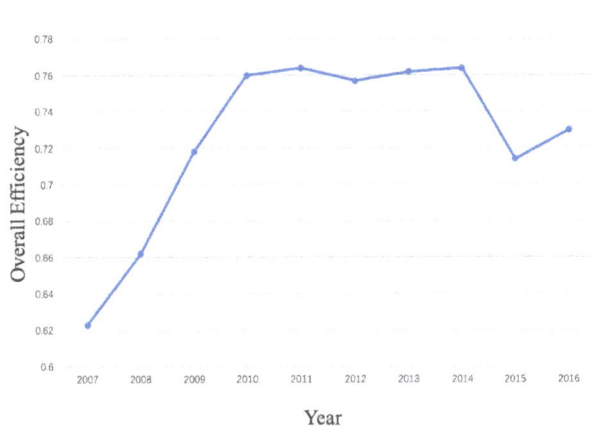

Figure 3. Overall efficiency of Chinese local government health expenditures from 2007 to 2016.

Figure 3 shows the changing trend of the static overall GHE efficiency of 31 regions from 2007 to 2016. During these 10 years, it can be seen that the overall efficiency increased from 0.62 to 0.73.

As shown in Figure 4, we used the average overall efficiency of the local GHE from 2007 to 2016 as a representative to analyze the differences in the total efficiencies among different regions. From Figure 4, we can see that the lowest overall efficiency is in Guizhou and the highest is in Ningxia. Among them, the overall efficiencies of 22 regions are under 0.8, for example, in Guizhou, Inner Mongolia, and Heilongjiang. There are nine regions whose overall efficiencies are greater than 0.9. Furthermore, it is not difficult to see that the overall efficiencies of the eastern region are generally higher, while those of the northeast and central regions are generally lower.

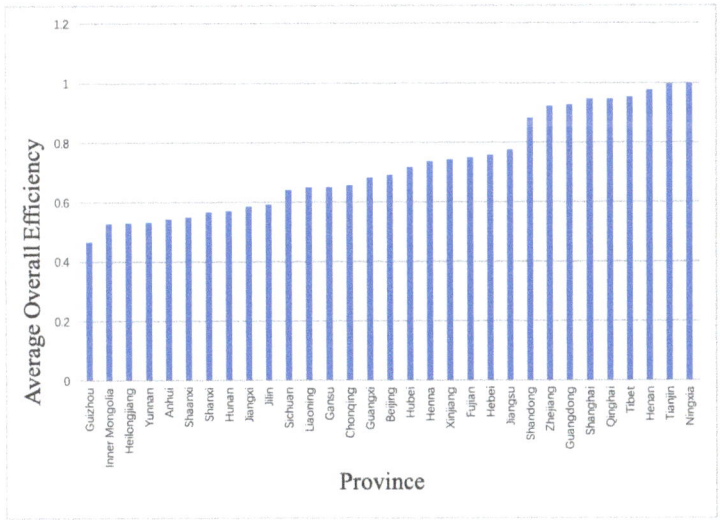

Figure 4. Ranking of the average overall efficiency of Chinese local government health expenditures from 2007 to 2016.

4.2. Spatial Spillover Effect Analysis of Local Government Health Expenditure

4.2.1. Global Moran Index Calculation

The efficiency of GHE is a multi-dimensional and comprehensive problem closely related to factors such as the economy, culture, population, and regional development. Moreover, factors such as economic development, population cluster, and other factors in neighboring regions may also have an impact on the efficiency of the local GHE. Therefore, theoretically speaking, the efficiency of the local GHE has spatial correlation. In order to verify this hypothesis, this paper used the Moran index.

In this paper, we used Stata software to test the global spatial autocorrelation of the static overall efficiency of the local GHE from 2007 to 2016. The results are shown in the following Table 3.

Table 3. Global spatial correlation test of static overall efficiency of government health expenditure.

Year	Moran's I Value	p-Value
2007	0.201	0.021
2008	0.22	0.016
2009	0.256	0.007
2010	0.22	0.017
2011	0.246	0.009
2012	0.255	0.008
2013	0.292	0.003
2014	0.336	0.001
2015	0.32	0.001
2016	0.315	0.002

Table 3 shows that the Moran's I value of the static overall efficiency of the local GHE from 2007 to 2016 is positive. Moreover, from the test of the 5% significance level, the efficiency of the local GHE is shown to have a positive spatial correlation in the past 10 years, that is, the efficiency of local GHE is spatial agglomeration. At the same time, we can see from the changing trend of the Moran's I value that the spatial correlation degree of the Chinese local GHE became stronger and stronger from 2007 to 2014 and slightly declined from 2015 to 2016.

4.2.2. Local Moran Index Calculation

The results of the global Moran index show that the efficiency of the local GHE has a positive spatial correlation from 2007 to 2016. However, it cannot reveal which regions are in high-cluster areas or low-cluster areas. In view of this, this paper chose the three years when China completed five key tasks of deepening the reform of medical and health systems from 2009 to 2011. We used Stata software to calculate the local Moran index of the local GHE efficiency, in order to further show whether there was a local spatial agglomeration phenomenon for the efficiency of the local GHE. In this paper, Arcmap 10.2 software was used to describe the distribution of Moran scatter plots. The results are shown in the following figures.

Figures 5–7 show that the positive spatial correlation regions are mainly concentrated in the northeastern, eastern, and western regions of China. Among them, the low-low cluster areas are mainly concentrated in Inner Mongolia, Liaoning, Jilin, and Heilongjiang in Northeastern China and Sichuan, Yunnan, Chongqing, Guizhou, Guangxi, etc. in Western China, belong to the low GHE efficiency regions. The high-high cluster areas, mainly concentrated in Beijing, Jiangsu, Shanghai, Zhejiang, etc. in Eastern China and Tibet and Qinghai in Western China, belong to the high GHE efficiency regions. Henan had a negative spatial correlation agglomeration in the past three years, showing high-low clustering phenomenon, which indicates that the GHE efficiency of its neighboring region is very low.

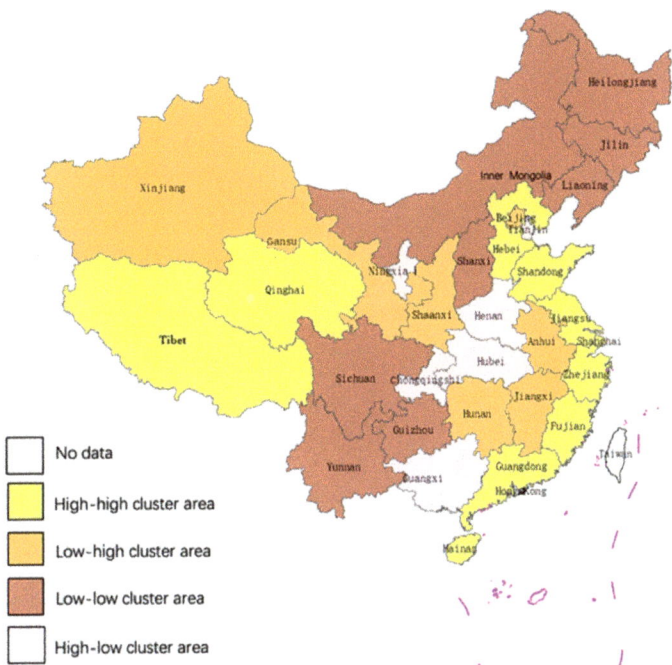

Figure 5. The spatial agglomeration of Chinese local government health expenditures overall efficiency in 2009.

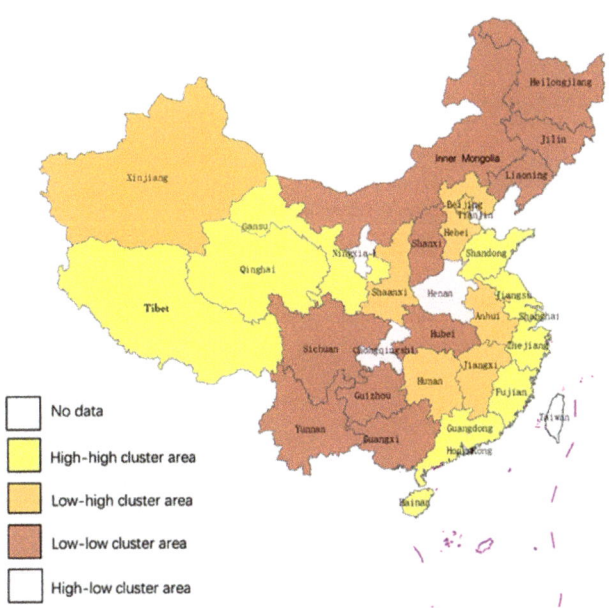

Figure 6. The spatial agglomeration of Chinese local government health expenditures overall efficiency in 2010.

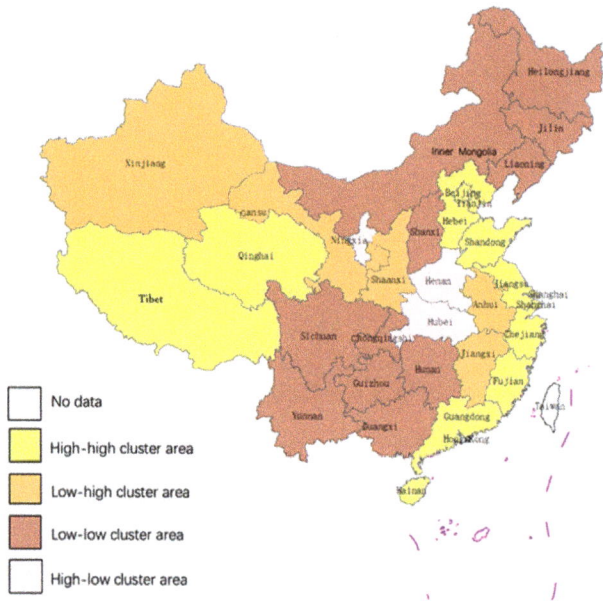

Figure 7. The spatial agglomeration of Chinese local government health expenditures overall efficiency in 2011.

4.2.3. Spatial Econometric Model Analysis

After verifying the spatial correlation of Chinese local GHE efficiency, we built a spatial panel econometric model to further analyze the impact of the proportion of urban population, illiteracy rate, the proportion of government health expenditure to fiscal expenditure, GDP per capita, and population density on the efficiency of the local GHE.

In this paper, the idea in [28] was used as a reference in choosing a spatial model, that is, an SDM model without any constraints was firstly estimated and then whether the SDM model can be simplified was tested. According to Equation (6), the SDM model estimation was first selected, then we processed the data using Stata software. Finally, Wald and likelihood ratio (LR) tests [29] were carried out to verify whether the SAR model and SEM model were nested in the SDM model. The results are shown in Table 4.

Table 4. Global spatial correlation test of static overall efficiency of government health expenditure.

Indicator Name	SDM Model Fixed Effect	SDM Model Random Effect
Proportion of urban population	0.0110 **	−0.00109
Illiteracy rate	−0.00698 *	−0.00628
Proportion of GHE to fiscal expenditure	0.0165 **	0.0177 **
GDP per capita	0.00000243	0.00000306 *
Fiscal decentralization	0.473 *	0.373
Population density	0.000984 ***	0.000132
rho	0.519 ***	0.517 ***
Hausman test	0.000	
Wald test	chi2(5) = 18.3 Prob > chi2 = 0.0000	
LR test	chi2(5) = 25.96 Prob > chi2 = 0.0001	
	AIC	BIC
SDM model	−687.2068	−634.8948
SAC model	−841.149	−811.2564

Note: *, **, *** indicate significant levels at 10%, 5%, and 1%, respectively.

From Table 4, the results of Wald and LR tests show that the hypothesis of $\tau = 0$ and $\delta = 0$ or $\tau = \rho = 0$ and $\delta = 0$ is negated. The SAC model and SDM model were further tested to see which was more suitable. The results showed that the absolute values of the Akaike information criterion (AIC) and Bayesian information criterion (BIC) of the SDM model were less than those of the SAC model, so the SDM model was more suitable for this paper. The Hausman test of the SDM model had a p-value of $0.000 < 0.05$, which indicated that the random effect model hypothesis was rejected at the 5% significance level. Therefore, the fixed effect model of SDM was more suitable.

On the other hand, we can see that the spatial lag coefficient (rho) of explanatory variables is not significantly zero according to the estimation results of SDM. LeSage and Pace (2009) proposed that there will be systematic errors in measuring the spillover effect using the coefficient of SDM when the spatial lag term coefficient of the explanatory variables is not significantly zero [27]. In this case, the spatial effect of SDM should be further decomposed to accurately reflect the direction and extent of the impact of each explanatory variable on the GHE efficiency in the local and neighboring regions [27]. In view of this, this paper decomposed the SDM to obtain the total, direct, and indirect effects of each explanatory variable, as shown in Table 5.

Table 5. Spatial spillover effect decomposition with SDM Model.

Indicator Name	Total Effect	Direct Effect	Indirect Effect
Proportion of urban population	−0.0032115 ***	−0.0019761 ***	−0.0012354 ***
Illiteracy rate	−0.0016742 ***	−0.0010302	−0.000644
Proportion of GHE to fiscal expenditure	0.0078264 ***	0.0048158 ***	0.0030106
GDP per capita	1.33 ***	8.21 ***	5.13 ***
Fiscal decentralization	−0.115438 ***	−0.0710317	−0.0444063
Population density	0.0000458 ***	0.0000282 ***	0.0000176 ***

Note: *, **, *** indicate significant levels at 10%, 5%, and 1%, respectively.

From Table 5, we can see that the total, direct, and indirect effects of the proportion of the urban population are significantly negative among the factors affecting the local GHE efficiency. It is also shown that, with the increase of the proportion of the urban population, both the local and neighboring GHE efficiencies decrease. The reason is that, with the increase of the urbanization proportion, people's healthcare needs increase correspondingly. However, with the increasingly convenient transportation and health services, people choose much more developed regions or countries for their healthcare service, which leads to a decline in the GHE efficiency.

The total, direct, and indirect effects of the illiteracy rate are all negative, but the direct and indirect effects have not passed the significant level test. This shows that the increase of the illiteracy rate will lead to a decrease of the local GHE efficiency, but the influence of spatial decomposition effect on the local and neighboring regions is very small. This may be due to the lower cultural quality of residents, because they know less about the transmission and prevention of some common diseases and are more likely to get sick. Moreover, the lower the education level of residents, the more difficult it will be to communicate with hospitals, ask for medical and health services, choose the right medical institutions, and obtain accurate healthcare information when they are sick. In addition, it will have some influence on people's awareness of the need to cooperate with the government's healthcare supervision, which will also decrease GHE efficiency.

The total and direct effects of the proportion of GHE to fiscal expenditure are significantly positive, while the indirect effects are negative and do not pass the significant level test. This shows that the increase of the proportion of GHE to fiscal expenditure will have a positive impact on the local GHE efficiency. The greater local governments' input in the field of healthcare, the higher the GHE efficiency will be. The reason is that, with the increase of local government input in the field of healthcare, it will be possible to provide better health services and thus improve the GHE efficiency.

The total, direct, and indirect effects of GDP per capita are all significantly positive, which indicates that the improvement of GDP per capita will improve the local GHE efficiency. This influence is reflected not only in improving the local GHE efficiency, but also the significant promotion effect on neighboring regions. This can be explained by the fact that residents in rich regions have a higher demand for high-quality health services, which may put more pressure on local governments to improve their health expenditure efficiency by increasing the health service level.

The total effect of fiscal decentralization is negative and has passed the significance level test, while the direct and indirect effects are negative but not significant. This indicates that the greater the degree of fiscal decentralization, the less the local GHE efficiency will be improved. This may be due to government competition caused by fiscal decentralization, which may lead to an inadequate provision of public goods by local governments and the reduction of the GHE scale, decreasing the efficiency of health expenditure.

The total, direct, and indirect effects of the population density are all significantly positive. The higher the population density, the higher the GHE efficiency. We believe that a higher population density can reduce the cost of government management and supervision and thus help to improve the GHE efficiency.

5. Discussion

In this paper, after using the DEA, spatial Moran's I value, and SDM model to measure the GHE efficiency and its spatial spillover effect from 2007 to 2016, we found that there are obvious differences in the local GHE efficiency due to the different levels of economic development and the high or low foundation of medical and health industry among different regions of China. We also found that the GHE efficiency in China increased year by year from 2007 to 2014, decreased slightly in 2015, and continued to increase in 2016. Finally, we found that the GHE efficiency has a significant positive spatial spillover. The proportion of GHE to fiscal expenditure, GDP per capita, and population density have a positive impact on the GHE efficiency. Their growth will promote the GHE efficiency in the local region and adjacent areas. Conversely, the proportion of urban population, illiteracy rate, and fiscal decentralization have a negative impact on the GHE efficiency. Their growth will reduce the efficiency in the local region and adjacent areas.

The strength of this study is to consider the spatial spillover effect in terms with realistic meaning. The results obtained can be used as a reference for optimizing the structure and improving the efficiency of government health inputs. It breaks the government's GDP-only theory-based assessment system and helps to improve it by assessing the GHE efficiency. On the other hand, our study makes a significant contribution to the literature on public health services with spatial spillover effect.

Based on the obtained results and analysis, we have some suggestions and policy recommendations, which are as follows:

Develop a reasonable health insurance system. In the current context of aging and urbanization, China should formulate a scientific and reasonable healthcare insurance system, which can not only minimize the waste of health resources, but also improve the efficiency of the local GHE.

Improve the fiscal decentralization system. China should strengthen the supervision and management of financial expenditure in various regions, so as to improve the efficiency of the local GHE.

Reduce the regional unbalance. From the calculation and analysis of the local Moran index of the GHE efficiency, the GHE efficiency of Beijing, Jiangsu, Shanghai, and Zhejiang in the eastern region and Tibet and Qinghai in the western region is high, showing a high-high cluster. Conversely, the GHE efficiency of Inner Mongolia, Liaoning, Jilin, and Heilongjiang in the northeastern region and Sichuan, Yunnan, Chongqing, Guizhou, and Guangxi in the western region is generally low, showing a low-low cluster. Henan Province in the middle region shows negative spatial correlation, which is a high-low cluster area. The central part is located in the east–west junction grounding zone, which is driven, to a certain extent, by the developed areas in the east, but the development is still lagging behind.

Therefore, the overall economic development pattern of China is not coordinated and is unbalanced among different regions. Correspondingly, the GHE efficiency is also unbalanced in terms of regional development. In order to maximize the GHE efficiency, we should vigorously implement the strategy of regional coordinated development, strengthen the health construction in the central and western regions, improve the level of health efficiency, and induce regional spillover of the GHE efficiency.

Strengthen the health cooperation. It is very important to strengthen the overall coordination among different regions and cross-administrative health cooperation. We should standardize inter-regional health rules and policies, improve the formulation and implementation of inter-regional environmental policies, reduce vicious competition in health expenditure efficiency and avoid blind competition and excessive competition. For the eastern region, which is in a high-high cluster area, regional exchanges and cooperation can be promoted to achieve coordinated development and common progress among regions. In order to reduce the efficiency of health expenditure and improve the "free-rider" behavior, it is necessary to establish standardized and unified health regulations and standards for the western and northeastern regions in low-low cluster areas.

Utilize the spatial spillover effect. Chinese GHE has a significant spatial spillover effect. In order to promote the coordinated development of the regional economy, the government should guide the flow of health resources in the region through fiscal and tax policies and optimize the layout of regional health centers. On the other hand, the government can fully utilize the spatial spillover effect of the health expenditure efficiency through the rational layout of regional health centers in order to promote regional development. In addition, we can use the spatial spillover effect to break down administrative barriers. Local government health services should break down the administrative barriers between regions, to make it convenient for people to enjoy the healthcare services in different places. At the same time, we need to strengthen the healthcare exchanges and cooperation with neighboring regions and make full use of regional spillover effect mechanism in order to better realize the effective supply of local basic healthcare services.

Optimize the urban population structure. China should rationally optimize the urban population structure, promote population aggregation, and play its role in improving the efficiency of health expenditure in local region and adjacent areas. Moreover, we need to accelerate the balanced development of the regional economy. From the analysis results concerning the spatial measurement of the health expenditure efficiency in China, the impact of Chinese economic development on the efficiency of health expenditure is obviously unbalanced. The growth of economics and the proportion of GHE to financial expenditure have promoted the efficiency of health expenditure in local regions and adjacent areas, while fiscal decentralization has inhibited it. The government can further adjust the proportion of GHE to financial expenditure to maintain economic growth and promote health expenditure efficiency. In order to comprehensively promote the construction of social education and improve people's cultural quality, the government needs to further promulgate policies to promote the development of Chinese education. The efficiency of health expenditure can be significantly improved if the illiteracy rate is reduced.

6. Conclusions

In this paper, the DEA and spatial regression models are used to measure the local GHE efficiency and its spatial spillover effect in 31 provinces (municipalities and autonomous regions) of China from 2007 to 2016. The conclusions are summarized as follows.

Due to the different levels of economic development and the high or low foundation of the medical and health industry in various regions of China, there are obvious differences in the local GHE efficiency.

As far as individual regions are concerned, the overall efficiency of local GHE in Shandong, Zhejiang, Guangdong, Shanghai, Qinghai, Tibet, Hainan, Tianjin, and Ningxia is higher than 0.8. However, the overall efficiency of other regions is generally not high, which indicates that there is a large waste of GHE in these regions.

The results of the global Moran index calculations show that there is a positive spatial correlation between the local GHE efficiency from 2007 to 2016, that is, the efficiency of the local GHE is a spatial agglomeration. At the same time, we can also see from the trend of the Moran index that the spatial correlation degree of the local GHE from 2007 to 2014 shows an upward trend, while the spatial correlation degree between 2015 and 2016 slightly declines. At the same time, from 2007 to 2016, the proportion of the urban population, the illiteracy rate, the proportion of GHE to fiscal expenditure, the GDP per capita, fiscal decentralization, and population density are the main factors affecting the efficiency of the local GHE and they are all spatially correlated.

The calculation results of the local Moran index show that the positive spatial correlation regions are mainly concentrated in the northeast, east, and west of China. Among them, the low-low cluster areas are mainly concentrated in Inner Mongolia, Liaoning, Jilin, and Heilongjiang in the northeast region and Sichuan, Yunnan, Chongqing, Guizhou, Guangxi, etc. in the western region. High-high cluster areas are mainly concentrated in Beijing, Jiangsu, Shanghai, Zhejiang, etc. in the eastern region and Tibet and Qinghai in the western region. Henan is a spatial negative correlation cluster region, showing a high-low clustering phenomenon.

The results of the spatial econometric model in this paper show that, from the perspective of total, direct, and indirect effects, the proportion of GHE to fiscal expenditure and GDP per capita are two important indicators representing economic factors and the population density represents the population factors. They have a positive impact on the health and financial expenditure efficiency of local government and their growth will improve the efficiency of the local and neighboring regions, while the three indicators of the proportion of urban population, illiteracy rate, and fiscal decentralization have a negative impact on the health and financial expenditure efficiency of local governments and their growth will reduce the efficiency of local and neighboring regions.

Author Contributions: M.W. and C.T. conceived and designed the study; M.W. collected and analyzed the data and drafted the paper; M.W. and C.T. read and revised the draft critically. All authors read and approved the final manuscript.

Funding: This research is funded by the National Social Science Foundation of China (Grant No. 16BTJ004; 14BJY160), the Bidding Project of Cooperative Innovation Center of Jiangxi University of Finance and Economics, "Research on Development of Biomedical Industry and Policy Support" (Grant No. 2016-03), Special Project of the National Social Science Foundation of China (Grant No. 18VSJ016), and the National Natural Science Foundation of China (Grant No. 81760619).

Acknowledgments: We would like to thank Lisu Yu and Xiaohui Liu for their help to improve the paper.

Conflicts of Interest: The authors declare no conflict of interest.

References

1. Ping, X.; Bai, J. Fiscal decentralization and local public good provision in China. *J. Financ. Trade Econ.* **2006**, *2*, 49–55.
2. Fu, Y. *Chinese Decentralization, Local Fiscal Models and Public Goods Supply: Theoretical and Empirical Research*; Fudan University: Shanghai, China, 2007.
3. Lv, W.; Wang, W. Research on the equalization of basic public service providing in China-based on the analysis of public demand and government ability. *J. Public Financ. Res.* **2008**, *5*, 10–18.
4. Liu, Z.; Tang, T.; Yang, W. Efficiency measurement of provincial expenditure: DEA technique. *J. Econ. Theor. Bus. Manag.* **2009**, *7*, 50–56.
5. Farrell, M.J. The measurement of technical efficiency. *J. R. Stat. Soc. Ser. Ageneral* **1957**, *30*, 1078–1092.
6. Charnes, A.; Cooper, W.W.; Rhodes, E. Measuring the efficiency of decision-making units. *Eur. J. Oper. Res.* **1978**, *2*, 429–444. [CrossRef]
7. Afonso, A.; Fernandes, S. Measuring local government spending efficiency: Evidence for the Lisbon region. *Reg. Stud.* **2006**, *40*, 39–53. [CrossRef]
8. Hadad, S.; Hadad, Y.; Tuval, T.S. Determinants of healthcare systems efficiency in OECD countries. *Eur. J. Health Econ.* **2013**, *14*, 253–265. [CrossRef]

9. Han, H.; Miao, Y. Calculation of local health expenditure efficiencies and empirical study on influencing factors: DEA-Tobit analysis based on panel data of 31 provinces in China. *J. Financ. Econ.* **2010**, *5*, 4–15.
10. Luo, H. Empirical study on fiscal spending efficiency on healthcare and its influencing factors. *J. Chin. Health Econ.* **2012**, *31*, 13–15.
11. Guan, Y.; Liu, J.; Wang, B. A study of dynamic evaluation on the efficiency of provincial public healthcare expenditure in China-based on the perspective of health system reform. *J. Guizhou Univ. Financ. Econ.* **2014**, *1*, 89–97.
12. Jing, R.; Song, X. Performance analysis of Chinese public health expenditure in the background of new medical reform-an empirical study based on DEA and Malmquist productivity index. *J. Public Financ. Res.* **2012**, *9*, 54–60.
13. Wang, Y.; Fan, J.; Zhao, J.; Dong, Y.; Wang, Y. Taking Shandong province as an example to explore the spatial analysis of utilization efficiency of health resource allocation. *J. Chin. Health Econ.* **2015**, *32*, 1056–1058.
14. Han, Y.; Hu, Q.; Wang, L.; Shao, Y.; Wang, Z.; Han, X. Analysis of the inter-provincial differences of the health resource allocation efficiency in China. *Chin. J. Soc. Med.* **2016**, *33*, 86–89.
15. Gu, J. A spatial study on the allocation of healthcare resource. *J. Chin. Health Econ.* **2014**, *31*, 21–23.
16. Retzlaff-Roberts, D.; Chang, C.F.; Rubin, R.M. Technical efficiency in the use of health care resources: A comparison of OECD countries. *J. Health Policy* **2004**, *69*, 55–72. [CrossRef]
17. Liu, Z.; Zhang, X.; Yang, D. Research on Efficiency Change of Chinese Government Health Investment: Based on Panel Three Stage DEA model. *J. Cent. Univ. Financ. Econ.* **2014**, *1*, 97–104.
18. Xiao, H.; Cao, T.; Tang, L. Measurement and analysis of government health expenditures and health efficiency. *Chin. J. Health Policy* **2014**, *7*, 71–77.
19. Tu, Y. Study on government health input's efficiency in China. *J. Chin. Health Econ.* **2012**, *9*, 62–66.
20. Li, Y.; Wang, Y. A study on healthcare expenditure efficiencies of China's local governments and their influencing factors. *J. Humanit. Soc. J. Hainan Univ.* **2015**, *5*, 41–49.
21. National Bureau of Statistics of China. *China Statistical Yearbook*; National Bureau of Statistics of China: Beijing, China, 2008–2017.
22. National Health Commision of the People's Republic of China. *China Health Statistical Yearbook*; National Health Commision of the People's Republic of China: Beijing, China, 2008–2017.
23. National Bureau of Statistics of China. *China Financial Yearbook*; National Bureau of Statistics of China: Beijing, China, 2008–2017.
24. Banker, R.D.; Charnes, A.; Cooper, W.W. Some models for estimating technical and scale inefficiencies in data envelopment analysis. *Manag. Sci.* **1984**, *30*, 1078–1092. [CrossRef]
25. Tobler, W. The First Law of Geography: A computer movie simulating urban growth in the Detroit region. *Econ. Geogr.* **1970**, *46*, 234–240. [CrossRef]
26. Viton, P.A. Notes on spatial econometric models. *City Reg. Plan.* **2010**, *870*, 2–17.
27. LeSage, J.; Pace, R.K. *Introduction to Spatial Econometrics*; Chapman and Hall/CRC: Boca Raton, FL, USA, 2009.
28. Ertur, C.; Koch, W. Growth, technological interdependence and spatial externalities: Theory and evidence. *J. Appl. Econom.* **2007**, *22*, 1033–1062. [CrossRef]
29. Engle, R.F. Wald, likelihood ratio, and Lagrange multiplier tests in econometrics. *Handb. Econom.* **1984**, *2*, 775–826.

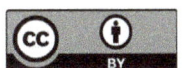

© 2019 by the authors. Licensee MDPI, Basel, Switzerland. This article is an open access article distributed under the terms and conditions of the Creative Commons Attribution (CC BY) license (http://creativecommons.org/licenses/by/4.0/).

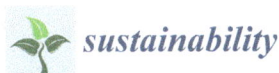

Article

Depression, Acculturative Stress, and Social Connectedness among International University Students in Japan: A Statistical Investigation

Minh Hoang Nguyen [1], Tam Tri Le [1] and Serik Meirmanov [2,*]

1. International Cooperation Policy, Graduate School of Asia Pacific Studies, Ritsumeikan Asia Pacific University, Beppu, Oita 874-8577, Japan; minhhn17@apu.ac.jp (M.H.N.); tamtle17@apu.ac.jp (T.T.L.)
2. Public Health Management Division, Graduate School of Asia Pacific Studies, Ritsumeikan Asia Pacific University, Beppu, Oita 874-8577, Japan
* Correspondence: serikmed@apu.ac.jp

Received: 23 December 2018; Accepted: 3 February 2019; Published: 8 February 2019

Abstract: (1) This study aims to examine the prevalence of depression and its correlation with Acculturative Stress and Social Connectedness among domestic and international students in an international university in Japan. (2) Methods: A Web-based survey was distributed among several classes of students of the university, which yielded 268 responses. On the survey, a nine-item tool from the Patient Health Questionnaire (PHQ-9), the Social Connectedness Scale (SCS) and Acculturative Stress Scale for International Students (ASSIS) were used together with socio-demographic data. (3) Results: The prevalence of depression was higher among international than domestic students (37.81% and 29.85%, respectively). English language proficiency and student age (20 years old) showed a significant correlation with depression among domestic students ($\beta = -1.63$, $p = 0.038$ and $\beta = 2.24$, $p = 0.048$). Stay length (third year) also displayed a significant correlation with depression among international students ($\beta = 1.08$, $p = 0.032$). Among international and domestic students, a statistically significant positive correlation between depression and acculturative stress, and negative associations of social connectedness with depression and acculturative stress were also found. (4) Conclusions: The high prevalence of depression, and its association with Acculturation stress and Social Connectedness, among the students in this study highlight the importance of implementing support programs which consider the role of Acculturation and Social Connectedness.

Keywords: depression; acculturation stress; social connectedness; international students; university students; ASSIS; Mindsponge; multicultural

---

1. Introduction

The rapid spread of globalization has made countries worldwide increasingly interconnected in many aspects, including in education. The number of globally mobile students increased by 25.3% from 2012 to 2017 [1]. Understanding the mental health condition among international students will help sustain the development of the social public health system, especially in countries with a high number of international students.

Depressive disorder is a major public health concern which affects 322 million people globally. In 2015, global depression prevalence was 4.4%. Together with HIV/AIDS and heart disease, depression was projected to be one of the three leading causes of burden of disease until 2030 [2]. If becoming too severe, depression can lead to suicide—the second leading cause of death for people aged 15–29 [3].

High depression prevalence (4.2%) is a serious problem to the sustainable public health development in Japan [3]. In 2008, depression entailed a substantial burden to the Japanese economy by costing approximately $11 billion [4]. Depressive disorder was also among the top causes of suicide in Japan [5,6].

Depression is more prevalent in university students compared to the general population [7], even in Japan. Major depressive disorder prevalence among first-year university students in Japan was reported at 20.7%, 53.4%, and 23.3% according to three different measurements [8]. Another paper found that around 30% of university students in Japan had depressive state [9]. As the number of international students in Japan increased rapidly by 45% in the last 3 years (from 184,155 in 2014 to 267,042 in 2017) [10], the mental health of international students has become a major concern. The prevalence of depression of international students in Japan was 41% [11]. A proportion of 34% of students visiting the mental health service at Tsukuba University health center informed being depressed [12].

Studies of factors contributing to depression in university students vary among countries regarding their findings [13–19]. For instance, a study in Kenya showed significant correlations between higher depression and year of study, academic performance, religion, age [14], while another study in Malaysia indicated significant associations of depression with age, gender, and economic status [15].

There were several studies on the predictors of depressive disorder in Japan. For instance, personality traits, such as self-directedness and harm avoidance, were significantly correlated with major depressive disorder in Japanese university students [20]. Negative automatic thought was found to be positively corelated with depression [21]. University life satisfaction and lifestyle (irregularity of meal and wake-up time) also contributed to depression among Japanese students. Meanwhile, gender, course category, and residential arrangement significantly correlated with depression among international students in Japan [11]. Overall, few studies about predictors of depression among domestic and international students in Japan have been conducted.

The results of cultural and psychological changes from moving to a foreign country or living in a new cultural environment are known as acculturation [22]. As international students start living in a new environment, intercultural contacts can cause acculturative stress, so they need to adapt to harmonize potential conflicts. Findings of many studies showed a significantly positive correlation between acculturative stress and depression [23–26]. Knowing more how acculturative stress is linked to depression in an international university will help improve the support systems for student's mental health. Findings of research about acculturation are mostly about acculturative stress, psychological adjustment, social belonging, depression, and anxiety [27]. While there are plenty of studies about acculturative stress in general immigrants [23,25,26] and international students in the US [28–30], the amount of studies on students in an international university in other country is still limited. University students have a worse quality of life [31]. The mental health condition of international university students needs special attention, especially considering the challenges they need to overcome when living in a new environment.

Social connectedness reflects an individual's opinion of themselves in relation to other people within a social context [32]. When the sense of connectedness of a person declines, that person starts to feel distant and different from other people and recall where it belongs [32]. Social connectedness is a predictor of depression among college students [33] and acculturative stress among international students [34]. International students who leave their home country to study in an entirely new environment become disconnected with their old relationships and connections. These losses might pose threat to student's mental health, such as depression. However, studies regarding the association between social connectedness and depression among students at an international university remain limited.

An international university is where students and faculties from different societies and cultural background are placed together. According to the Times Higher Education, the international outlook of a university is assessed based on three factors: the proportion of international students, the proportion of international staffs, and its international collaboration [35]. As a result, the greater the proportion of international students and faculties from various countries and regions is, the more multicultural the international university becomes.

It is worth nothing that studying in an international university is a double-edged experience. On the one hand, individuals being in a multicultural environment might receive many positive outcomes, for example, having a higher degree of cultural additivity [36] and behaving appropriately under multiple cultural contexts [37]. On the other hand, living in a multicultural environment could lead to problems of acculturation, such as feeling being rejected from multiple cultural contexts [38]. Not only international but even domestic students might experience difficulties in adjusting to the environment of international university. This is why it is important to understand the impact of acculturation and an individual's sense of connectedness on depression level in an international university.

To our knowledge, there was no comparative study concerning depression, acculturative stress, and social connectedness among domestic and international students in Japan. Since the literature about depression prevalence and the association of depression with acculturative stress and social connectedness in an international university is still limited, this study aims to examine: (1) the prevalence and predictors of depression and (2) the hypotheses of associations of depression with acculturative stress and social connectedness among domestic and international students at an international university. On the basis of the examined literature, the study seeks to answer the following research questions (RQ1 and RQ2) and hypotheses (H1 and H2) based on data collected from an international university in Japan:

RQ1: What is the prevalence of depression among domestic and international students?

RQ2: What are the socio-demographic predictors of depression among domestic and international students?

H1: Acculturative stress will be significantly positively associated with depression in both domestic and international students. Students in an international university were expected to have higher depression levels due to extensive conflicts during acculturation process.

H2: Social connectedness will be significantly negatively associated with depression in both domestic and international students. A greater sense of connectedness with others will make individual feel more comfortable and confident within a social context, which will prevent depression.

2. Materials and Methods

2.1. Study Site

In this study, we selected Ritsumeikan Asia Pacific University (APU), which is situated at Beppu City, Oita Prefecture in southern Japan, as our study area because it is Japan's first truly international university and is currently the most diverse university in Japan in terms of international faculty and student [39]. As of 2017, the number of international students and faculties on APU campus consisted of 50.1% of total 5,887 students and 49.4% of 166 faculty members, respectively [40]. The diversity of this university is not only limited to the proportion of students and faculties but also their variety of origins. According to official statistics of the university in 2018, international students came from 86 countries and regions, while the faculty members are from 22 different countries and regions [41]. The diversity of APU made an appropriate site for studying students in a multicultural environment—a subject found to be limited within the extant scholarship.

2.2. Participants

The study collected web-based questionnaires (Google Forms) of 268 students from a variety of countries who are currently studying at APU. A proportion of 75% of the number of participants were international students (N = 201), while domestic students accounted for 25% (N = 67). Among 201 international students, the highest percentages of students were from South East Asia (75%), including Vietnam, Indonesia, Thailand, and Malaysia. Students originating from East Asia, which consists of

China Korea, and Taiwan, accounted for 25%. Students from South Asia and other areas accounted for 9% and 5%, respectively.

Participants consisted of 170 females (63.4%) and 98 males (36.6%), with half of them being freshmen or who had been staying in APU within one year (see Table 1). As for language proficiency, around 76% of international students could speak English with high proficiency, whereas most of the native students acquired medium English proficiency and only 20% of them could use English fluently. The rate of international students able to speak the Japanese language fluently was quite low with only 12.6%, and almost half of them informed acquiring low Japanese proficiency. More than half of the participants, both domestic and international students, reported that they had no intimate partner at the time of filling the questionnaire (seven participants failed to report whether they had an intimate partner). The number of international students reported being religious was higher than that domestic students (37.31% compared to 23.88%).

Table 1. Socio-demographic characteristics of domestic and international students.

	Domestic Students			International Students		
	Total (N = 67) Weighted %	Male (N = 25) Weighted %	Female (N = 42) Weighted %	Total (N = 201) Weighted %	Male (N = 73) Weighted %	Female (N = 128) Weighted %
Age						
17–19	28.36	20.00	33.33	35.82	31.51	38.28
20	25.37	40.00	16.67	16.92	10.96	20.31
>20	46.27	40.00	50.00	47.26	57.53	41.41
Length of stay						
Freshman	29.85	24.00	33.33	47.26	45.21	48.44
2 years	19.40	24.00	16.67	19.40	16.44	21.09
3 years	34.33	28.00	38.10	22.89	23.29	22.66
>3 years	16.42	24.00	11.90	10.45	15.07	7.81
English Proficiency						
Low	22.39	20.00	23.81	3.48	2.74	3.91
Average	58.21	60.00	57.14	20.40	15.07	23.44
High	16.42	16.00	16.67	58.71	67.12	53.91
Native	2.99	4.00	2.38	17.41	15.07	18.75
Japanese Proficiency						
Low	1.49	4.00	—	45.27	41.10	47.66
Average	5.97	8.00	4.76	42.29	42.47	42.19
High	1.49	4.00	—	11.94	16.44	9.38
Native	91.04	84.00	95.24	0.50	—	0.78
Intimate partner						
Yes	40.30	40.00	40.48	37.81	30.14	42.19
No	59.70	60.00	59.52	58.21	60.27	57.03
Religion						
Yes	23.88	24.00	23.81	37.31	45.21	32.81
No	76.12	76.00	76.19	62.69	54.79	67.19

2.3. Instruments

2.3.1. Measures of Depression

The PHQ-9, a nine-item tool from the Patient Health Questionnaire (PHQ), was used to measure Depression. The questionnaire consists of 9 questions based on the Diagnostic and Statistical Manual for Mental Disorders—4th edition (DSM-IV) criteria for diagnosis depression. With only nine questions, the PHQ-9 can be used for dual purposes, being the diagnosis of depressive disorder and grade depressive symptom severity [42]. By asking the participants about the frequency of various symptoms over the past two weeks, the study then categorized the respondents as having major depressive disorder or other depressive disorder. The respondents are diagnosed positive to major depressive disorder or other depressive disorder if 5 or 2 depressive symptoms respectively present at least "more than half of the days" over the past two weeks, and one of the symptoms needs to be depressed mood or anhedonia [43]. Notably, the symptom "thoughts that you would be better off dead or of hurting yourself in some way" is counted regardless of the duration. To estimate the severity of depression, the DSM-IV criteria are scored as "0" (not at all) to "3" (nearly every day) in the PHQ-9, and thus the depressive severity score ranges from 0 to 27. The severity of depression is also categorized into five levels (minimal depression, mild depression, moderate depression, moderately severe depression, and severe depression) based on the score 1–4, 5–9, 10–14, 15–19, and 20–27 accordingly.

The validity of the PHQ-9 was tested for correlation with diagnosis by many mental health studies [44,45]. In the original study, Spitzer et al. acquired the validation of sensitivity and specificity at 73% and 98%, respectively, for significant depression among primary care patients [46]. The PHQ-9 was used to measure depression of not only patients but also a wide range of populations, including international students [44,45,47,48]. The Cronbach alpha measured in this study were 0.81 and 0.80 for international and domestic students respectively, which were acceptable.

2.3.2. Measures of Social Connectedness

The measure of Social Connectedness in this research was the Social Connectedness Scale (SCS) developed by Lee and Robbins to evaluate an individual's emotional distance or connectedness between themselves and other people [32]. The Social Connectedness Scale consists of 8 items representing three aspects of belongingness: Connectedness (4 items), Affiliation (3 items), and Companionship (1 item). Each item is rated on a 6-point Likert scale ranging from 1 (Strongly Disagree) to 6 (Strongly Agree). A sample is "I feel disconnected from the world around me". The total score is the sum of 8 items, with higher scores indicating higher social connectedness. The potential score of Social Connectedness ranges from 6 to 48.

In the original study of Social Connectedness scale, the internal reliability or coefficient of Cronbach's alpha estimated was 0.91 [32], whereas alpha coefficients in other studies ranged from 0.83 to 0.93 [34,49–52]. The Alpha Coefficient in this study of international and domestic students was similar with 0.95. The construct validity was also supported by a negative association with anxiety, a positive association with self-esteem [53], and a negative correlation with acculturative stress [34].

2.3.3. Measures of Acculturative Stress

This study measured acculturative stress using the Acculturative Stress Scale for International Students (ASSIS) developed by Sandhu and Asrabadi [54]. The ASSIS, a 36-item questionnaire about acculturative stress of international students, covers 7 major factors: Perceived Discrimination (8 items), Homesickness (4 items), Perceived Hatred (5 items), Fear (4 items), Culture Shock (3 items), Guilt (2 items), and Miscellaneous (10 items). Each item is scored on a 5-point Likert scale ranging from 1 (strongly disagree) to 5 (strongly agree). The sum of all 7 major factors represents the total score of acculturative stress. The higher the total score, the higher the degree of acculturative stress international students undergo. However, since this study was conducted in an English-speaking campus in a country where English is not the native language, the survey was modified suitably for the study area. Specifically, based on the item "I feel nervous to communicate in English", there was on additional item related to student's Japanese proficiency: "I feel nervous to communicate in Japanese." On the other hand, as the factor related to social connectedness was covered in the SCS, the item "I feel intimidated to participate in social activities" was omitted to keep the total score from 36 to 180.

In other research, the alpha coefficient for acculturative stress total score ranged from 0.92 to 0.95 for international students [28,29,34,50]. In this study, the alpha coefficient was 0.95 for both international students and domestic students, indicating a high average inter-item correlation. The construct validity of ASSIS was supported by the positive correlation with depression [28,29] and mental health [55], and the negative correlation with condom-use intentions [55].

2.4. Procedure

The questionnaire was approved by the Ethical Committee Board of APU. Google Forms was selected as the platform to conduct the questionnaire because it is common and easy to manage. After a brief explanation of the project, the link to the questionnaire was distributed in several classes and among the APU Vietnamese community from the end of 2018. We chose the Vietnamese community as two authors are originally from Vietnam. After the announcement, survey was available online and students had the chance to answer the survey at their convenience (campus, home, library, etc.). The total response rate was 40.05% (268/669).

Informed consent was obtained from each participant: after following the survey link, each participant read the informed consent text together with an explanation on the research's goals (based on APU regulations), below which the participants had the choice to participate or not by choosing "Agree" or "Not agree." The participants had an option to quit survey by choosing "Not agree" or any time later, just by not submitting the survey. In the case of agreeing to participate, each participant was shown the list of questions to which he/she needs to answer.

2.5. Statistical Analysis

The statistical analysis of the research consists of two main parts. The first part is for estimating the prevalence of depression and potential socio-demographic predictor of depression, whereas the second part is to test the association of two predictors (social connectedness and acculturative stress) with the severity of depression.

The correlations between depression and socio-demographic factors, such as, gender, age, length of stay, language proficiency, e.g., were examined to find out potential predictors of depression. People who suffered from major or other depressive disorder were considered as being depressed. Dichotomous logistic regression was used as a statistical analysis tool for testing the potential socio-demographic predictor, because of three main points: (1) predetermined number of variables was comprised in the model making it show each variable's significance more clearly; (2) the model can indicate all odd ratios simultaneously between dependent variable and other categories [56]; and (3) binary logistic regression was widely used in other studies with the same topic [45,57–59]. Thus, the examined model of being depressed as dependent variables was presented as follows:

$$\begin{aligned} \ln\left(\tfrac{p}{1-p}\right)_{depression} &= \ln(Odd\ Ratios)_{depression} \\ &= \alpha + \beta_{1j}gender_{1j} + \beta_{2j}age_{2j} + \beta_{3j}stay_{3j} + \beta_{4j}Eng_{4j} + \beta_{5j}Jap_{5j} \\ &\quad + \beta_{6j}partner_{6j} + \beta_{7j}religion_{7j} + e, \end{aligned}$$

with

p: the probability of being depressed
α: intercept
β: coefficient which is the logarithm of Odd Ratios
j: categorical factor of independent variables
gender, age, etc.: independent variables
e: error term.

The binary logistic model was applied to both domestic and international students for comparative purpose. However, as no domestic students reported low Japanese proficiency and very few reported average Japanese proficiency, Japanese proficiency variable was omitted when the model was employed on the data set of domestic students.

Pearson Correlation Coefficient (PCC) analysis was first employed to look at the correlation among main variables used in the study for two reasons: (1) PCC indicates the strength of linear relationship of two variables [60]; and (2) PCC was widely used in studies in the same field [61–64]. According to the Cauchy-Schwartz inequality, PCC (r) has a value of between -1 and $+1$, where $+1$

indicates total positive linear correlation, 0 indicates no linear correlation, and −1 shows total negative linear correlation [65]. Next, to test the two hypotheses H1 and H2, multiple regression analysis was conducted to explore the contribution of main variables on predicting depression severity. Multiple regression analysis has been widely used in many other studies of the same field [23,25,66].

Raw data were cleaned in MS Excel and saved as CSV files. The data were then transferred into the database of STATA statistical software (version 15.1) to run statistical analysis. STATA statistical software was used for running dichotomous logistic regression, Pearson Correlation Coefficient, and multiple regression analysis. Additionally, robust statistics was also comprised in the dichotomous logistic regression model to omit outliners [67]. The p-value indicated the significance of independent variables in the models. It is conventional to choose p-value < 0.05 as a required statistical significance [68].

3. Results

3.1. Descriptive Results

According to the PHQ-9, 37.81% of international students and 29.85% of domestic students were found to be positive with depression (see Table 2). The proportion of depressed international students was higher than that of domestic students by almost 8%. While international students possessed a lower rate of major depressive disorder (14.93%) than other depressive disorder (22.89%), major depressive disorder (17.91%) was more significant than other depressive disorder (11.94%) among domestic students. Among the depressed domestic students, there was not much difference between males and females. On the other hand, international female students (39.84%) had a higher rate of depression than male international students (34.25%).

Table 2. Prevalence of depression.

	Domestic Students			International Students		
	Total (N = 67) Weighted %	Male (N = 25) Weighted %	Female (N = 42) Weighted %	Total (N = 201) Weighted %	Male (N = 73) Weighted %	Female (N = 128) Weighted %
Type of depression	**29.85**	**28.00**	**30.95**	**37.81**	**34.25**	**39.84**
Other depression	11.94	8.00	14.29	22.89	19.18	25.00
Major depression	17.91	20.00	16.67	14.93	15.07	14.84
Level of depression	**100.00**	**100.00**	**100.00**	**100**	**100**	**100**
Minimal depression	20.90	24.00	19.05	25.37	34.25	20.31
Mild depression	38.81	32.00	42.86	40.30	36.99	42.19
Moderate depression	29.85	32.00	28.57	26.37	20.55	29.69
Moderately severe depression	5.97	8.00	4.76	5.47	4.11	6.25
Severe depression	4.48	4.00	4.76	2.49	4.11	1.56

Among international students, the percentage of students being depressed varied according to their regions of origin. International students who were originally from South East Asia had the highest percentage of depression (39.34%), while students from South Asia possessed the lowest rate of depression (27.78%), which was even lower than domestic students (29.85%). Students from other regions had relatively similar rates of depression at 38%. Similar to domestic students, students from South Asia suffered from major depression (16.67%) more than other depression (11.11%).

Of the 67 domestic students and 201 international students, more than half of them only reported minimal depression or mild depression. More domestic students (40.3%) indicated suffering moderate depression or higher, compared to international students (34.33%). A higher percentage of moderate and more severe depression was reported in domestic male students (44%) than in domestic female students (38.09%). On the contrary, the number of international female students (37.5%) undergoing moderate to severe depression exceeded the number of international male students (28.77%)

Based on the PHQ-9, ASSIS, and SCS, the average total scores of each concept was presented in Figure 1. As can be seen, domestic students (8.61) had higher average stress level compared to that of international students (8.04), but the difference was negligible. Domestic and international students shared a relatively same level of social connectedness. The result also indicated that acculturative stress was perceived more strongly among international students (75.56) than domestic students (62.88).

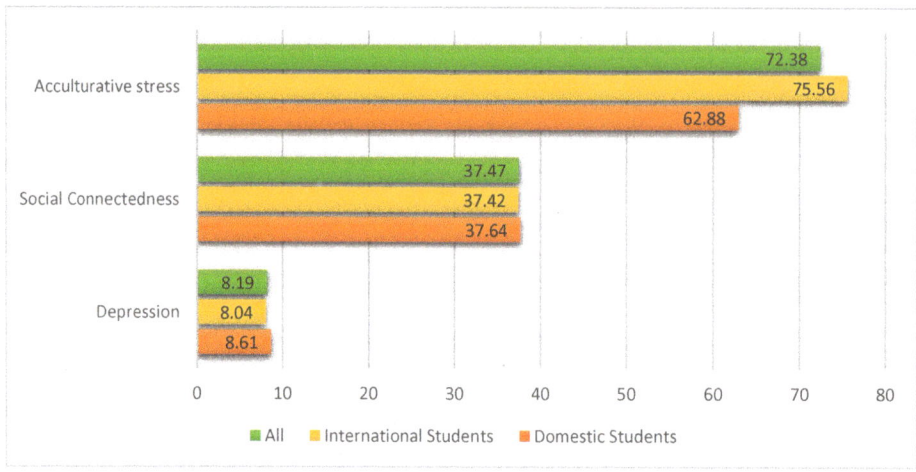

Figure 1. The total scores for depression, social connectedness, and acculturative stress among international and domestic students.

3.2. Main Analysis

3.2.1. Binary Logistic Regression Analysis

The results of the dichotomous logistic regression with the dependent variable "depression" on the independent socio-demographic variables were displayed in Table 3. In Table 3, there are also the estimated coefficients and the *p*-value of each variable for both domestic students and international students (with the coefficient being the logarithm of Odd Ratio).

The results showed multiple socio-demographic characteristics predicting the depression in domestic students at *p*-value < 0.05, whereas only one potential predictor can be found in international students. Domestic students in the age of 20 were more likely to have depression than those with ages from 17 to 19 ($\beta = 2.24$, $p = 0.048$). Another predictor of depression among domestic students was English proficiency. Domestic students speaking average English had a lower rate of being depressed than those who acquired low English proficiency ($\beta = -1.63$, $p = 0.038$). On the other hand, the only predictor for international students was the length of stay. International students living in Japan for three years suffered from a higher risk of being depressed than first-year students ($\beta = 1.08$, $p = 0.032$).

Table 3. Coefficient (β) and p-value for predictors of depression.

	Domestic Students		International Students	
	β	p-Value	β	p-Value
Gender: Male				
Female	0.24	0.721	0.05	0.879
Age: 17–19				
20	2.24	0.048 *	−0.87	0.129
>20	2.24	0.104	−0.59	0.216
Length of stay: Freshman				
2 years	−1.46	0.190	0.80	0.103
3 years	−2.63	0.063	1.08	0.032 *
>3 years	−2.87	0.096	1.04	0.106
English Proficiency: Low				
Average	−1.63	0.038 *	−0.03	0.968
High	−1.33	0.112	−0.27	0.720
Native	−	−	0.40	0.621
Japanese Proficiency: Low				
Average	−	−	−0.04	0.910
High	−	−	−0.25	0.638
Native	−	−	−	−
Intimate partner: No				
Yes	0.42	0.549	0.20	0.55
Religion: No				
Yes	−0.91	0.255	−0.45	0.180

Note: * and *** are statistically significant at 0.05 and 0.001, respectively.

3.2.2. Pearson Coefficient Correlation Analysis

In pairwise correlation analysis (see Tables 4 and 5), all relationships were found to be statistically significant at p-value < 0.001 for both international and domestic students. According to the finding, our hypotheses were confirmed that social connectedness significantly negatively correlated with depression in both domestic and international students (r = −0.6 and r = −0.54, respectively), and that acculturative stress significantly positively corresponded with depression in international students (r = 0.41). In other words, students with high social connectedness would be more likely to have higher depression levels, while international students with higher acculturative stress levels reported higher depression levels.

Table 4. Correlational relationship among Depression, Acculturative Stress, and Social Connectedness (Domestic students).

Pearson Correlation (Domestic Student)	1	2	3
1. Depression	1.00		
2. Acculturative stress	0.45 ***	1.00	
3. Social Connectedness	−0.60 ***	−0.55 ***	1.00

Note: * and *** are statistically significant at 0.05 and 0.001, respectively.

Table 5. Correlational relationship among Depression, Acculturative Stress, and Social Connectedness (International students).

Pearson Correlation (International Student)	1	2	3
1. Depression	1.00		
2. Acculturative stress	0.41 ***	1.00	
3. Social Connectedness	−0.54 ***	−0.58 ***	1.00

Note: * and *** are statistically significant at 0.05 and 0.001, respectively.

The finding also indicated a significantly negative relationship between social connectedness and acculturative stress in international students (r = −0.58). International students suffering from high acculturative stress reported lower sense of connectedness with surroundings. Additionally, there were statistically significant correlations of acculturative stress with depression and social connectedness estimated among domestic students (r = 0.45 and r = −0.55, respectively). The decrease of acculturative stress corresponded with the decrease of depression among domestic students, whereas the growing feeling of being connected to others correlated with less stress occurring during acculturation.

3.2.3. Multiple Regression Analysis

The normality of the dependent variable was first evaluated using the Skewness and Kurtosis normality test to make sure the variable was normally distributed. The Skewness and Kurtosis of international students were 0 and 0.06, respectively, indicating a normal distribution. On the other hand, those of domestic students were 0.14 and 0.41, indicating a mild nonnormality [28]. Therefore, we used square-root transformation for the dependent variable of domestic student [69]. After transformation, the Skewness and Kurtosis of domestic students were 0 and 0.15, indicating a normal distribution similar to those of international students. The transformed dependent variable of domestic students was used in the remaining of the analysis.

Domestic students. Regressing two main variables on transformed depression, results showed that the model accounted for 35.7% (R^2 = 0.357) of the variance (see Table 6). The F value of the model, $F(2,64)$ = 17.77 was statistically significant at p-value < 0.001. Both of the main predictors had statistically significant association with depression. Social connectedness was negatively correlated with depression (β = −0.044, p-value < 0.01). This indicated that people with stronger feeling of connectedness were likely to have lower severity of depression. Meanwhile, acculturative stress had a positively significant relationship with level of depression (β = 0.014, p-value < 0.05). In other words, domestic students with higher acculturative stress would likely suffer from more severe depression.

Table 6. Multiple regression analyses.

	Domestic Students		International Students	
	β	*p*-Value	β	*p*-Value
Social connectedness	−0.044	0.001 **	−0.241	0.000 ***
Acculturative stress	0.014	0.026 *	0.033	0.037 *
R^2	0.357		0.303	
F (df)	F (2,64) = 17.77 ***		F (2,198) = 43.15 ***	

Note: * and *** are statistically significant at 0.05 and 0.001, respectively.

International students. The regression analysis of the international student sample showed similar results to the domestic student sample. The goodness of fit of the international sample (R^2 = 0.303) was smaller than that of domestic samples, while the F value was still significant at p-value < 0.001 with F (2,198) = 43.15. All two main variables significantly predicted depression level. International students feeling connected to surrounding people were more likely to have low depression level (β = 0.033, p-value < 0.001). Higher acculturative stress could also predict more serious depression in international students (β = 0.033, p-value < 0.05).

The results from both domestic and international students implied the impact of social connectedness and acculturative stress on depression. According to the correlational results from the PCC test, social connectedness and acculturative stress were negatively correlated, social connectedness and acculturative stress might have not only direct impacts but also indirect impacts on the level of depression. Social connectedness could possibly directly affect depression levels and indirectly increase depression levels through escalating acculturative stress, and vice versa for acculturative stress.

4. Discussion and Conclusions

By collecting questionnaires from both domestic and international students at APU, the current study presents a primary investigation on depression, social connectedness, and acculturative stress in a multicultural environment. In the cross-sectional questionnaire of 67 domestic students and 201 international students, the study found that 29.85% of domestic students and 37.81% of international students were positive to major depressive disorder or other depressive disorder. In addition, the findings also highlight several socio-demographic predictors (age, English proficiency, and length of stay) and main associations (social connectedness and acculturative stress) of depression. The Mindsponge concept [70] was used to explain the findings.

4.1. Prevalence of Depression

According to this study, 30% of domestic students at APU had depression. This figure is quite common among studies of depression prevalence of students in Japan. In a study using The Center for Epidemiologic Studies Depression Scale (CES-D), one third of the total 105 students reported having mild depression and higher [9]. Based on The Zung Self-Rating Depression Scale (SDS), a study in 2011 also showed 30% of 2197 of Japanese dental college students having symptoms of moderate or severe depression [71]. As can be seen, the depression rate of Japanese college students was around 30%, which was close to the prevalence of depression among university students (30.6%) reported in a systematic review of 11 countries [7].

The depression prevalence of international students in this study was 37.81%, while 34% of international students who visited a mental health service at Tsukuba University health care were found to be depressed [12]. Another study employing the Center for Epidemiologic Studies Depression Scales reported 41% of 480 international respondents to be depressed [11]. In all cases, the situations of international students were more serious than those of domestic students, which required policy makers, schools, or anyone in charge to pay more attention to the mental health of international students.

The fact that more international students suffer from depression than domestic students can be the consequence of multiple sources. First, international students at an international university received higher level of acculturative stress (see Figure 1), which elevated the risk of being depressed [28–30,55]. Second, international students have lower access to mental health support than domestic students [44,72]. Third, international students have fewer choices of help-seeking sources than their domestic counterparts. For example, it is difficult for international students to seek help from parents and relatives due to the geographical distance [73].

Compared to the depression of students in other countries, the depression prevalence at APU and in Japan, in general, was not high. For example, a study in India employing the University Student Depression Inventory (USDI) showed 53.2% of students being positive to depression [13]. Using Depression Anxiety Stress Scale-21 (DASS-21), 60.8% of Egyptian students, 37.2% of Malaysian students, and 33% American students reported being depressed [15,19,74]. A web-based questionnaire among 4330 students using BAPI depression scale showed that 28.25% of Turkish students exhibited symptoms of depression [17].

Different levels of prevalence among countries are attributable to several reasons. Different types of questionnaire were used to measure depression (PHQ-9, The Center for Epidemiologic Studies Depression Scale (CES-D) [9], The Zung Self-Rating Depression Scale (SDS) [71], the University Student Depression Inventory (USDI) [13], Depression Anxiety Stress Scale-21 (DASS-21) [15,19,74], and BAPI depression scale [17]). Moreover, the difference might also result from macro-scale, micro-scale, and personal-scale factors. Among the macro-scale factors, depression can be influenced by a socio-economic background in which the university is located, such as income inequality and cultures [75], while the micro-scale factors, which include the living arrangement on campus and academic environment, might play an essential role in driving depression [13]. Apart from that, personal activities, beliefs, and issues might also be crucial contributors to depression [13,75].

Different levels of prevalence by gender were also noted. In both international and domestic students, a higher proportion of female students was found to be depressed than that of male. This difference might be explained by the fact that female students seem to have higher emotional, physiological, and behavioral reactions to stressors [76].

4.2. Socio-Demographic Factors Associated with Depression

In this study, socio-demographic data such as age, gender, length of stay in a new environment, and language proficiency, e.g., were selected to examine the association with depression using dichotomous logistic regression. Compared to another finding of the depression among international students [11], the results here confirmed that age and Japanese language proficiency were not potential predictors of depression among international students in Japan. On the other hand, studies of international students in the United States [77] revealed English proficiency as a predictor for depression. Along this note, the current study did confirm English proficiency as a predictor of depression among the Japanese students. A high percentage of foreign staffs and students, and mandatory English-based subjects for domestic students might be the answers.

Apart from English proficiency, the results also showed two other statistically significant predictors for depression among domestic students. First, age was a significant predictor for depression. Domestic students aged 20 reported having higher rate of being depressed than students with ages between 17 and 19. This finding was consistent with the findings in Kenya and Malaysia [14,15], while the fact that depression did not vary according to age was pointed out in another study in the U.S. [78]. Thus, it might depend on the cultural and social context of the study site to say whether age can be a predictor. In this case, Japanese teenagers were afraid of becoming adults [79], and when Japanese teenagers become 20, they will be considered as adults after the Coming of Age Day (*Seijin no Hi*). As a result, depression might be more likely to occur among 20-year-old Japanese students.

Another notable result in this study was that third-year international students had a higher chance of being depressed than first-year students. There are several possible explanations: (1) third-year students at APU need to take major courses which are more difficult than the introductory and basic courses in the first and second years; (2) the end of the third year is the period that students have to think about their career paths, and career indecision was positively correlated with depression [80,81].

Findings that age and length of stay were contributors to depression provided some insights of emerging adulthood theory [82] in an Asian country, a topic that has not been explored much. Some people in their late teens to their mid-to late 20s experience serious mental health problem as they do not want to take adult responsibilities and obligations [82,83]. Additionally, facing difficulties and lacking educational information when entering into the labor market might be very stressful for emerging adult students [84,85]. In general, depression related to the fear of being an adult or career indecision during the emerging adulthood period does not happen only in Western countries, but also in the Asian settings.

4.3. Mindsponge Theory as an Explaination for Depression, Social Connectedness and Acculturation

Findings of the current study confirmed the two main hypotheses that (H1) acculturative stress was significantly positively associated with depression, and (H2) social connectedness was significantly negatively correlated with depression among both domestic and international students. The Mindsponge concept [70] could serve as an explanation for the underlying mechanism among depression, social connectedness, and acculturation among students from a multicultural aspect.

Mindsponge is a concept designed to illustrate the mechanism of how a person absorbs and integrates new cultural values into a his/her own mindset and the reverse of ejecting inappropriate core values (see Figure 1 in the work of Vuong & Napier [70]).

Acculturative stress. This study found a positive correlation between acculturative stress and depression among domestic and international students. This judgement was supported by similar findings from other studies [23–26,28,29]. Acculturative stress happens during the acculturation process as a result of an individual facing various unfamiliar aspects in his/her daily life while trying to adapt to the new environment. Here, students studying in a new environment are prone to acculturative stress, especially those living in a multicultural environment (e.g., climate, food, language, race, landscape, culture) [86].

Living in different environments means facing different cultural and ideological values. Studying in a multicultural environment, students are more likely to be exposed to many new cultural values, which requires adjustment and adaptation. However, it is not easy to for the mindset to integrate and absorb new values. From the external environment to the core value, new cultural values need to get through points of filter. During the filtering process, old and new values are evaluated, connected, and compared [87] to integrate, synthesize, and incorporate values that are compatible or eject waning values. The filtering process is also where the acculturative conflict takes place and causes acculturative stress [22].

The extent to which an individual trusts a new value to be compatible with his/her mindset is the key in the filtering process. Living among new cultural values that an individual has not yet trusted will lead to sustained stress, which may cause brain dysfunction (certain types of depression) [88]. As the conflict becomes more serious, similar to the natural resistance of a human body, the filtering membrane of an individual might receive signal from the mindset to grow thicker to protect the old core values. This, in turn, makes the core values become even more distant with the external values, which greatly raises the level of distrust, intensifies the stress level, and eventually escalates the depression level. For example, low language proficiency makes an individual unable to communicate. Without communication, new cultural values cannot be interpreted, which may lead to distrust of new values, conflict and stress. Eventually, that may give rise to depression.

Social connectedness. The negative association between social connectedness and depression was found in the current study. In other words, social connectedness may help lessen the negative impacts of depression in a multicultural context. The social connectedness reflects "one's opinion of self in relation to other people" in term of emotional distance [32]. When students start to live in a new environment, their social networks begin to change. Living in a new environment where the ideological setting and surrounding people are different, students have to adapt and make new friends. This process can also be explained by the Mindsponge concept.

Assuming the self of an individual is also his/her own mindset. Making new friends is equivalent to accepting new values, so it requires a point of filter. At that point, a friend's personality, perception, and opinion will need to get through a filtering process to make sure whether a self/mindset trusts its new friend/value. If a new friend/value is trustworthy, it can possibly come closer to the self/mindset. This is when a student has a high sense of connectedness. On the other hand, if a new friend/value is in conflicts with the self/mindset, it will be considered as untrustworthy. Functionally, the filter will become thicker, increase the emotional distance from self/mindset to a new friend/value. In other words, feeling difficult to have new friends, students may have no sense of connectedness which may result in strong feeling of hopelessness [89,90] and gradually contribute to loneliness [91]. As loneliness is among the top predictors of depression [91–94] and hopelessness is also positively correlated with depression [95], the lower social connectedness, the higher depression will be. This way of explanation may also be compatible with the association between social connectedness and depression in other population.

In addition, social connectedness under a multicultural context may also have a buffering effect on acculturative stress [34]. As discussed, the mindset increasingly distrusts new value, the distance between mindset and new cultural value is widened due to the rising acculturative conflicts. Social connectedness may contribute to enhance trust of mindset toward new cultural values, which may facilitate the acculturation process. Eventually, since acculturation happens more smoothly, acculturative stress decreases, depression is less likely to happen.

5. Recommendations for School Policy

Based on the above findings, the study suggested some recommendations to have a healthier and more sustainable educational environment in international universities.

- Having a warmer, more close-knit, and friendly education atmosphere is good to enhance trust among students, staffs, and university. By doing so, students will feel more connected to new environment and suffer less from acculturative stress.
- Empowering community-based activities is a potential bottom-up approach for increasing social connectedness, as well as reducing difficulties from acculturation.
- Depression during the emerging adulthood period might be indispensable [82]. Thus, providing appropriate mental and physical supports is necessary. Consultancy or seminar integrating scientific findings [96–98] on the matter of emerging adulthood could be added.

6. Limitation and Recommendation for Further Research

This paper has some limitations. In the data collection process, the team used sampling and needed to modify the model questionnaire slightly. In addition, findings were based on self-reported measures.

Regarding of the results on depression, the comparison with the prevalence in other studies might not be precise due to different types of questionnaire used in each study. The questionnaire was collected between November and January, when winter signs were apparent, so depression might be affected by seasonality, primarily when a large number of students originated from tropical areas. The impacts of seasonality on depression were confirmed in other studies [99,100]. Besides that, the current study had higher proportion of females than males, while depression among female students was more prevalent than among male students. The gender disparity in sampling might, therefore, leads to a higher percentage of depression.

The imbalances between the numbers of international and domestic students might be a limitation of this study. Besides that, different proportions of students from different origins might cause the results to have a regional bias among the surveyed international students.

There is a need to find out cause-effect relationships among the correlation, as well as for qualitative studies to provide more in-depth information. The study also recommend a meta-analysis for the mental health of international students in Japan like the following work [101]. This will increase the integration and synthesis of mental health research in Japan. Moreover, the Mindsponge concept was recommended to explain results in mental health study.

Author Contributions: Conceptualization, M.H.N., T.T.L. and S.M.; methodology, M.H.N. and S.M.; software, M.H.N.; validation, M.H.N. and S.M.; formal analysis, M.H.N.; investigation, M.H.N and T.T.L.; resources, M.H.N., T.T.L., and S.M.; data curation, M.H.N.; writing—original draft preparation, M.H.N. and T.T.L.; writing—review and editing, M.H.N. and S.M.; visualization, M.H.N.; supervision, S.M.; project administration, M.H.N. and S.M.; funding acquisition, S.M.

Funding: This research received no external funding.

Acknowledgments: We thank Ho Manh Tung (Ritsumeikan Asia Pacific University) and Nguyen To Hong Kong (Vuong & Associates) for giving advices and comments that greatly help us during the course of this research. We would also like to show our gratitude to the Research Office of Ritsumeikan Asia Pacific University for facilitating our research process.

Conflicts of Interest: The authors declare no conflict of interest.

References

1. UNESCO. Education: Outbound Internationally Mobile Students by Host Region. 2019. Available online: http://data.uis.unesco.org/Index.aspx?queryid=172# (accessed on 26 January 2019).
2. Mathers, C.D.; Loncar, D. Projections of Global Mortality and Burden of Disease from 2002 to 2030. *PLoS Med.* **2006**, *3*, e442. [CrossRef] [PubMed]

3. *Depression and Other Common Mental Disorders: Global Health Estimates*; World Health Organization: Geneva, Switzerland, 2017.
4. Okumura, Y.; Higuchi, T. Cost of Depression among Adults in Japan. *Prim. Care Companion CNS Disord.* **2011**, *13*. [CrossRef]
5. Rupert, W. Hayes Why Does Japan Have Such a High Suicide Rate? *BBC News*, 2015. Available online: https://www.bbc.com/news/world-33362387 (accessed on 29 January 2019).
6. The Free Library Suicides Due to Hardships in Life, Job Loss up Sharply in 2009. 17 May 2010. Available online: https://www.thefreelibrary.com/Suicidesduetohardshipsinlife,joblossupsharplyin2009.-a0226580269 (accessed on 29 January 2019).
7. Ibrahim, A.K.; Kelly, S.J.; Adams, C.E.; Glazebrook, C. A systematic review of studies of depression prevalence in university students. *J. Psychiatr. Res.* **2013**, *47*, 391–400. [CrossRef] [PubMed]
8. Tomoda, A.; Mori, K.; Kimura, M.; Takahashi, T.; Kitamura, T. One-year prevalence and incidence of depression among first-year university students in Japan: A preliminary study. *Psychiatry Clin. Neurosci.* **2000**, *54*, 583–588. [CrossRef] [PubMed]
9. Kawada, T.; Katsumata, M.; Suzuki, H.; Shimizu, T. Actigraphic predictors of the depressive state in students with no psychiatric disorders. *J. Affect. Disord.* **2007**, *98*, 117–120. [CrossRef] [PubMed]
10. *International Students in Japan*; Japan Student Services Organization: Tokyo, Japan, 2017.
11. Eskanadrieh, S.; Liu, Y.; Yamashina, H.; Kono, K.; Arai, A.; Lee, R.; Tamshiro, H. Depressive symptoms among international university students in northern Japan: Prevalence and associated factors. *J. Int. Health* **2012**, *27*, 165–170.
12. Takafumi, H.; Terumi, I.; Hirokazu, T.; Naoko, S.; Tadashi, T.; Takashi, A.; Adm Jon, L. An analysis of mental disorders of international students visiting the Mental Health Service at Tsukuba University Health Center. *Seishin shinkeigaku zasshi = Psychiatria et neurologia Japonica* **2012**, *114*, 3–12.
13. Deb, S.; Banu, P.R.; Thomas, S.; Vardhan, R.V.; Rao, P.T.; Khawaja, N. Depression among Indian university students and its association with perceived university academic environment, living arrangements and personal issues. *Asian J. Psychiatry* **2016**, *23*, 108–117. [CrossRef] [PubMed]
14. Othieno, C.J.; Okoth, R.O.; Peltzer, K.; Pengpid, S.; Malla, L.O. Depression among university students in Kenya: Prevalence and sociodemographic correlates. *J. Affect. Disord.* **2014**, *165*, 120–125. [CrossRef] [PubMed]
15. Shamsuddin, K.; Fadzil, F.; Ismail, W.S.W.; Shah, S.A.; Omar, K.; Muhammad, N.A.; Jaffar, A.; Ismail, A.; Mahadevan, R. Correlates of depression, anxiety and stress among Malaysian university students. *Asian J. Psychiatry* **2013**, *6*, 318–323. [CrossRef]
16. Sarokhani, D.; Delpisheh, A.; Veisani, Y.; Sarokhani, M.T.; Manesh, R.E.; Sayehmiri, K. Prevalence of Depression among University Students: A Systematic Review and Meta-Analysis Study. *Depression Res. Treat.* **2013**, *2013*, 1–7. [CrossRef] [PubMed]
17. Gulec Oyekcin, D.; Sahin, E.M.; Aldemir, E. Mental health, suicidality and hopelessness among university students in Turkey. *Asian J. Psychiatry* **2017**, *29*, 185–189. [CrossRef] [PubMed]
18. Jasso-Medrano, J.L.; López-Rosales, F. Measuring the relationship between social media use and addictive behavior and depression and suicide ideation among university students. *Comput. Hum. Behav.* **2018**, *87*, 183–191. [CrossRef]
19. Abdel Wahed, W.Y.; Hassan, S.K. Prevalence and associated factors of stress, anxiety and depression among medical Fayoum University students. *Alex. J. Med.* **2017**, *53*, 77–84. [CrossRef]
20. Mitsui, N.; Asakura, S.; Takanobu, K.; Watanabe, S.; Toyoshima, K.; Kako, Y.; Ito, Y.M.; Kusumi, I. Prediction of major depressive episodes and suicide-related ideation over a 3-year interval among Japanese undergraduates. *PLoS ONE* **2018**, *13*, e0201047. [CrossRef] [PubMed]
21. Tanaka, N.; Uji, M.; Hiramura, H.; Chen, Z.; Shikai, N.; Kitamura, T. Cognitive patterns and depression: Study of a Japanese university student population. *Psychiatry Clin. Neurosci.* **2006**, *60*, 358–364. [CrossRef] [PubMed]
22. Berry, J.W. Acculturation: Living successfully in two cultures. *Int. J. Intercult. Relat.* **2005**, *29*, 697–712. [CrossRef]
23. Hovey, J.D. Acculturative stress, depression, and suicidal ideation in Mexican immigrants. *Cult. Divers. Ethn. Minor. Psychol.* **2000**, *6*, 134–151. [CrossRef]

24. Tummala-Narra, P.; Alegria, M.; Chen, C.-N. Perceived discrimination, acculturative stress, and depression among South Asians: Mixed findings. *Asian Am. J. Psychol.* **2012**, *3*, 3–16. [CrossRef]
25. Revollo, H.-W.; Qureshi, A.; Collazos, F.; Valero, S.; Casas, M. Acculturative stress as a risk factor of depression and anxiety in the Latin American immigrant population. *Int. Rev. Psychiatry* **2011**, *23*, 84–92. [CrossRef]
26. Park, H.-S.; Rubin, A. The mediating role of acculturative stress in the relationship between acculturation level and depression among Korean immigrants in the U.S. *Int. J. Intercult. Relat.* **2012**, *36*, 611–623. [CrossRef]
27. Brunsting, N.C.; Zachry, C.; Takeuchi, R. Predictors of undergraduate international student psychosocial adjustment to US universities: A systematic review from 2009-2018. *Int. J. Intercult. Relat.* **2018**, *66*, 22–33. [CrossRef]
28. Wei, M.; Heppner, P.P.; Mallen, M.J.; Ku, T.-Y.; Liao, K.Y.-H.; Wu, T.-F. Acculturative stress, perfectionism, years in the United States, and depression among Chinese international students. *J. Couns. Psychol.* **2007**, *54*, 385–394. [CrossRef]
29. Constantine, M.G.; Okazaki, S.; Utsey, S.O. Self-Concealment, Social Self-Efficacy, Acculturative Stress, and Depression in African, Asian, and Latin American International College Students. *Am. J. Orthopsychiatr.* **2004**, *74*, 230–241. [CrossRef] [PubMed]
30. Lee, J.-S.; Koeske, G.F.; Sales, E. Social support buffering of acculturative stress: A study of mental health symptoms among Korean international students. *Int. J. Intercult. Relat.* **2004**, *28*, 399–414. [CrossRef]
31. Ribeiro, Í.J.S.; Pereira, R.; Freire, I.V.; de Oliveira, B.G.; Casotti, C.A.; Boery, E.N. Stress and Quality of Life Among University Students: A Systematic Literature Review. *Health Prof. Educ.* **2018**, *4*, 70–77. [CrossRef]
32. Lee, R.M.; Robbins, S.B. Measuring belongingness: The Social Connectedness and the Social Assurance scales. *J. Couns. Psychol.* **1995**, *42*, 232–241. [CrossRef]
33. Williams, K.L.; Galliher, R.V. Predicting Depression and Self–Esteem from Social Connectedness, Support, and Competence. *J. Soc. Clin. Psychol.* **2006**, *25*, 855–874. [CrossRef]
34. Yeh, C.J.; Inose, M. International students' reported English fluency, social support satisfaction, and social connectedness as predictors of acculturative stress. *Couns. Psychol. Q.* **2003**, *16*, 15–28. [CrossRef]
35. Times Higher Education World University Rankings 2019: Methodology 2018. Available online: https://www.timeshighereducation.com/world-university-rankings/methodology-world-university-rankings-2019#survey-answer (accessed on 28 January 2019).
36. Vuong, Q.-H.; Bui, Q.-K.; La, V.-P.; Vuong, T.-T.; Nguyen, V.-H.T.; Ho, M.-T.; Nguyen, H.-K.T.; Ho, M.-T. Cultural additivity: Behavioural insights from the interaction of Confucianism, Buddhism and Taoism in folktales. *Palgrave Commun.* **2018**, *4*, 143. [CrossRef]
37. Pekerti, A.A.; Thomas, D.C. n-Culturals: Modeling the multicultural identity. *Cross Cult. Strateg. Manag.* **2016**, *23*, 101–127. [CrossRef]
38. Pekerti, A.A.; Vuong, Q.H.; Napier, N.K. Double edge experiences of expatriate acculturation: Navigating through personal multiculturalism. *J. Glob. Mobil.* **2017**, *5*, 225–250. [CrossRef]
39. APU. *Awards and Rankings*; APU: Oita, Japan, 2018; Available online: http://en.apu.ac.jp/home/about/content177/ (accessed on 23 December 2018).
40. APU. *APU Student Numbers as of May 2017*; APU: Oita, Japan, 2017; Available online: http://en.apu.ac.jp/home/news/article/?storyid=2865 (accessed on 23 December 2018).
41. APU. *APU Outline*; APU: Oita, Japan, 2018; Available online: http://en.apu.ac.jp/home/about/content55/ (accessed on 23 December 2018).
42. Kroenke, K.; Spitzer, R.L. The PHQ-9: A New Depression Diagnostic and Severity Measure. *Psychiatr. Ann.* **2002**, *32*, 509–515. [CrossRef]
43. Kroenke, K.; Spitzer, R.L.; Williams, J.B.W. The PHQ-9: Validity of a brief depression severity measure. *J. Gen. Intern. Med.* **2001**, *16*, 606–613. [CrossRef] [PubMed]
44. Eisenberg, D.; Golberstein, E.; Gollust, S.E. Help-Seeking and Access to Mental Health Care in a University Student Population. *Med. Care* **2007**, *47*, 594–601. [CrossRef] [PubMed]
45. Eisenberg, D.; Gollust, S.E.; Golberstein, E.; Hefner, J.L. Prevalence and correlates of depression, anxiety, and suicidality among university students. *Am. J. Orthopsychiatr.* **2007**, *77*, 534–542. [CrossRef] [PubMed]
46. Spitzer, R.L. Validation and Utility of a Self-report Version of PRIME-MDThe PHQ Primary Care Study. *JAMA* **1999**, *282*, 1737. [CrossRef]

47. Han, X.; Han, X.; Luo, Q.; Jacobs, S.; Jean-Baptiste, M. Report of a Mental Health Survey Among Chinese International Students at Yale University. *J. Am. Coll. Health* **2013**, *61*, 1–8. [CrossRef]
48. Eisenberg, D.; Hunt, J.; Speer, N.; Zivin, K. Mental Health Service Utilization Among College Students in the United States. *J. Nerv. Ment. Dis.* **2011**, *199*, 301–308. [CrossRef]
49. Hendrickson, B.; Rosen, D.; Aune, R.K. An analysis of friendship networks, social connectedness, homesickness, and satisfaction levels of international students. *Int. J. Intercult. Relat.* **2011**, *35*, 281–295. [CrossRef]
50. Cao, C.; Meng, Q.; Shang, L. How can Chinese international students' host-national contact contribute to social connectedness, social support and reduced prejudice in the mainstream society? Testing a moderated mediation model. *Int. J. Intercult. Relat.* **2018**, *63*, 43–52. [CrossRef]
51. Lee, R.M.; Keough, K.A.; Sexton, J.D. Social Connectedness, Social Appraisal, and Perceived Stress in College Women and Men. *J. Couns. Dev.* **2002**, *80*, 355–361. [CrossRef]
52. Lee, R.M.; Robbins, S.B. Understanding Social Connectedness in College Women and Men. *J. Couns. Dev.* **2000**, *78*, 484–491. [CrossRef]
53. Lee, R.M.; Robbins, S.B. The relationship between social connectedness and anxiety, self-esteem, and social identity. *J. Couns. Psychol.* **1998**, *45*, 338–345. [CrossRef]
54. Sandhu, D.S.; Asrabadi, B.R. Development of an Acculturative Stress Scale for International Students: Preliminary Findings. *Psychol. Rep.* **1994**, *75*, 435–448. [CrossRef] [PubMed]
55. Yang, N.; Xu, Y.; Chen, X.; Yu, B.; Yan, H.; Li, S. Acculturative stress, poor mental health and condom-use intention among international students in China. *Health Educ. J.* **2018**, *77*, 142–155. [CrossRef]
56. Vuong, Q.-H.; Ho, T.-M.; Nguyen, H.-K.; Vuong, T.-T. Healthcare consumers' sensitivity to costs: A reflection on behavioural economics from an emerging market. *Palgrave Commun.* **2018**, *4*, 70. [CrossRef]
57. Hefner, J.; Eisenberg, D. Social support and mental health among college students. *Am. J. Orthopsychiatr.* **2009**, *79*, 491–499. [CrossRef]
58. Keyes, C.L.M.; Eisenberg, D.; Perry, G.S.; Dube, S.R.; Kroenke, K.; Dhingra, S.S. The Relationship of Level of Positive Mental Health with Current Mental Disorders in Predicting Suicidal Behavior and Academic Impairment in College Students. *J. Am. Coll. Health* **2012**, *60*, 126–133. [CrossRef]
59. Marconi, A.; Ranum, N.; Van Orman, S.; Hanson, B.; Donovan, V.; Borenitsch, E. Demographic differences in response rates for PHQ9 in a university student population. *J. Am. Coll. Health* **2018**, 1–7. [CrossRef]
60. Benesty, J.; Chen, J.; Huang, Y.; Cohen, I. Pearson Correlation Coefficient. In *Noise Reduction in Speech Processing*; Springer: Berlin/Heidelberg, Germany, 2009; Volume 2, pp. 1–4. ISBN 978-3-642-00295-3.
61. Ogunsanya, M.E.; Bamgbade, B.A.; Thach, A.V.; Sudhapalli, P.; Rascati, K.L. Determinants of health-related quality of life in international graduate students. *Curr. Pharm. Teach. Learn.* **2018**, *10*, 413–422. [CrossRef] [PubMed]
62. Dogra, S.; MacIntosh, L.; O'Neill, C.; D'Silva, C.; Shearer, H.; Smith, K.; Côté, P. The association of physical activity with depression and stress among post-secondary school students: A systematic review. *Ment. Health Phys. Act.* **2018**, *14*, 146–156. [CrossRef]
63. Lex, H.; Ginsburg, Y.; Sitzmann, A.F.; Grayhack, C.; Maixner, D.F.; Mickey, B.J. Quality of life across domains among individuals with treatment-resistant depression. *J. Affect. Disord.* **2019**, *243*, 401–407. [CrossRef] [PubMed]
64. Md, T.L.; Mb, C.J.; Mm, Y.-F.P.; Mb, W.Z.; Mb, X.F. Correlation between premature ejaculation and psychological disorders in 270 Chinese outpatients. *Psychiatry Res.* **2019**, *272*, 69–72. [CrossRef] [PubMed]
65. Lee Rodgers, J.; Nicewander, W.A. Thirteen Ways to Look at the Correlation Coefficient. *Am. Stat.* **1988**, *42*, 59–66. [CrossRef]
66. Mui, A.C.; Kang, S.-Y. Acculturation Stress and Depression among Asian Immigrant Elders. *Soc. Work* **2006**, *51*, 243–255. [CrossRef]
67. Rousseeuw, P.J.; Hubert, M. Robust statistics for outlier detection: Robust statistics for outlier detection. *WIREs Data Min. Knowl. Discov.* **2011**, *1*, 73–79. [CrossRef]
68. Vuong, Q.H.; Napier, N.K.; Tran, T.D. A categorical data analysis on relationships between culture, creativity and business stage: The case of Vietnam. *Int. J. Transit. Innov. Syst.* **2013**, *3*, 4. [CrossRef]
69. Cohen, J.; Cohen, J. (Eds.) *Applied Multiple Regression/Correlation Analysis for the Behavioral Sciences*, 3rd ed.; L. Erlbaum Associates: Mahwah, NJ, USA, 2003; ISBN 978-0-8058-2223-6.

70. Vuong, Q.H.; Napier, N.K. Acculturation and global mindsponge: An emerging market perspective. *Int. J. Intercult. Relat.* **2015**, *49*, 354–367. [CrossRef]
71. Takayama, Y.; Miura, E.; Miura, K.; Ono, S.; Ohkubo, C. Condition of depressive symptoms among Japanese dental students. *Odontology* **2011**, *99*, 179–187. [CrossRef]
72. Hyun, J.; Quinn, B.; Madon, T.; Lustig, S. Mental Health Need, Awareness, and Use of Counseling Services Among International Graduate Students. *J. Am. Coll. Health* **2007**, *56*, 109–118. [CrossRef] [PubMed]
73. Wilson, C.J.; Deane, F.P.; Ciarrochi, J.V.; Rickwood, D. Measuring help seeking intentions: Properties of the General Help Seeking Questionnaire. *Can. J. Couns.* **2005**, *39*, 15–28.
74. Beiter, R.; Nash, R.; McCrady, M.; Rhoades, D.; Linscomb, M.; Clarahan, M.; Sammut, S. The prevalence and correlates of depression, anxiety, and stress in a sample of college students. *J. Affect. Disord.* **2015**, *173*, 90–96. [CrossRef] [PubMed]
75. Steptoe, A.; ardle, J.; Tsuda, A.; Tanaka, Y. Depressive symptoms, socio-economic background, sense of control, and cultural factors in University students from 23 Countries. *Int. J. Behav. Med.* **2007**, *14*, 97–107. [CrossRef] [PubMed]
76. Misra, R.; Crist, M.; Burant, C.J. Relationships among Life Stress, Social Support, Academic Stressors, and Reactions to Stressors of International Students in the United States. *Int. J. Stress Manag.* **2003**, *10*, 137–157. [CrossRef]
77. Sümer, S.; Poyrazli, S.; Grahame, K. Predictors of Depression and Anxiety among International Students. *J. Couns. Dev.* **2008**, *86*, 429–437. [CrossRef]
78. Lester, D. Depression and suicide in college students and adolescents. *Person. Individ. Differ.* **1990**, *7*, 757–758. [CrossRef]
79. Mathews, G.; White, B. (Eds.) *Japan's Changing Generations: Are Young People Creating a New Society?* Japan Anthropology Workshop Series; Routledge Curzon: London, UK; New York, NY, USA, 2004; ISBN 978-0-415-32227-0.
80. Saunders, D.E.; Peterson, G.W.; Sampson, J.P.; Reardon, R.C. Relation of Depression and Dysfunctional Career Thinking to Career Indecision. *J. Vocat. Behav.* **2000**, *56*, 288–298. [CrossRef]
81. Rottinghaus, P.J.; Jenkins, N.; Jantzer, A.M. Relation of Depression and Affectivity to Career Decision Status and Self-Efficacy in College Students. *J. Career Assess.* **2009**, *17*, 271–285. [CrossRef]
82. Arnett, J.J. Emerging Adulthood: What Is It, and What Is It Good For? *Child Dev. Perspect.* **2007**, *1*, 68–73. [CrossRef]
83. Levine, M.D. *Ready or Not, Here Life Comes*; Simon & Schuster: New York, NY, USA, 2006.
84. Hamilton, S.F.; Hamilton, M.A. School, Work, and Emerging Adulthood. In *Emerging Adults in America: Coming of Age in the 21st Century*; Arnett, J.J., Tanner, J.L., Eds.; American Psychological Association: Washington, DC, USA, 2006; pp. 257–277. ISBN 978-1-59147-329-9.
85. Côté, J.E. *Arrested Adulthood: The Changing Nature of Maturity and Identity*; New York University Press: New York, NY, USA, 2000; ISBN 978-0-8147-1598-7.
86. Smith, R.A.; Khawaja, N.G. A review of the acculturation experiences of international students. *Int. J. Intercult. Relat.* **2011**, *35*, 699–713. [CrossRef]
87. Vuong, Q.H.; Napier, N.K. Making creativity: The value of multiple filters in the innovation process. *Int. J. Transit. Innov. Syst.* **2014**, *3*, 294. [CrossRef]
88. Van Praag, H.M. Can stress cause depression? *World J. Biol. Psychiatry* **2005**, *6*, 5–22. [CrossRef] [PubMed]
89. Eraslan-Capan, B. Social Connectedness and Flourishing: The Mediating Role of Hopelessness. *Univers. J. Educ. Res.* **2016**, *4*, 933–940. [CrossRef]
90. Rice, K.G.; Leever, B.A.; Christopher, J.; Porter, J.D. Perfectionism, stress, and social (dis)connection: A short-term study of hopelessness, depression, and academic adjustment among honors students. *J. Couns. Psychol.* **2006**, *53*, 524–534. [CrossRef]
91. Furr, S.R.; Westefeld, J.S.; McConnell, G.N.; Jenkins, J.M. Suicide and depression among college students: A decade later. *Prof. Psychol. Res. Pract.* **2001**, *32*, 97–100. [CrossRef]
92. Wilbert, J.R.; Rupert, P.A. Dysfunctional attitudes, loneliness, and depression in college students. *Cognit. Ther. Res.* **1986**, *10*, 71–77. [CrossRef]
93. Rich, A.R.; Scovel, M. Causes of Depression in College Students: A Cross-Lagged Panel Correlational Analysis. *Psychol. Rep.* **1987**, *60*, 27–30. [CrossRef]

94. Wei, M.; Russell, D.W.; Zakalik, R.A. Adult Attachment, Social Self-Efficacy, Self-Disclosure, Loneliness, and Subsequent Depression for Freshman College Students: A Longitudinal Study. *J. Couns. Psychol.* **2005**, *52*, 602–614. [CrossRef]
95. Rosembaum Asarnow, J.; Guthrite, D. Suicidal Behavior, Depression, and Hopelessness in Child Psychiatric Inpatients: A Replication and Extension. *J. Clin. Child Psychol.* **1989**, *18*, 129–136. [CrossRef]
96. Vuong, Q.H. Impacts of geographical locations and sociocultural traits on the Vietnamese entrepreneurship. *SpringerPlus* **2016**, *5*, 1189. [CrossRef] [PubMed]
97. Aryee, S.; Debrah, Y.A. A cross-cultural application of a career planning model. *J. Organ. Behav.* **1993**, *14*, 119–127. [CrossRef]
98. Krumboltz, J.D. Integrating Career and Personal Counseling. *Career Dev. Q.* **1993**, *42*, 143–148. [CrossRef]
99. Lyall, L.M.; Wyse, C.A.; Celis-Morales, C.A.; Lyall, D.M.; Cullen, B.; Mackay, D.; Ward, J.; Graham, N.; Strawbridge, R.J.; Gill, J.M.R.; et al. Seasonality of depressive symptoms in women but not in men: A cross-sectional study in the UK Biobank cohort. *J. Affect. Disord.* **2018**, *229*, 296–305. [CrossRef]
100. Oyane, N.M.F.; Bjelland, I.; Pallesen, S.; Holsten, F.; Bjorvatn, B. Seasonality is associated with anxiety and depression: The Hordaland health study. *J. Affect. Disord.* **2008**, *105*, 147–155. [CrossRef] [PubMed]
101. Vuong, Q.-H.; La, V.-P.; Vuong, T.-T.; Ho, M.-T.; Nguyen, H.-K.T.; Nguyen, V.-H.; Pham, H.-H.; Ho, M.-T. An open database of productivity in Vietnam's social sciences and humanities for public use. *Sci. Data* **2018**, *5*, 180188. [CrossRef] [PubMed]

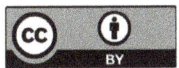

© 2019 by the authors. Licensee MDPI, Basel, Switzerland. This article is an open access article distributed under the terms and conditions of the Creative Commons Attribution (CC BY) license (http://creativecommons.org/licenses/by/4.0/).

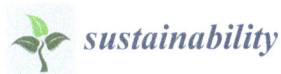

Article

Sex Differences and Psychological Factors Associated with General Health Examinations Participation: Results from a Vietnamese Cross-Section Dataset

Quan-Hoang Vuong [1,2,*], Kien-Cuong P. Nghiem [3], Viet-Phuong La [1,2], Thu-Trang Vuong [4], Hong-Kong T. Nguyen [5], Manh-Toan Ho [1,2], Kien Tran [6,7], Thu-Hong Khuat [6] and Manh-Tung Ho [1,2,*]

[1] Centre for Interdisciplinary Social Research, Phenikaa University, Yen Nghia, Ha Dong, Ha Noi 100803, Vietnam; phuong.laviet@phenikaa-uni.edu.vn (V.-P.L.); toan.homanh@phenikaa-uni.edu.vn or tung.homanh@phenikaa-uni.edu.vn (M.-T.H.)
[2] Faculty of Economics and Finance, Phenikaa University, Yen Nghia, Ha Dong, Hanoi 100803, Vietnam
[3] Vietnam-Germany Hospital, 16 Phu Doan street, Hoan Kiem district, Hanoi 100000, Vietnam; kimcuongvd@gmail.com
[4] Campus Dijon, Sciences Po, 75337 Paris, France; thutrang.vuong@sciencespo.fr
[5] AI for Social Data Lab, Vuong & Associates, 3/161 Thinh Quang, Dong Da, Hanoi 100000, Vietnam; htn2107@caa.columbia.edu
[6] Institute for Social Development Studies - ISDS, Suite 1804, PH Floor, The Garden Building, Me Tri Road, Tu Liem District, Hanoi 100000, Vietnam; trankien@vnu.edu.vn (K.T.); hongisds@gmail.com (T.-H.K.)
[7] School of Law, Vietnam National University, Hanoi 100803, Vietnam
* Correspondence: hoang.vuongquan@phenikaa-uni.edu.vn (Q.-H.V.); tung.homanh@phenikaa-uni.edu.vn (M.-T.H.)

Received: 4 December 2018; Accepted: 14 January 2019; Published: 18 January 2019

Abstract: This study focuses on the association of sex differences and psychological factors with periodic general health examination (GHE) behaviors. We conducted a survey in Hanoi and the surrounding areas, collecting 2068 valid observations; the cross-section dataset was then analyzed using the baseline category logit model. The study shows that most people are afraid of discovering diseases through general health examinations (76.64%), and the fear of illness detection appears to be stronger for females than for males ($\beta_{1(male)} = -0.409, p < 0.001$). People whose friends/relatives have experienced prolonged treatment tend to show more hesitation in participating in physical check-ups ($\beta_2 = 0.221, p < 0.05$). On the ideal frequency of GHEs, 90% of the participants agree on once or twice a year. The probability of considering a certain period of time as an appropriate frequency for GHEs changes in accordance with the last doctor visit (low probability of a health examination every 18 months) and one's fear of potential health problems post-checkup (no fear raises probability of viewing a health examination every 6 months by 9–13 percentage points). The results add to the literature on periodic GHE in particular and on preventive health behaviors in general.

Keywords: periodic general health examination; fear of illness detection; sex; Vietnam

1. Introduction

1.1. On General Health Examinations

Periodic general health examination (GHE) is expected to be an effective method of helping people improve their health [1,2]. One of the first mentions of periodic health examination was by Dobell in 1861: he advocated for such examinations as a method of following up on the health status of tuberculosis patients [3]. From the 1920s until the 1970s, many medical institutions in the U.S systematically encouraged and advised citizens to take periodic health checkups [4,5]. In earlier surveys, over 90% of participants thought they should check their blood pressure, heart, lungs and stomach regularly [6]. Many studies have suggested more efficient use of healthcare resources on the grounds that periodic GHEs may help reduce the actual mortality rate [1,7–10].

Yet, it is important to note that this practice is not widely followed across the world. This study looks at the case of Vietnam, a developing country with a per capita income of approximately USD2000 and a large population facing diverse health issues [11]. In terms of periodic GHE, Vietnam's healthcare lacks sustainability on both the institutional and individual levels. First, there is little regulation in this area. Most governmental efforts focus on health insurance, namely the expansion of insurance coverage, the positive effects of which have been debated and refuted [12]. Otherwise, health-related programs mostly concern health communication—often at a rather rudimentary level such as education on basic hygiene—and improvement of infrastructure. This mostly applies to rural areas in order to compensate for the fact that the health system is still largely centralized, with many rural patients risking destitution to travel to larger cities to receive treatment [13]. This could result in overpopulation of central hospitals in large cities, especially during disease outbreaks, which clogs the flow of patients and leads to lower treatment quality—characteristics of an unsustainable health system [14].

Second, on the individual level, employers are required to organize at least one GHE every six months for heavy manual workers and every year for other employees [15]. People are, however, skeptical about the quality of these enforced check-ups [16] and for a good reason: no regulations exist regarding GHE, creating legal loopholes for employers to cut down on costs by organizing inadequate check-ups. This means that the only health checkups that should "count" are those taken by people on their own initiative. Yet most people only willingly perform health examinations when they suspect they have a health-related condition, which may lead to late discovery of illness and higher treatment costs later, exacerbating the risk of financial difficulty for individuals from rural areas.

1.2. Sex and Psychological Differences Involved in Health Behaviors

Although there are doubts over the relationship between gender and periodic health examination [17], numerous reports provide evidence that women have more healthy habits and use health services more often than men do [18–25]. In the U.S, several survey results have concluded that men have higher mortality rates [26–28] despite overestimating their own health status [29]. This behavior was also observed among male university students in Canada, the majority of whom rated their health status as "very good", whereas female students admitted their health to be just "good", or lower [30].

While several reasons ranging from personality to actual health conditions could account for such behavior, the differences of the sexes undoubtedly provide some explanation [17,19,31]. Women may be more sensitive and able to perceive more subtle signals from their own body [32]. With a positive attitude towards healthcare and diseases prevention, women tend to detect health problems early on, while men mostly perform medical examinations when obliged to, such as for work purposes or during the process of acquiring insurance [33,34]. Aside from the biological differences of the two sexes, social factors might also explain the diverging behaviors of men and women regarding healthcare. For instance, in traditional views, men tend to (falsely) think of themselves as less susceptible to injuries or illness [29,35]. This mentality may be rooted in traditional gender roles: A man is the family's breadwinner and usually accepts higher workplace risks while a woman has a higher priority for health matters of the family, which includes that of her own [30,36]; nevertheless, perceptions of healthcare might vary under the effects of marriage [37]. Considering the influence of family members' health status on the decisions regarding GHEs, there is evidence showing that women tend to spend less money on GHE than men and will consider GHE fees before deciding to participate [7,38–42]. But if a family member is seriously sick or dying, women's anxiety over health status will significantly increase and affect their healthcare decisions [43].

The survey of related literature shows a considerable difference in healthcare decision-making between the sexes. However, it is still not clear, for example, how the differences in men and women's GHEs participation are associated with psychological factors such as a family member suffering from prolonged treatment or the fear of finding out one's own illness.

1.3. Psychological Factors and GHEs Participation

The voluminous literature on health beliefs has long explored the complex relationship between psychological factors and healthcare behaviors [44,45]. For example, a study finds people who feel healthy at the moment as one of the reasons for not attending GHEs [46], another shows that non-attenders tend not to value health as strongly, have low self-efficacy, feel less in control of their health and be less likely to believe in the efficacy of health checks [47]. In contrast, it is known that those with a relatively good health condition, taking medical examinations and receiving advice from health experts about diseases prevention tend to improve their health status, helping to reduce the number of visits to health professionals [48]. In addition, as periodic GHEs only perform a number of standard tests for early symptoms, they should not cause a build-up of psychological hesitations [12,17,49].

Studies confirm that spending money on preventive health practice such as general physical examinations is a complicated decision, in particular when psychological factors are taken into account. However, the literature seems to overlook the influence of the fear of finding out one's own illness and the experience of having one's family members or close relatives going through long-term medical treatment. This study will (i) demonstrate the correlation among the sexes, the health status of relatives/friends and people's reluctance to take health checkups due to worries over potential discovery of illness; and (ii) provide empirical evidence on the association between the time gap since the last health checkup and the fear of uncovering any health problems with the propensity of taking up GHEs.

2. Materials and Methods

2.1. Sample

The dataset of the study was collected in various clinics, hospitals, companies, schools and households in Hanoi and its surrounding areas. It was conducted by the Vuong & Associates research team during the last quarter of 2016, under the ethical standards and institutional approval numbered V&A/07/2016 (12 September 2016), following which a statement of research ethics is provided at the end of each questionnaire (the participants will be anonymized; all information collected will be used for only research purposes; the participants are free to leave the interview at any point of their own choosing). Overall, the survey team approached 2479 people; one out of six declined to take part in the study. The time for each interview was 10–15 min/questionnaire. In the end, the final sample size was 2068 subjects. The data descriptor of the final dataset has been approved by Nature Research [50,51] and it was deposited at both Open Science Framework and Harvard's Dataverse [51] according to the principle of open data and scientific transparency [52].

2.2. Procedures

Raw data are entered in MS Excel then converted into CSV. Data treatment and categorical structuring for multi-way contingency data tables are performed in R 3.3.1. The actual estimating of statistical coefficients, and computing relevant test statistics, employs the baseline-categorical logit (BCL) model, enabling the exploring of possible relationships among the concerning variables through different specifications depending upon choices of response and predictor variables [46]. The following passages give an overview of the descriptive statistics.

Among 2068 respondents, the percentage of young people (<30 years old) accounts for the majority (63.15%), and the proportion of respondents aged 50 or more ($\geq$50 years) is very small, only about 5.67% (Table 1). It is worth noting that 64.08% respondents were female, which was significantly skewed compared to the man-to-woman ratio of 97.5:100 for the entire country and 96.7:100 for Hanoi (2017 preliminary statistics provided by the General Statistics Office of Vietnam—citation later). Women appear to have accepted interviews more often than men; this observation shall be further discussed later in this article.

Table 1. Descriptive statistics.

Characteristics	N	Percentage (%)
Age		
<30	1306	63.15
30–49	643	31.09
≥50	119	5.76
Sex ("Sex")		
Male	728	35.2
Female	1340	64.8
Hesitation due to possible discovery of diseases ("DiscDisease")		
Yes	483	23.36
No	1585	76.64
Time since the most recent visit to doctor ("RecExam")		
Less than 12 months	1373	66.39
From 12 to 24 months	200	9.67
Above 24 months	125	6.05
Unknown	370	17.89
Having friends under long-term treatments ("AcqTrmt")		
Yes	917	44.34
Never	1151	55.66
Perceived suitable periodic GHE frequency ("SuitFreq")		
Every 6 months	1238	59.86
Every 12 months	638	30.85
≥18 months	192	9.28

More than 3/4 of the survey respondents said they were not concerned about participating in periodic GHEs due to possible disease detection but rather due to other causes: too time-consuming (51.69%), financially costly (37.23%), low confidence in the quality of service (26.78%), or feeling that GHEs aren't urgent or important (51.89%).

Notably, about 2/3 of the respondents had their most recent check-up less than 12 months ago (66.39%) with the main reasons being early symptoms of a health problem (35.30%) and at the request of the employers (35.11%). The remaining reasons are due to public rumors or unofficial information about some epidemic or disease outbreaks (4.74%), and self-perceived needs of health checkups (24.85%).

Concerning health status of relatives/friends of the participants, 44.34% had friends or relatives who had been or were currently under long-term treatment, while the remainder had relatives/friends in good health and who had never received long-term treatment. In addition, over 90% of those interviewed said that if they had enough time and money, GHEs should be taken once or twice a year. Still 9.28% thought that attending GHEs should take place every 18 months or even longer. The hesitation toward GHE due to possible discovery of diseases in relation to the appropriate examination time is described in Figure 1.

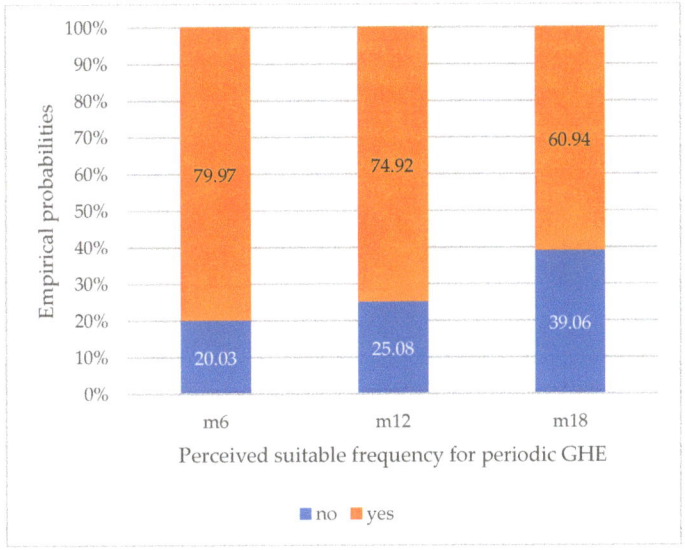

Figure 1. Relationship between fear of illness detection and perceived suitable GHE frequency (date from Table S1).

In Figure 1, it can be seen that the proportion of people afraid of detecting illnesses through periodic GHE ("yes") at the appropriate time of 6 months ("m6") is the highest, and this percentage decreases as the time gap since the participant's most recent GHE increases.

2.3. Measures

Specifically, in this article, two kinds of probability will be measured:

(i) The probability of a person hesitant to take periodic general health examination due to fear of discovering one's disease (coded as "DiscDisease") against sex ("Sex") and whether their friends or family have gone through long-term treatment ("AcqTrmt");
(ii) The probability of perceived appropriate periodic GHE frequency (6 months, 12 months, ≥18 months) ("SuitFreq") against the time since their last visit to a doctor ("RecExam") and the fear of diseases detection ("DiscDisease").

2.4. Analysis

The baseline-categorical logit model has been employed in order to investigate the probability of the dependent variable against both independent variables simultaneously.

The estimated coefficients in multivariable logistic models are used to calculate the empirical probabilities. The statistical significance of predictor variables in the model are determined based on z-value and p-value (p); with $p < 0.05$ being the conventional level of statistical significance required for a positive result. The general equation of the baseline-categorical logit model is:

$$\ln(\pi_j(\mathbf{x})/\pi_J(\mathbf{x})) = \alpha_j + \boldsymbol{\beta}_j^T \mathbf{x}, j = 1, \ldots, J-1.$$

in which $\mathbf{x}$ is the independent variable; and $\pi_j(\mathbf{x}) = P(Y = j \mid \mathbf{x})$ its probability. Thus $\pi_j = P(Y_{ij} = 1)$ with Y being the dependent variable [53].

In the logit model, the probability of an event, among a distribution $\{\pi_j(\mathbf{x})\}$, is computed as:

$$\pi_j(\mathbf{x}) = \exp(\alpha_j + \boldsymbol{\beta}_j^T \mathbf{x}) / (1 + {}^{J-1}\sum_{(h-1)} \exp(\alpha_j + \boldsymbol{\beta}_j^T \mathbf{x}))$$

with $\sum_j \pi_j(x) = 1$; $\alpha_j = 0$ and $\beta_j = 0$; in which n is the number of observations in the sample, j the categorical values of an observation i, and h a row in basic matrix Xi. Estimated probabilities can be used to predict the possibilities of Y in different conditions of Xi [13,50,51,53,54].

Applying the regression model, first, the relationship between hesitation towards GHE due to fear of disease discovery associated with sex differences and health status of friends/relatives. The dependent variable is "DiscDisease" (hesitation due to possible disease detection) with two categories "Yes" and "No". The dependent variables are "Sex", having values of "Male" and "Female"; and "AcqTrmt" (the status of the respondents having friends/relatives undertaking a long-term medical treatment), which can be true ("Yes") or false ("Never"). The results give statistically significant ($p < 0.0001$) coefficients which help to establish an empirical relationship as provided in Table 2.

Table 2. Estimation results of the response "DiscDisease" and the predictor "Sex" and "AcqTrmt".

	Intercept	"Sex"	"AcqTrmt"
		"Male"	"Yes"
	β_0	β_1	β_2
logit(yes | no)	−1.155 ***	−0.409 ***	0.221 *
	(−14.573)	(−3.602)	(2.110)

Significance codes: 0 '***' 0.001 '**' 0.01 '*'; z-value in square brackets; baseline category for: "Sex" = "Female"; and "AcqTrmt" = "Never". Log-likelihood: −12.89 on 1 degree of freedom (d.f.). Residual deviance: 0.68 on 1 d.f.

From the results above, the regression equation (Equation (1)) is derived.

$$\ln(\pi_{yes}/\pi_{no}) = -1.155 - 0.409 \times \text{male.Sex} + 0.221 \times \text{yes.AcqTrmt} \qquad (1)$$

According to Equation (1), in order to calculate the probability of a man being afraid of GHE and having friends/relatives experiencing long-term treatment, the following formula is employed:

$$\pi_{yes} = e^{-1.155-0.409+0.221}/(1 + e^{-1.155-0.409+0.221}) = 0.207$$

Next, periodic GHE behaviors are assessed through the dependent variable—the perceived suitable frequencies of GHE ("SuitFreq"): every 6 months ("m6"), every 12 months ("m12"), and every 18 months or more ("m18"). The first factor that is supposed to have an impact on the people's behavior is the fear of diseases, represented by the variable of "DiscDisease", having one of the two categorical values: "Yes" and "No". The second factor, the time since a respondent's most recent medical examination ("RecExam"), is also taken into account and divided into four categories: <12 months ("less12"), 12–24 months ("b1224"), more than 24 months ("g24"), and forgotten/never attending ("unknown"). Actual estimations for logistic regression models report that almost all estimate coefficients are highly significant with <0.01. Detailed results are presented in Table 3.

Table 3. Estimating the response "SuitFreq" against the predictor "RecExam" and "DiscDisease".

	Intercept	"RecExam"			"DiscDisease"
		"less12"	"g24"	"unknown"	"Yes"
	β_0	β_1	β_2	β_3	β_4
logit(m6 | m18)	2.026 ***	0.854 **	−0.588	−1.085 ***	−0.838 ***
	(7.495)	(2.937)	(−1.620)	(−3.741)	(−4.862)
logit(m12 | m18)	1.793 ***	0.277	−0.865 *	−1.553 ***	−0.594 **
	(6.540)	(0.937)	(−2.307)	(−5.170)	(−3.276)

Significance codes: 0 '***' 0.001 '**' 0.01 '*' 0.05 '.' 0.1 ' ' 1; z-value in square brackets; baseline category for: "RecExam" = "b1224"; and "DiscDisease" = "No". Log-likelihood: −44.58 on 6 d.f. Residual deviance: 10.73 on 6 d.f.

The equations of Equations (2) and (3) below help to quantify the influence of the time since the participant's most recent doctor visit and psychological concerns to diseases on perceivably appropriate GHE frequency.

$$\ln(\pi_{m6}/\pi_{m18}) = 2.026 + 0.854 \times \text{less12.RecExam} - 0.588 \times \text{g24.RecExam} \\ - 1.085 \times \text{unknown.RecExam} - 0.838 \times \text{yes.DiscDisease} \quad (2)$$

$$\ln(\pi_{m12}/\pi_{m18}) = 1.793 + 0.277 \times \text{less12.RecExam} - 0.865 \times \text{g24.RecExam} \\ - 1.553 \times \text{unknown.RecExam} - 0.594 \times \text{yes.DiscDisease} \quad (3)$$

Modifying Equations (2) and (3), we can obtain π_{m6} on the conditions of "RecExam" = "less12" and "DiscDisease" = "Yes" according to the following formula:

$$\pi_{m6} = e^{2.026 + 0.854 - 0.838}/(1 + e^{2.026 + 0.854 - 0.838} + e^{1.793 + 0.277 - 0.594}) = 0.589$$

3. Results

3.1. Fear of Disease Detection in GHE Decisions

Other conditional probabilities are computed likewise, with the empirical results being reported in Table 4.

Table 4. Probability of hesitation toward GHE due to disease detection as influenced by the sex and health status of friends or relatives.

"DiscDisease"	"Yes"		"No"	
"AcqTrmt" | "Sex"	"Male"	"Female"	"Male"	"Female"
"Yes"	0.207	0.282	0.793	0.718
"Never"	0.173	0.240	0.827	0.760

It is clear from Table 4 that both men and women are significantly more likely not to be afraid of finding out their own health problems through GHEs (from nearly 72% to 83% probability) whether they have friends or family members who go through long-term medical treatment or not.

For people afraid of discovering their own diseases, women are about 7–8 percentage points more likely to be reluctant to attend a health exam. By contrast, the probability of being afraid of disease detection in GHE is lower in men. It is of interest to observe the calculated coefficients as they evaluate the extent to which psychological factors affect participants' hesitation toward periodic GHE (Equation (1)). Notably, the coefficient of the variable "Sex" at "male" is negative ($\beta_1 = -0.409$ with $p < 0.001$), meaning that π_{yes} of male participants is smaller than that of females. This is also confirmed by the probabilities in Table 3. However, the difference between men and women is not too large.

Table 3 also reveals that those who have friends or relatives who used to suffer from long-time treatment are more likely to fear disease detection as a reason to their hesitation toward periodic GHE. For example, if a woman has relatives or friends who have experienced long-time therapy, the probability of her hesitating to take periodic GHE is 28.2%, but this figure will drop to 24% if her friends or relatives have good health.

3.2. Correlates of Perception on the Appropriate GHE Frequencies

Table 5 below shows the probability of selecting the appropriate periodic GHE frequencies controlling the time since the most recent doctor visit and the fear of detecting diseases through check-ups.

Table 5. Probabilities of periodic GHE frequencies perceived as suitable based on the time since the participant's most recent doctor visits and the fear of detecting disease through check-ups.

"SuitFreq"		"m6"			
"DiscDisease" | "RecExam"		"less12"	"b1224"	"g24"	"unknown"
"yes"		0.589	0.432	0.432	0.394
"no"		0.666	0.520	0.544	0.530
"SuitFreq"		"m12"			
"DiscDisease" | "RecExam"		"less12"	"b1224"	"g24"	"unknown"
"yes"		0.334	0.437	0.331	0.250
"no"		0.296	0.412	0.327	0.263
"SuitFreq"		"m18"			
"DiscDisease" | "RecExam"		"less12"	"b1224"	"g24"	"unknown"
"yes"		0.077	0.131	0.237	0.356
"no"		0.038	0.068	0.129	0.207

Table 5 shows that participants are most inclined to attend a regular health check every 6 months regardless of having fear of finding out their own health problems or visiting the doctor recently (from 39.4% to 66.6%). Opinions on a checkup every 12 months appear neutral, fluctuating from 25% to 43.7%. By contrast, the frequency of every 18 months marks the widest range of probability, from 3.8% up to 35.6%.

Looking at the finer details, one can see that regardless of the fear of discovering one's own illness, those who have visited the doctor within the last two years tend to have a very low probability of seeing 18 months as an appropriate frequency for GHE uptake (3.8–13.1%).

The probability of a person seeing every six months as an appropriate frequency for GHE is shown to increase from 9 to 13 percentage points if the person is not afraid of discovering one's own illness. The pattern reverses for the 12 months and 18 months frequency.

When it comes to people's behaviors toward periodic GHEs, from Equations (2) and (3), it can be seen that apart from intercepts, the coefficient at "unknown" of "RecExam" has the largest absolute value ($\beta_3 = -1.085$ with p-value < 0.001 at Equation (2) and $\beta_3 = -1.553$ with p-value < 0.001 at Equation (3)). Thus, out of all the time values since the patient's most recent doctor visit, it is in reality the "unknown" variable that has a significant impact on the likelihood of people believing that periodic GHE should be taken every 6 or 12 months. Figure 2 depicts the impact tendencies of "RecExam" and "DiscDisease" on participants' perception of suitable GHE frequencies.

Figure 2a depicts changes in the preferred periodic GHE frequencies of those who last visited doctors two years ago. It can be easily observed that the line of "m6" goes upward and "m18" downward as they move from "yes.DiscDisease" (afraid of detecting disease) to "no.DiscDisease" (not afraid). In other words, people without the fear of detecting their own illness through GHE are more likely to perceive every six months as the appropriate frequency for the service and less likely to perceive every 18 months as appropriate. For the frequency of every 12 months, the line "m12" lays nearly horizontal, showing that both ready patients and hesitating patients have nearly the same propensity to take periodic GHE every 12 months.

Figure 2b presents the changes in suitable periodic GHE frequencies as perceived by those who are afraid of figuring out diseases through periodic physical exams. It can be remarked that when moving from the point "less12" to "unknown", the probability line of "m6" goes downward from nearly 60% to almost 40%, whereas the "m18" has an opposite slope from 7.7% to nearly 36%. In particular, the "m12" line is broken at the point "b1224" but then continues going down. In summary, the longer the time since the last doctor visit, the less likely that a person would accept attending periodic GHE every six or 12 months.

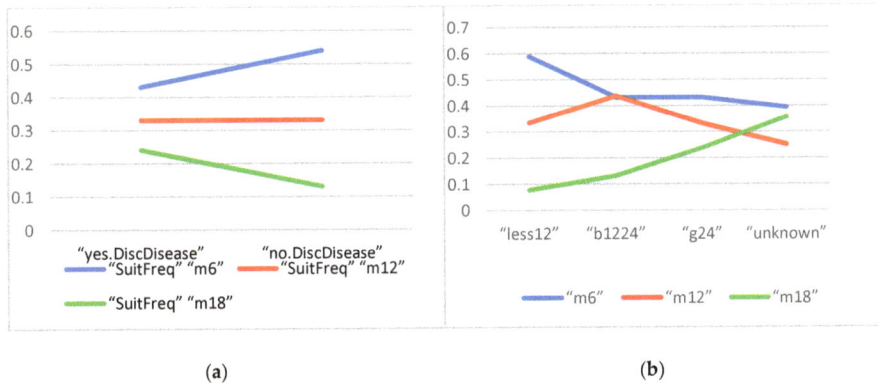

Figure 2. (a) Changes in preferred periodic GHE frequencies of those who last visited doctors 2 years ago; (b) Changes in preferred periodic GHE frequencies as perceived by those who are afraid of figuring out diseases through periodic GHEs (data from Tables S2 and S3).

4. Discussion

This study has shown the high probability of a person, regardless of his or her sex, *not* to be afraid of finding out his or her own health problems through GHEs (from nearly 72% to 83% probability), regardless of having friends or family who go through long-term medical treatment. This result is not surprising given that most people often cited reasons of a practical nature for not attending health examination, such as a lack of time or hindrances at work [46,47]. However, reluctance toward regular health checks doesn't only stem from concerns over a lack of resources, such as time or money [55]; psychological factors, such as the fear of discovering a potential negative health condition, as this study has shown, could also influence people's decision-making regarding the services. Among the notable results, the probability of hesitating to take GHE due to the fear of discovering diseases is about 7–8 percentage points higher in women, while the pattern reverses for men. In other words, women are more likely than men to be reluctant to take GHE due to the fear of potential illness detection. This behavioral pattern is attributable to the viewpoint that in a society such as Vietnam, women are traditionally viewed as more vulnerable. However, the literature in Western countries seems to show women to be more likely to use health screening services [19,20,47,51], thus suggesting the result obtained in this study might only be generalizable in patriarchal cultures.

Another counter-intuitive result is the hesitation toward periodic health check-ups among those whose friends or relatives used to suffer from long-term treatment. One would expect someone who knows how taxing illnesses can be through witnessing experiences of their closed ones to be more careful and inclined towards having periodic GHE. This behavior, driven by the fear of detecting one's potential illness, might be explained by a number of factors: the trauma caused by witnessing the long-term medical treatment of family friends, or perhaps, the financial constraints when the ill person happens to be dependent on a respondent to some degree [6,10,55–57].

The study also confirms that the average person is most likely to see "every six months" as an appropriate frequency for GHE, regardless of their fear of finding out their own health problems, and of the length of time since their most recent doctor visit. However, when looking at more details, the probability of a person seeing "every six months" as an appropriate frequency for GHE is shown to increase slightly if the person is *not* afraid of the potential of detecting an illness. This pattern is the opposite for the 12 months and 18 months frequency. That means having fear of facing the possibility of discovering illness through GHEs is associated with a higher probability of delaying GHE and widening the gap between each check-up. This procrastination is interesting given the literature on the subject tends to focus on the binary choice of attending or not-attending [8,19,31,47]. In fact, this touches upon a new dimension of the quality and effectiveness of periodic GHE that had not been discussed in the extant literature, which is its frequency. This is especially important as some countries have regulations concerning periodic GHE and its frequency while others might not.

Regarding how the time since the most recent doctor visit is associated with the perceived appropriate frequency of GHE, those who have visited the doctor within the last two years tend to have a very low probability of seeing every 18 months as an appropriate frequency (3.8–13.1%). This might just be because they are still being monitored by professional healthcare personnel, either in treatment or post-treatment recovery. But their higher level of concerns over health matters can also be due to their past experience with being ill: they pay more attention to healthcare because they understand the importance of having check-ups regularly. In other words, they have "learned their lesson," and are much more willing to take GHE on a regular basis. This result is intuitive and, interestingly, in stark contrast with the behavior of those who have witnessed friends or relatives cope with diseases. It seems that for more sustainable health behaviors such as more frequent GHE, firsthand experience with illness is more motivating factor compared with merely witnessing health struggles.

Although this study has offered some insights into the behaviors and psychology of GHE decision-making, it is not without limitations. First, regarding the sample itself, the survey is limited to the vicinity of Hanoi, Vietnam, thus, the results presented here should be interpreted with care. The sample is also skewed in regards to biological sex, with over 64 percent participants being female, hence, this skewness's effect on the representativeness should be taken into account when conducting any analysis of the dataset. Second, there are other psychological factors that are involved in health-related behaviors that the paper has not been able to examine. For example, there can be certain misconceptions about the utility and purpose of the health check-up [2,5,6] that might make people less inclined to take up the service. There can be a central role for the view of a person on uncertainty in the decision of attending a GHE or not [51]. Finally, it is arguable that health behaviors are influenced by cultural factors, for example, people in different cultures might have different patterns in spending, reasoning or procrastinating, etc. [58]. Hence, future studies should take into account cultural differences in health behaviors.

5. Conclusions

This paper has presented a statistical analysis using the baseline-category logit model to explore how the factors of sex differences and having family members/friends going through a long-term medical treatment are associated with the fear of discovering one's own illness through GHEs. Results confirm that the majority of participants do not hesitate to take periodic GHE out of fear of discovering illnesses. However, being a woman and having family members or friends going through a long-term medical treatment are factors that are shown to increase the probability of reluctance towards periodic GHE due to that fear. This clashes with the extant literature dominated by studies done in developed Western countries as well as with rationality and perhaps implies that it is a feature unique to Vietnam and similar countries.

The paper also investigates how the fear of discovering one's own illness and the time since the most recent doctor visit are associated with the perception of appropriate frequency for GHE. The most notable result is that fear of illness discovery will increase the probability of widening the gap between each GHE. In addition, having had a doctor visit within two years is associated with a very low probability of perceiving a large time gap between general health check-ups as appropriate. The results are shown to add to the literature on GHE decision-making, which seems to dominantly focus on the binary choice of participation or non-participation in GHE and still has a gap regarding the associated psychological factors in preventive health behaviors.

Supplementary Materials: The following are available online at http://www.mdpi.com/2071-1050/11/2/514/s1, Table S1: Distribution of patients against psychological hesitation towards periodic GHE due to diseases discovering and perceivably suitable periodic GHE frequency (Data used for Figure 1), Table S2: Changes in probability of perceivably suitable periodic GHE frequency of those having the last doctor visit 2 years ago (Data used for Figure 2a), Table S3: Changes in probability of perceivably suitable periodic GHE frequency of those who have hesitation towards GHE due to disease identification (Data used for Figure 2b).

Author Contributions: Conceptualization, Q.-H.V.; methodology, Q.-H.V.; validation, T.-H.K. and K.T.; formal analysis, T.-T.V. and V.-P.L.; investigation, K.-C.N.P., V.-P.L. and T.-T.V.; data curation, K.-C.N.P. and T.-T.V.; writing—original draft preparation, T.T.V., M.-T.H., and H.K.T.N.; writing—review and editing, Q.H.V., T.-T.V., M.-T.H., and H.-K.T.N.; visualization, T.-T.V. and K.-C.P.N.; supervision, Q.-H.V.; project administration, Q.H.V. and K.T.

Funding: The research was conducted independently and received no funding from any public or private institutions. The authors were responsible for all expenditures during the investigation.

Acknowledgments: The authors would like to express a deep sense of gratitude towards the respondents of the study, without whom, this research cannot be done. The authors would like to thank several people at Vuong & Associates for their assistance in collecting the data, particularly Dam Thu Ha, Do Thu Hang, Do Phuong Ngoc, Nguyen Thi Phuong, Mai Anh Tuan.

Conflicts of Interest: The authors declare no conflict of interest.

Data availability: The description of how the datasets of this study were generated and processed could be found at [50]. The complete datasets could be found in Open Science Framework: https://osf.io/afz2w/ and Harvard Dataverse: https://doi.org/10.7910/DVN/CWHOIC.

References

1. Holland, W. Periodic health examination: History and critical assessment. *EuroHealth* **2009**, *15*, 16–20.
2. Roberts, N.T. The values and limitations of periodic health examinations. *J. Chronic Dis.* **1959**, *9*, 95–116. [CrossRef]
3. Dobell, H. Lectures on the Germs and Vestiges of Disease, and on the Prevention of the Invasion and Fatality of Disease by Periodical Examinations. Available online: https://www.ncbi.nlm.nih.gov/pmc/articles/PMC5180312/pdf/brforeignmcrev72757-0171.pdf (accessed on 18 January 2018).
4. Emerson, H. Periodic medical examinations of apparently healthy persons. *JAMA J. Am. Med. Assoc.* **1923**, *80*, 1376. [CrossRef]
5. Han, P.K.J. Historical Changes in the Objectives of the Periodic Health Examination. *Ann. Intern. Med.* **1997**, *127*, 910. [CrossRef]
6. Oboler, S.K.; Prochazka, A.V.; Gonzales, R.; Xu, S.; Anderson, R.J. Public Expectations and Attitudes for Annual Physical Examinations and Testing. *Ann. Intern. Med.* **2002**, *136*, 652. [CrossRef]
7. Zielhuis, G.A. Are periodic school health examinations worthwhile? *Health Policy* **1985**, *5*, 241–253. [CrossRef]
8. Wu, H.-Y.; Yang, L.-L.; Zhou, S. Impact of periodic health examination on surgical treatment for uterine fibroids in Beijing: A case-control study. *BMC Health Serv. Res.* **2010**, *10*. [CrossRef]
9. Burton, L.C.; Steinwachs, D.M.; German, P.S.; Shapiro, S.; Brant, L.J.; Richards, T.M.; Clark, R.D. Preventive services for the elderly: Would coverage affect utilization and costs under Medicare? *Am. J. Public Health* **1995**, *85*, 387–391. [CrossRef] [PubMed]
10. Nakanishi, N.; Tatara, K.; Fujiwara, H. Do preventive health services reduce eventual demand for medical care? *Soc. Sci. Med.* **1996**, *43*, 999–1005. [CrossRef]
11. Vuong, Q. The financial economy of Viet Nam in an age of reform, 1986–2016. In *Routledge Handbook of Banking and Finance in Asia*; Volz, U., Morgan, P., Yoshino, N., Eds.; Routledge T&F: London, UK, 2019.
12. Vuong, Q.-H.; Vu, Q.-H.; Vuong, T.-T. What makes Vietnamese (not) attend periodic general health examinations? A 2016 cross-sectional study. *Osong Public Health Res. Perspect.* **2017**, *8*, 147–154. [CrossRef] [PubMed]
13. Vuong, Q.H. Be rich or don't be sick: Estimating Vietnamese patients' risk of falling into destitution. *SpringerPlus* **2015**, *4*. [CrossRef] [PubMed]
14. Fineberg, H.V. A Successful and Sustainable Health System—How to Get There from Here. *N. Engl. J. Med.* **2012**, *366*, 1020–1027. [CrossRef] [PubMed]
15. International Cooperation Department. *Labour Codes, General Labour and Employment Acts*; Ministry of Labour, Official Gazette: Hanoi, Vietnam, 2012; Volume 2012, pp. 48–78.
16. LĐO. Kham Suc Khoe Dinh Ky Cho Vui [Periordic Health Check-Ups for Fun]. Available online: https://laodong.vn/suc-khoe/kham-suc-khoe-dinh-ky-cho-vui-584383.ldo (accessed on 25 December 2018).
17. Nupponen, R. Client views on periodic health examinations: Opinions and personal experience. *J. Adv. Nurs.* **1996**, *23*, 521–527. [CrossRef] [PubMed]

18. Liang, W. A population-based study of age and gender differences in patterns of health-related behaviors. *Am. J. Prev. Med.* **1999**, *17*, 8–17. [CrossRef]
19. Pinkhasov, R.M.; Wong, J.; Kashanian, J.; Lee, M.; Samadi, D.B.; Pinkhasov, M.M.; Shabsigh, R. Are men shortchanged on health? Perspective on health care utilization and health risk behavior in men and women in the United States. *Int. J. Clin. Pract.* **2010**, *64*, 475–487. [CrossRef]
20. Waldron, I. Sex differences in illness incidence, prognosis and mortality: Issues and evidence. *Soc. Sci. Med.* **1983**, *17*, 1107–1123. [CrossRef]
21. Cleary, P.D.; Mechanic, D.; Greenley, J.R. Sex Differences in Medical Care Utilization: An Empirical Investigation. *J. Health Soc. Behav.* **1982**, *23*, 106. [CrossRef] [PubMed]
22. Hibbard, J.H.; Pope, C.R. Gender roles, illness orientation and use of medical services. *Soc. Sci. Med.* **1983**, *17*, 129–137. [CrossRef]
23. Verbrugge, L.M.; Wingard, D.L.; Features Submission, H.C. Sex Differentials in Health and Mortality. *Women Health* **1987**, *12*, 103–145. [CrossRef]
24. Courtenay, W.H. Constructions of masculinity and their influence on men's well-being: A theory of gender and health. *Soc. Sci. Med.* **2000**, *50*, 1385–1401. [CrossRef]
25. Woodwell, D. National Ambulatory Medical Care Survey, 1996. In *ICPSR Data Holdings*; Inter-University Consortium for Political and Social Research (ICPSR): California, CA, USA, 1998.
26. United Nations Statistics Division. Demographic Yearbook 2003. Available online: https://unstats.un.org/unsd/demographic-social/products/dyb/dybsets/2003%20DYB.pdf (accessed on 18 January 2019).
27. Kung, H.-C.; Hoyert, D.L.; Xu, J.; Murphy, S.L. Deaths: Final data for 2005. *Natl. Vital. Stat. Rep.* **2008**, *56*, 1–120. [PubMed]
28. Publications S.S.O.A. Actuarial Studies. Available online: http://www.ssa.gov/OACT/NOTES/actstud.html (accessed on 24 May 2018).
29. Davies, J.; McCrae, B.P.; Frank, J.; Dochnahl, A.; Pickering, T.; Harrison, B.; Zakrzewski, M.; Wilson, K. Identifying Male College Students' Perceived Health Needs, Barriers to Seeking Help, and Recommendations to Help Men Adopt Healthier Lifestyles. *J. Am. Coll. Health* **2000**, *48*, 259–267. [CrossRef] [PubMed]
30. Dawson, K.A.; Schneider, M.A.; Fletcher, P.C.; Bryden, P.J. Examining gender differences in the health behaviors of Canadian university students. *J. R. Soc. Promot. Health* **2007**, *127*, 38–44. [CrossRef] [PubMed]
31. Jepson, R.; Clegg, A.; Forbes, C.; Lewis, R.; Sowden, A.; Kleijnen, J. The determinants of screening uptake and interventions for increasing uptake: A systematic review. *Health Technol. Assess* **2000**, *4*, 1–133.
32. Van Wijk, C.M.T.G.; Kolk, A.M. Sex differences in physical symptoms: The contribution of symptom perception theory. *Soc. Sci. Med.* **1997**, *45*, 231–246. [CrossRef]
33. Franks, P.; Clancy, C.M.; Gold, M.R.; Nutting, P.A. Health insurance and subjective health status: Data from the 1987 National Medical Expenditure survey. *Am. J. Public Health* **1993**, *83*, 1295–1299. [CrossRef]
34. Sullivan, T.J.; Andersen, R.; Lion, J.; Anderson, O.W. Two Decades of Health Services: Social Survey Trends in Use and Expenditure. *Soc. Forces* **1978**, *56*, 970. [CrossRef]
35. Addis, M.E.; Mahalik, J.R. Men, masculinity, and the contexts of help seeking. *Am. Psychol.* **2003**, *58*, 5–14. [CrossRef]
36. Mahedy, L.; Todaro-Luck, F.; Bunting, B.; Murphy, S.; Kirby, K. Risk factors for psychological distress in Northern Ireland. *Int. J. Soc. Psychiatry* **2012**, *59*, 646–654. [CrossRef]
37. Vuong, Q.-H.; Vuong, T.-T.; Ho, T.; Nguyen, H. Psychological and Socio-Economic Factors Affecting Social Sustainability through Impacts on Perceived Health Care Quality and Public Health: The Case of Vietnam. *Sustainability* **2017**, *9*, 1456. [CrossRef]
38. Ladwig, K.-H.; Marten-Mittag, B.; Formanek, B.; Dammann, G. Gender differences of symptom reporting and medical health care utilization in the German population. *Eur. J. Epidemiol.* **2000**, *16*, 511–518. [CrossRef]
39. Jianakoplos, N.A.; Bernasek, A. Are women more risk averse? *Econ. Inq.* **1998**, *36*, 620–630. [CrossRef]
40. Croson, R.; Gneezy, U. Gender Differences in Preferences. *J. Econ. Lit.* **2009**, *47*, 448–474. [CrossRef]
41. Donna, R. Women Are Better Retirement Savers than Men, But Still Have a Lot Less Money. Available online: http://time.com/money/3911377/retirement-401ks-women-men/ (accessed on 18 January 2019).
42. Lucy, B. The Truth about Our Economy's Gender Divide? Women Are Saving More Money—But They Won't Invest. Available online: http://www.independent.co.uk/voices/the-truth-about-our-economys-gender-divide-women-save-more-money-but-they-wont-invest-a6942596.html (accessed on 21 May 2018).

43. Wennman-Larsen, A.; Tishelman, C. Advanced home care for cancer patients at the end of life: A qualitative study of hopes and expectations of family caregivers. *Scand. J. Caring Sci.* **2002**, *16*, 240–247. [CrossRef]
44. Rosenstock, I.M. The Health Belief Model and Preventive Health Behavior. *Health Educ. Monogr.* **1974**, *2*, 354–386. [CrossRef]
45. Skinner, C.; Tiro, J.; Champion, V. The health belief model. In *Health Behavior: Theory, Research, and Practice*, 5th ed.; Glanz, K., Rimer, B., Viswanath, K., Eds.; Jossey-Bass: San Francisco, CA, USA, 2015.
46. Wall, M.; Teeland, L. Non-participants in a preventive health examination for cardiovascular disease: Characteristics, reasons for non-participation, and willingness to participate in the future. *Scand. J. Prim. Health Care* **2004**, *22*, 248–251. [CrossRef]
47. Dryden, R.; Williams, B.; McCowan, C.; Themessl-Huber, M. What do we know about who does and does not attend general health checks? Findings from a narrative scoping review. *BMC Public Health* **2012**, *12*. [CrossRef]
48. Burton, L.C.; German, P.S.; Shapiro, S. A Preventive Services Demonstration. *Med. Care* **1997**, *35*, 1149–1157. [CrossRef]
49. Boland, B.J.; Wollan, P.C.; Silverstein, M.D. Yield of laboratory tests for case-finding in the ambulatory general medical examination. *Am. J. Med.* **1996**, *101*, 142–152. [CrossRef]
50. Vuong, Q.-H. Survey data on Vietnamese propensity to attend periodic general health examinations. *Sci. Data* **2017**, *4*, 170142. [CrossRef]
51. Vuong, Q.-H.; Ho, T.-M.; Nguyen, H.-K.; Vuong, T.-T. Healthcare consumers' sensitivity to costs: A reflection on behavioural economics from an emerging market. *Palgrave Commun.* **2018**, *4*. [CrossRef]
52. Vuong, Q.-H.; La, V.-P.; Vuong, T.-T.; Ho, M.-T.; Nguyen, H.-K.T.; Nguyen, V.-H.; Pham, H.-H.; Ho, M.-T. An open database of productivity in Vietnam's social sciences and humanities for public use. *Sci. Data* **2018**, *5*, 180188. [CrossRef] [PubMed]
53. Agresti, A. *Categorical Data Analysis*; John Wiley & Sons, Inc.: New York, NY, USA, 2002.
54. Vuong, Q.; Nguyen, T. Vietnamese patients' choice of healthcare provider: In search of quality information. *Int. J. Behav. Healthcare Res.* **2015**, *5*, 184–212. [CrossRef]
55. Kuo, R.N.; Lai, M.-S. The influence of socio-economic status and multimorbidity patterns on healthcare costs: A six-year follow-up under a universal healthcare system. *Int. J. Equity Health* **2013**, *12*, 69. [CrossRef] [PubMed]
56. Sun, X.; Chen, Y.; Tong, X.; Feng, Z.; Wei, L.; Zhou, D.; Tian, M.; Lv, B.; Feng, D. The use of annual physical examinations among the elderly in rural China: A cross-sectional study. *BMC Health Serv. Res.* **2014**, *14*. [CrossRef] [PubMed]
57. Horner, S.D.; Ambrogne, J.; Coleman, M.A.; Hanson, C.; Hodnicki, D.; Lopez, S.A.; Talmadge, M.C. Traveling for Care: Factors Influencing Health Care Access for Rural Dwellers. *Public Health Nurs.* **1994**, *11*, 145–149. [CrossRef]
58. Vuong, Q.-H.; Bui, Q.-K.; La, V.-P.; Vuong, T.-T.; Nguyen, V.-H.T.; Ho, M.-T.; Nguyen, H.-K.T.; Ho, M.-T. Cultural additivity: Behavioural insights from the interaction of Confucianism, Buddhism and Taoism in folktales. *Palgrave Commun.* **2018**, *4*, 143. [CrossRef]

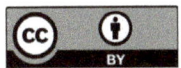

© 2019 by the authors. Licensee MDPI, Basel, Switzerland. This article is an open access article distributed under the terms and conditions of the Creative Commons Attribution (CC BY) license (http://creativecommons.org/licenses/by/4.0/).

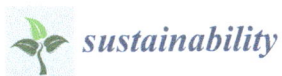

Article

Sleep Duration and Sleep Quality as Predictors of Health in Elderly Individuals

Lovro Štefan [1,*], Vlatko Vučetić [1], Goran Vrgoč [2] and Goran Sporiš [1]

1. Faculty of Kinesiology, University of Zagreb, 10 100 Zagreb, Croatia; vlatko.vucetic@kif.hr (V.V.); sporis.79@gmail.com (G.S.)
2. Clinical Hospital Center 'Sveti Duh', 10 000 Zagreb, Croatia; gvrgoc@gmail.com
* Correspondence: lovro.stefan1510@gmail.com; Tel.: +385-098-9177-060

Received: 4 October 2018; Accepted: 26 October 2018; Published: 28 October 2018

Abstract: The main purpose of the present study was to explore the associations of sleep duration and sleep quality with self-rated health. In this cross-sectional study, participants were 894 elderly individuals. Self-rated health, sleep duration, and sleep quality were self-reported. The associations were examined using multiple logistic regression analyses.After adjusting for sex, physical activity, smoking consumption, alcohol consumption, psychological distress, socioeconomic status, and chronic disease/s, sleeping <6 h (OR (Odds ratio) = 3.21; 95% CI (95 percent confident interval) 1.61 to 6.39), 6–7 h (OR = 2.47; 95% CI 1.40 to 4.36), 8–9 h (OR = 3.26; 95% CI 1.82 to 5.83), and >9 h (OR = 3.62; 95% CI 1.57 to 8.34) and having 'poor' sleep quality (≥5 points; OR = 2.33; 95% CI 1.46 to 3.73) were associated with 'poor' self-rated health. When sleep duration and sleep quality were entered simultaneously into the model, the same associations remained. Our findings provide evidence that both 'short' and 'long' sleep and 'poor' sleep quality are associated with 'poor' self-rated health. Thus, interventions that promote healthy sleep hygiene in the elderly are warranted.

Keywords: sleep hygiene; health; old people; association; logistic regression

1. Introduction

Sleep duration is an important factor that contributes to overall health status [1]. It has been reported that extreme values of sleep duration (both short and long sleep) are associated with higher levels of mortality rates [2,3] and increased incidence of cardiovascular [4] and metabolic [5] diseases. Along with sleep duration, sleep quality is also a part of sleep hygiene that is remotely associated with health [6]. Specifically, a study by Hulvej Rod et al. [7] showed that men and women with sleep disturbances were more likely to develop cardiovascular and metabolic diseases, yet men with ≥3 types of sleep disturbances had a higher risk of committing suicide.

Self-rated health has become an increasingly common tool for measuring a subjective perception of health [1]. Previous studies have shown that self-rated health serves as a good predictor of objective health status [8] and is associated with health outcomes [9].

Associations between sleep duration and self-rated health have been well-documented in young [10,11] and general populations [12,13]. In both groups, studies have shown a U-shaped association between sleep duration and self-rated health, that is, both short and long sleep are associated with 'poor' self-rated health. Only a handful of studies examined the same associations in the elderly [6,14] and showed similar results, where both 'short' and 'long' sleep duration were associated with reporting 'poor' self-rated health. However, studies examining the associations between sleep quality and self-rated health are lacking, especially in the elderly population.

In general, the elderly experience many physical and psychological changes, of which sleep duration and sleep quality play an important role [15]. Studies have also shown that sleep disturbances increase with age [16] and the prevalence of such disturbances is higher than 50% in community-dwelling elderly people [17]. On the other hand, self-rated health in the elderly is driven by numerous factors, of which sleep hygiene is an important determinant of such perception. That being said, it is necessary to explore the associations of both sleep duration and sleep quality with self-rated health in the elderly in order to create effective strategies and policies that would leverage good sleep hygiene and lead to higher levels of health.

Therefore, the main purpose of the present study was to explore the associations of sleep duration and sleep quality with self-rated health. We hypothesized that both 'short' and 'long' sleep duration and 'poor' sleep quality, entered separately and simultaneously into the models, would be associated with 'poor' self-rated health in elderly individuals.

2. Materials and Methods

2.1. Study Participants

In this cross-sectional study, participants were elderly individuals (mean age 80±3 years; 56.0% of women) from the city of Zagreb. In the city of Zagreb, there are in total of 10 nursing homes with approximately 4000 users. At the first stage, we randomly selected five out of ten nursing homes, with 2000 users. At the second stage, we contacted principles, head nurses, and social workers of each home to help us organize the protocol. At the time this study was conducted, each nursing home had 250–300 users and the univariate analysis revealed no statistical differences in the size of the nursing homes ($p = 0.897$). Data collection in each home was done in groups of 15–20 people. The criteria for selecting participants were: Age ≥ 65, free of cognitive disabilities, and physically independent. First, we explained the main purpose of the study and possible reasons for conducting a study. Second, we briefly explained the risks of the study. Out of 2000 users, we collected the data from 1187 users. However, by checking the data, we extracted those with missing data ($N = 153$) and those who did not want to participate in the study ($N = 140$). Our final sample was based on 894 (894/1187; 75% response rate) elderly individuals from all five nursing homes. All the procedures were anonymous and in accordance with the Declaration of Helsinki and approved by the Institutional Review Board of the Faculty of Kinesiology. Additionally, before the study began, each participant had given their written informed consent to participate in the study and the approval to use the obtained data for scientific contribution. All the data will be provided to others by reasonable request from the corresponding author.

2.2. Outcome Variable

We used oneitem question to assess self-rated health: 'How would you rate your health'? Answers were arranged along a Likert-type scale as follow: (1) Very poor, (2) poor, (3) fair, (4) good, and (5) excellent. We dichotomized the outcome variable into 'good' (fair, good, and excellent) vs. 'poor' (poor and very poor) self-rated health. Previous studies have shown that self-rated health is a reliable measure to assess overall health status and is associated with mortality [18].

2.3. Independent Variables

Sleep duration was assessed by asking participants the following question: 'On average, how many hours of sleep do you get in a 24-h period'? The response was a numerical variable. Finally, we categorized the response into 5 groups for the current analysis: ≤ 6 h, 6–7 h, 7–8 h, 8–9 h, and >9 h.

To assess sleep quality, we used the Pittsburgh Sleep Quality Index (PSQI) [19]. It is composed of 19 questions, which create 7 major components [19]. All seven components are then summed up to create a scale from 0 to 21 points. Buysee et al. [19] proposed that the score of <5 denoted 'good' sleep quality, while ≥ 5 denoted 'poor' sleep quality.

2.4. Covariates

To assess PA (Physical activity) in the last 7 days, we used the adapted version of the International Physical Activity Questionnaire-short form, a reliable and valid instrument designed to measure physical activity in respondents aged ≥65 [20]. The questionnaire provides information about the time and number of days spent in light, moderate, and vigorous intensity physical activity. For each participant, we calculated the time spent in moderate and vigorous physical activity. According to the World Health Organization [21], elderly people aged ≥65 should participate in 'at least 150 min of moderate-intensity aerobic PA throughout the week or do at least 75 min of vigorous-intensity aerobic PA throughout the week or an equivalent combination of both'. Thus, we categorized the participants who met the aforementioned recommendation as 'sufficiently' active compared with the participants who did not meet the recommended levels as 'insufficiently' active. Smoking status was categorized as: (1) Nonsmoker/former smoker vs. (2) present smoker. Alcohol consumption was used as a covariate and was assessed by one question: "In the past week, did you consume an alcoholic drink?" with 'Yes' and 'No' answers. Psychological distress was assessed using Kessler's six-item questionnaire [22]. The questionnaire has been described elsewhere [22]. Each question is scored from 0 (none of the time) to 4 (all of the time). Scores of each question are summed up between 0 and 24, with a lower score indicating a lower level of psychological distress. Kessler et al. [22] showed that responses <13 points vs. ≥13 points discriminated participants without and with psychological distress. Internal consistency for the questionnaire in our study was satisfactory (Cronbach's alpha = 0.76). Socioeconomic status was assessed by oneitem question: 'How would you perceive your socioeconomic status'? Responses were arranged along a three-item scale as follows: (1) Below average, (2) average, and (3) above average. The presence or absence of a chronic disease was asked by oneitem question: 'Have you ever been told by a doctor, that you suffer from any kind of chronic disease?' with 'Yes' and 'No' answers. Sex (men and women) was entered in as a covariate.

2.5. Data Analysis

Basic descriptive statistics of the study participants are presented as frequencies (n) and percentages (%). Differences between categorical variables were analyzed using the Chi-square test. To examine the associations of sleep duration and sleep quality with self-rated health, we used multiple logistic regression analysis by using subcommand contrast. Additionally, we tested the variables for multicollinearity using variance inflation factors (VIF), normality of residuals using the normal probability plot, and histogram of residuals and heteroscedasticity using the standardized residuals versus predicted plot. The VIF ranged between 1.10 and 1.63, showing no multicollinearity, and other assumptions were also met. In model 1, we examined the association between sleep duration (7–8 h as referent value) and 'poor' self-rated health. In model 2, we examined the association between sleep quality ('good' as referent value) and 'poor' self-rated health. Finally, we entered sleep duration and sleep quality simultaneously into model 3, to examine the associations with 'poor' self-rated health. All three models were adjusted for sex, physical activity, smoking consumption, alcohol consumption, psychological distress, socioeconomic status, and chronic disease/s. Significance was set at $\alpha = 0.05$ and it was two-sided (2-sided). All the analyses were performed in the Statistical Package for Social Sciences Software, V.22 (IBM Corp, Armonk, New York, NY, USA).

3. Results

Basic descriptive statistics of the study participants are presented in Table 1. In general, a higher percentage of individuals sleeping 6 h, 6–7 h, 8–9 h, and >9 h reported having 'poor' self-rated health ($p < 0.001$). Also, a higher percentage of individuals who reported 'poor' sleep quality had 'poor' self-rated health ($p < 0.001$). Among the covariates, 'insufficiently' active participants who did smoke or consume alcohol and who had 'high' psychological distress reported 'poor' self-rated health. Finally, those individuals with the presence of chronic disease/s more frequently reported having 'poor' self-rated health, compared to those with no chronic disease/s ($p < 0.001$).

Table 1. Basic descriptive statistics of the study participants ($N = 894$).

Study Variables	Total (N = 894) N (%)	'Poor' Self-Rated Health (N = 132) N (%)	'Good' Self-Rated Health (N = 762) N (%)	p-Value *
Sleep duration				
<6 h	76 (8.5)	23 (17.4)	53 (7.0)	
6–7 h	150 (16.8)	29 (22.0)	121 (15.9)	
7–8 h	486 (54.4)	38 (28.8)	448 (58.8)	
8–9 h	132 (14.8)	31 (23.5)	101 (13.3)	
>9 h	50 (5.6)	11 (8.3)	39 (5.1)	<0.001
Sleep quality				
Poor	483 (54.0)	102 (77.3)	381 (50.0)	
Good	411 (46.0)	30 (22.7)	381 (50.0)	0.001
Sex				
Men	393 (44.0)	50 (37.9)	343 (45.0)	
Women	501 (56.0)	82 (62.1)	419 (55.0)	0.130
Physical activity				
Insufficiently	505 (56.5)	97 (73.5)	408 (53.5)	
Sufficiently	389 (43.5)	35 (26.5)	354 (46.5)	<0.001
Smoking consumption				
Yes	281 (31.4)	60 (45.5)	221 (29.0)	
No	613 (68.6)	72 (54.5)	541 (71.0)	<0.001
Alcohol consumption				
Yes	227 (25.4)	44 (33.3)	183 (24.0)	
No	667 (74.6)	88 (66.7)	576 (76.0)	0.030
Psychological distress				
High	124 (13.9)	56 (42.4)	68 (8.9)	
Low	770 (86.1)	76 (57.6)	694 (91.1)	<0.001
Socioeconomic status				
Low	33 (3.7)	7 (5.3)	26 (3.4)	
Middle/high	861 (96.3)	125 (94.7)	736 (96.6)	0.313
Chronic Disease/s				
Yes	115 (12.9)	44 (33.3)	71 (9.3)	
No	779 (87.1)	88 (66.7)	691 (90.7)	<0.001

* Chi-square test

The associations of sleep duration and sleep quality with 'poor' self-rated health are presented in Table 2. In model 1, sleeping <6 h (OR = 3.21; 95% CI 1.61 to 6.39), 6–7 h (OR = 2.47; 95% CI 1.40 to 4.36), 8–9 h (OR = 3.26; 95% CI 1.82 to 5.83), and >9 h (OR = 3.62; 95% CI 1.57 to 8.34) was associated with 'poor' self-rated health. In model 2, 'poor' sleep quality (OR = 2.33; 95% CI 1.46 to 3.73) was associated with 'poor' self-rated health. When sleep duration and sleep quality were entered simultaneously into model 3, sleeping <6 h (OR = 2.60; 95% CI 1.29 to 5.23), 6–7 h (OR = 2.04; 95% CI 1.14 to 3.64), 8–9 h (OR = 3.18; 95% CI 1.77 to 5.74), and >9 h (OR = 3.59; 95% CI 1.53 to 8.41) and having 'poor' sleep quality (OR = 2.06; 95% CI 1.26 to 3.38) remained associated with 'poor' self-rated health.

Table 2. The associations of sleep duration and sleep quality with 'poor' self-rated health in the study participants (N = 894).

Study Variables	Model 1	Model 2	Model 3
	OR (95% CI)	OR (95% CI)	OR (95% CI)
Sleep duration			
<6 h	3.21 (1.61 to 6.39) ***		2.60 (1.29 to 5.23) **
6–7 h	2.47 (1.40 to 4.36) ***		2.04 (1.14 to 3.64) *
7–8 h	Ref.		Ref.
8–9 h	3.26 (1.82 to 5.83) ***		3.18 (1.77 to 5.74) ***
>9 h	3.62 (1.57 to 8.34) **		3.59 (1.53 to 8.41) **
Sleep quality			
Good		Ref.	Ref.
Poor		2.33 (1.46 to 3.73) ***	2.06 (1.26 to 3.38) **
Sex			
Men	Ref.	Ref.	Ref.
Women	0.81 (0.52 to 1.27)	0.94 (0.61 to 1.46)	0.85 (0.54 to 1.35)
Physical activity			
Sufficiently	Ref.	Ref.	Ref.
Insufficiently	1.80 (1.12 to 2.90) **	1.61 (1.01 to 2.56) *	1.70 (1.05 to 2.75) *
Smoking consumption			
No	Ref.	Ref.	Ref.
Yes	1.70 (1.09 to 2.65) *	1.65 (1.07 to 2.56) *	1.65 (1.06 to 2.57) *
Alcohol consumption			
No	Ref.	Ref.	Ref.
Yes	1.55 (0.97 to 2.46)	1.59 (1.00 to 2.53) *	1.65 (1.03 to 2.64) *
Psychological distress			
Low	Ref.	Ref.	Ref.
High	5.89 (3.67 to 9.48) ***	5.09 (3.18 to 8.14) ***	5.08 (3.12 to 8.26) ***
Socioeconomic status			
Middle/high	Ref.	Ref.	Ref.
Low	0.77 (0.27 to 2.19)	0.97 (0.36 to 2.67)	0.75 (0.26 to 2.14)
Chronic disease/s			
No	Ref.	Ref.	Ref.
Yes	3.57 (2.16 to 5.89) ***	3.95 (2.42 to 6.43) ***	3.51 (2.12 to 5.81) ***

Model 1: Examine the association between sleep duration and 'poor' self-rated health adjusted for sex, physical activity, smoking consumption, alcohol consumption, psychological distress, socioeconomic status, and chronic disease/s.; **Model 2:** Examine the association between sleep quality and 'poor' self-rated health adjusted for sex, physical activity, smoking consumption, alcohol consumption, psychological distress, socioeconomic status, and chronic disease/s; **Model 3:** Examine the associations of sleep duration and sleep quality with 'poor' self-rated health adjusted for sex, physical activity, smoking consumption, alcohol consumption, psychological distress, socioeconomic status, and chronic disease/s; * $p < 0.05$; ** $p < 0.01$; *** $p < 0.001$.

4. Discussion

The main purpose of the present study was to explore the associations of sleep duration and sleep quality with self-rated health. Our study shows that both 'short' and 'long' sleep duration and 'poor' sleep quality were associated with 'poor' self-rated health, after adjusting for numerous covariates.

Previous studies have also shown that 'short' sleep duration is associated with 'poor' self-rated health in the populations of young adults [11], adults [12,13], and the elderly [6,14]. Contrary to our findings, Steptoe et al. [10] showed that only 'short' sleep duration was associated with 'poor' self-rated health in a sample of 17,456 university students. Even no association between sleep duration and self-rated health was found [23]. In general, evidence shows that both short and long sleep duration are associated with increased rates of mortality [2,3] and higher incidence of cardiovascular and metabolic diseases [4,5]. Additionally, short and long sleep duration impair mood and cognitive functioning [24], increase daytime fatigue [25], and are associated with numerous negative health outcomes, such as impaired glucose intolerance [26] and increased risk for chronic diseases [4,5]. One previous study proposed an inverse association, that is, 'poor' self-rated health led to 'short' and 'long' sleep duration [12]; yet we are unable to make such a conclusion, due to the cross-sectional nature of our data. However, it is possible that the association between 'short' and 'long' sleep duration and 'poor' self-rated health is bidirectional.

Our results also showed that 'poor' sleep quality was associated with 'poor' self-rated health, independently of 'short' and 'long' sleep duration. When sleep duration and sleep quality were entered simultaneously into the model, both variables remained associated with 'poor' self-rated health. To the best of the authors' knowledge, this is the first exploration of the associations of both sleep duration and sleep quality with self-rated health in a sample of elderly individuals. Since this is the first of such studies, our results were explained in the highlights of similar studies [27,28]. Specifically, Paunio et al. [27] and Rissanen et al. [28] showed that 'poor' sleep quality was associated with 'poor' life satisfaction in the general population. Our results could be explained by the fact that life satisfaction was strongly associated with self-rated health in previous studies [29]. Moreover, previous studies have shown that both 'poor' self-rated health and 'poor' life satisfaction' are associated with negative health outcomes [30]. Thus, although we did not use the same variables, our study shows a strong association between 'poor' sleep quality and 'poor' self-rated health in a relatively large sample of elderly individuals.

This study has several strengths. First, we randomly selected five nursing homes and conducted a study among a relatively high number of individuals ($N = 894$), minimizing the risk of measurement bias. Second, we used previously validated questionnaires to assess PA, sleep duration, and sleep quality. Third, all three models were adjusted for sex, physical activity, smoking consumption, alcohol consumption, psychological distress, socioeconomic status, and chronic disease/s.

However, our study has several limitations. Due to a cross-sectional design, the associations between sleep duration and sleep quality with self-rated health must be interpreted with caution. It is possible that 'poor' self-rated health led to both 'short' and 'long' sleep duration and 'poor' sleep quality. Although we used validated questionnaires, our second limitation was the usage of self-reported measures. Third, we were lacking in collecting information about physiological parameters and daylight exposure, even though daylight exposure has a beneficial effect on well-being and psychological functioning [31]. Fourth, we based our sample only on elderly individuals situated in nursing homes in the city of Zagreb. However, free-living individuals might have had different levels of self-rated health and sleep, leading to different associations. Future studies should use objective methods (accelerometry, polysomnography) and follow-up methodology in order to better capture and understand the causality between sleep hygiene and self-rated health.

In conclusion, our study shows that 'short' and 'long' sleep duration and 'poor' sleep quality were associated with 'poor' self-rated health in a sample of elderly individuals living in nursing homes. Thus, special policies and strategies that promote sleep hygiene in order to increase self-rated health are warranted.

Author Contributions: Conceptualization: L.Š., Data curation: V.V., G.V., and G.S., Formal analysis: L.Š., Funding acquisition:/Investigation: L.Š., Methodology: L.Š., V.V., G.V., and G.S., Project administration: L.Š., Resources: L.Š., Software: L.Š. and G.S., Supervision: G.S., Validation: V.V., G.S., Visualization: L.Š., Roles/Writing—original draft: L.Š., V.V., G.V., and G.S., Writing—review and editing: L.Š., V.V., G.V,. and G.S.

Funding: This research did not receive any specific grant from funding agencies in the public, commercial, or not-for-profit sectors.

Acknowledgments: We would like to thank all the participants, principles, social workers, and head nurses for their enthusiastic participation in the study.

Conflicts of Interest: The authors declare no conflict of interest.

References

1. Frange, C.; de Queiroz, S.S.; da Silva Prado, J.M.; Tufik, S.; de Mello, M.T. The impact of sleep duration on self-rated health. *Sleep Sci.* **2014**, *7*, 107–113. [CrossRef] [PubMed]
2. Tamakoshi, A.; Ohno, Y.; JACC Study Group. Self-reported sleep duration as a predictor of all-cause mortality: Results from the JACC study, Japan. *Sleep* **2004**, *27*, 51–54. [PubMed]
3. Heslop, H.; Smith, G.D.; Metcalfe, C.; Macleod, J.; Hart, C. Sleep duration and mortality: The effect of short or long sleep duration on cardiovascular and all-cause mortality in working men and women. *Sleep* **2002**, *3*, 305–314. [CrossRef]
4. Sabanayagam, C.; Shankar, A. Sleep duration and cardiovascular disease: Results from the National Health Interview Survey. *Sleep* **2010**, *33*, 1037–1042. [CrossRef] [PubMed]
5. Yaggi, H.K.; Araujo, A.B.; McKinlay, J.B. Sleep duration as a risk factor for the development of type 2 diabetes. *Diabetes Care* **2006**, *29*, 657–661. [CrossRef] [PubMed]
6. Magee, C.A.; Caputi, P.; Iverson, D.C. Relationships between self-rated health, quality of life and sleep duration in middle aged and elderly Australians. *Sleep Med.* **2011**, *12*, 346–350. [CrossRef] [PubMed]
7. Hulvej Rod, R.; Kumari, M.; Lange, T.; Kivimäki, M.; Shipley, M.; Ferrie, J. The joint effect of sleep duration and disturbed sleep o cause-specific mortality: Results from the Whitehall II cohort study. *PLoS ONE* **2014**, *9*, e91965.
8. Wu, S.; Wang, R.; Zhao, Y.; Ma, X.; Wu, M.; Yan, X.; He, J. The relationship between self-rated health and objective health status: A population-based study. *BMC Public Health* **2013**, *13*, 320. [CrossRef] [PubMed]
9. Miilunpalo, S.; Vuori, I.; Oja, P.; Pasanen, M.; Urponen, H. Self-rated health status as a health measure: The predictive value of self-reported health status on the use of physician services and on mortality in the working-age population. *J. Clin. Epidemiol.* **1997**, *50*, 517–528. [CrossRef]
10. Steptoe, A.; Peacey, V.; Wardle, J. Sleep duration and health in young adults. *Arch. Int. Med.* **2006**, *166*, 1689–1692. [CrossRef] [PubMed]
11. Štefan, L.; Juranko, D.; Prosoli, R.; Barić, R.; Sporiš, G. Self-reported sleep duration and self-rated health in young adults. *J. Clin. Sleep Med.* **2017**, *13*, 899–904. [CrossRef] [PubMed]
12. Shankar, A.; Charumathi, S.; Kalidindi, S. Sleep duration and self-Rated health: The National Health InterviewSurvey 2008. *Sleep* **2011**, *34*, 1173–1177. [CrossRef] [PubMed]
13. Kim, J.H.; Kim, K.R.; Cho, K.H.; Yoo, K.B.; Kwon, J.A.; Park, E.C. The association between sleep duration and self-rated health in the Korean general population. *J.Clin. Sleep Med.* **2013**, *9*, 1057–1064. [CrossRef] [PubMed]
14. Selvamani, Y.; Arokiasamy, P.; Chaudhari, M.; Himanshu, M. Association of sleep problems and sleep duration with self-rated health and grip strength among older adults in India and China: Results from the study on global aging and adult health (SAGE). *J. Public Health* **2018**. [CrossRef]
15. Espiritu, J.R. Aging-related sleep changes. *Clin. Geriatr. Med.* **2008**, *24*, 1–14. [CrossRef] [PubMed]
16. Ohayon, M.M. Epidemiology of insomnia: What we know and what we still need to learn. *Sleep Med. Rev.* **2002**, *6*, 97–111. [CrossRef] [PubMed]
17. Rao, V.; Spiro, J.R.; Samus, Q.M.; Rosenblatt, A.; Steele, C.; Baker, A.; Harper, M.; Brandt, J.; Mayer, L.; Rabins, P.V.; Lyketsos, C.G. Sleep disturbances in the elderly residing in assisted living: Findings from the Maryland Assisted Living Study. *Int. J. Geriatr. Med.* **2005**, *20*, 956–966. [CrossRef] [PubMed]
18. Eriksson, I.; Undén, A.L.; Elofsson, S. Self-rated health. Comparisons between three different measures. Results from a population study. *Int. J. Epidemiol.* **2001**, *30*, 326–333. [CrossRef] [PubMed]
19. Buysse, D.J.; Reynolds, C.F.; Monk, T.H.; Berman, S.R.; Kupfer, D.J. The Pittsburgh Sleep Quality Index: A new instrument for psychiatric practice and research. *Psychiatry Rev.* **1989**, *28*, 193–213. [CrossRef]
20. Hurtig-Wehnlöf, A.; Hagströmer, M.; Olsson, L.A. The International Physical Activity Questionnaire modified for the elderly: Aspects of validity and feasibility. *Public Health Nutr.* **2010**, *13*, 1847–1854. [CrossRef] [PubMed]
21. World Health Organization. *Global Recommendations on Physical Activity for Health*; World Health Organization: Geneva, Switzerland, 2010.
22. Kessler, R.C.; Barker, P.R.; Colpe, L.J.; Epstein, J.F.; Gfroerer, J.C.; Hiripi, E.; Howes, M.J.; Normand, S.L.; Manderscheid, R.W.; Walters, E.E.; et al. Screening for serious mental illness in the general population. *Arch. Gen. Psychiatry* **2003**, *60*, 184–189. [CrossRef] [PubMed]

23. Jean-Louis, G.; Kripke, D.F.; Ancoli-Israel, S. Sleep and quality of well-being. *Sleep* **2000**, *23*, 1115–1121. [PubMed]
24. Faubel, R.; Lopez-Garcia, E.; Guallar-Castillon, P.; Graciani, A.; Banegas, J.R.; Rodriguez-Artalejo, F. Usual sleep duration and cognitive function in older adults in Spain. *J. Sleep Res.* **2009**, *18*, 427–435. [CrossRef] [PubMed]
25. Goldman, S.E.; Ancoli-Israel, S.; Boudreau, R.; Cauley, J.A.; Hall, M.; Stone, K.L.; Rubin, S.M.; Satterfield, S.; Simonsick, E.M.; Newman, A.B. Health, Aging and Body Composition Study. Sleep problems and associated daytime fatigue in community-dwelling older individuals. *J. Gerontol. A Biol. Sci. Med. Sci.* **2008**, *63*, 1069–1075. [CrossRef]
26. Keckeis, M.; Lattova, Z.; Maurovich-Horvat, E.; Beitinger, P.A.; Birkmann, S.; Lauer, C.J.; Wetter, T.C.; Wilde-Frenz, J.; Pollmächer, T. Impaired glucose intolerance in sleep disorders. *PLoS ONE* **2010**, *5*, e9444. [CrossRef] [PubMed]
27. Paunio, P.; Korhonen, T.; Hublin, C.; Partinen, M.; Kivimäki, M.; Koskenvuo, M.; Kaprio, J. Longitudinal study on poor sleep and life dissatisfaction in a nationwide cohort of twins. *Am. J. Epidemiol.* **2009**, *169*, 206–213. [CrossRef] [PubMed]
28. Rissanen, T.; Lehto, S.M.; Hintikka, J.; Honkalampi, K.; Saharinen, T.; Viinamäki, H.; Koivumaa-Honkanen, H. Biological and other health related correlates of long-term life dissatisfaction burden. *BMC Psychiatry* **2013**, *13*, 202. [CrossRef] [PubMed]
29. Benyamini, Y.; Leventhal, H.; Leventhal, E.A. Self-rated oral health as an independent predictor of self-rated general health, self-esteem and life satisfaction. *Soc. Sci. Med.* **2004**, *59*, 1109–1116. [CrossRef] [PubMed]
30. Collins, A.L.; Glei, D.A.; Goldman, N. The role of life satisfaction and depressive symptoms in all-cause mortality. *Psychol. Aging* **2009**, *24*, 696–702. [CrossRef] [PubMed]
31. Youngstedt, S.D.; Freelove-Charton, J.D. Exercise and sleep. In *Exercise, Health and Mental Health*; Faulkner, G.E.J., Taylor, A.H., Eds.; Routledge: London, UK, 2005.

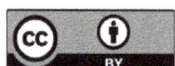

© 2018 by the authors. Licensee MDPI, Basel, Switzerland. This article is an open access article distributed under the terms and conditions of the Creative Commons Attribution (CC BY) license (http://creativecommons.org/licenses/by/4.0/).

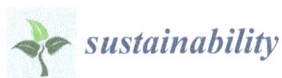

Article

Factors Associated with the Regularity of Physical Exercises as a Means of Improving the Public Health System in Vietnam

Quan-Hoang Vuong [1,*], Anh-Duc Hoang [2], Thu-Trang Vuong [1,3], Viet-Phuong La [4], Hong Kong T. Nguyen [4] and Manh-Tung Ho [1,5]

1. Centre for Interdisciplinary Social Research, Thanh Tay University, Yen Nghia, Ha Dong, Hanoi 100803, Vietnam; trang.vuong@thanhtay.edu.vn (T.-T.V.); tung.ho@thanhtay.edu.vn (M.-T.H.)
2. Academic Affairs, Gateway International School, Hanoi 100000, Vietnam; ducha.hoang@gmail.com
3. Sciences Po, 75337 Paris, France; thutrang.vuong@sciencespo.fr
4. Vuong & Associates Co., Hanoi 100000, Vietnam; lvphuong@gmail.com (V.-P.L.); htn2107@caa.columbia.edu (H.K.T.N.)
5. Ritsumeikan Asia Pacific University, Beppu, Oita 874-8577, Japan
* Correspondence: hoang.vuong@thanhtay.edu.vn

Received: 3 October 2018; Accepted: 22 October 2018; Published: 23 October 2018

Abstract: Being ranked among the most sedentary countries, Vietnam's social public health is challenged by the rising number of overweight people. This study aims to evaluate factors associated with the regularity of exercise and sports (EAS) among Vietnamese people living in the capital city of Hanoi, using data collected from a randomized survey involving 2068 individuals conducted in 2016. Physical exercises and daily sports are considered a major means for improving the Vietnamese social public health system by the government, families, and individuals. Applying the baseline-category logit model, the study analyzed two groups of factors associated with EAS regularity: (i) physiological factors (sex, body mass index (BMI)) and (ii) external factors (education, health communication, medical practice at home). Females with a university education or higher usually exercise less than those with lower education, while the opposite is true for males. The study also shows that those with a higher BMI tend to report higher activity levels. Additionally, improved health communication systems and regular health check-ups at home are also associated with more frequent EAS activities. These results, albeit limited to only one location in Vietnam, provide a basis for making targeted policies that promote a more active lifestyle. This, in turn, could help the country realize the goal of improving the average height of the population and reducing the incidents of non-communicable diseases.

Keywords: physical exercises and sports; sex; educational background; social public health; health communication

1. Background

Physical exercises and daily sports are considered a major means for improving the social public health system all over the world, including that in a developing country such as Vietnam. According to the first national estimates of physical activity for Vietnam, which used data (14,706 subjects) from a national population-based survey of risk factors for non-communicable diseases in SVietnam between 2009 and 2010, around 70% of adults aged 18–64 years meet the World Health Organization (WHO) recommendations for physical activity, but mainly from work activities [1]. The study also found the highest proportion of participation in leisure activity among Hanoi residents, who at the same time, spend the most time sitting [1]. In 2017, a team at Stanford University published a global study that analyzed daily step recordings on smartphones from over 717,000 anonymous users from 111 countries.

The results showed that Vietnamese people are among the most sedentary worldwide, with their daily steps averaging 3643—significantly below the global mean of 4961 steps [2,3]. Meanwhile, the amount of overweight individuals (body mass index (BMI) ≥ 25) has grown in Vietnam, especially in urban areas, over the past decade as the overall income levels rise [4–6].

Against this fact, Vietnamese society, as Craig pointed out in "Familiar Medicine", one of the first medical ethnographies to be written on contemporary Vietnam, has been very concerned with healthcare. The tropical climate in Vietnam, which brings about six months of hot and humid weather and another three of drizzle, and cold and dry spells, has contributed to the development of "a rich popular discourse and practice of everyday health and medicine" [7]. The local medical practice is strongly influenced by traditional Chinese medicine, but is also rooted in local ingredients, self-management, household care, and the inheritance of oral traditions and home-remedy recipes [7].

Given this background and previous studies that have described the lack of physical exercise among Vietnamese people, this study seeks, for the first time, to examine factors associated with the self-reported regularity of a specific form of physical activity, that is, exercise and sports (EAS), among people living in Hanoi, using a 2016 cross-section dataset. EAS is defined as leisure time physical activities ranging from moderate to vigorous intensity such as aerobics, walking, running, cycling, dancing, martial arts, and football, among others. The study chooses leisure time activities instead of work-related activities because most studies on the correlations of physical activity are focused on high-income countries or look only at activities associated with transport and occupation in developing countries [8]. With a population of 92 million and a low per capita gross domestic product (GDP) of approximately $2000, Vietnam is a developing country at the middle-income level. Thus, the study hopes to fill the gap in the literature.

Factors associated with the frequency and magnitude of an individual's physical training are often complex and diverse. Several studies have looked at the association between physical activity and a host of socio-demographic and lifestyle factors such as aging; sedentary behavior; nutrition; or the use of drugs such as cigarettes, alcohol, and others [8–11]; environmental components such as noises or availability of facilities are shown to affect physical activities [12–14]. This study takes another approach by applying a baseline category logit model to assess two groups of factors specifically associated with the self-reported regularity of physical exercise in Hanoi, namely (i) physiological factors (sex, body mass index or BMI) and (ii) external factors (education, health communication, medical practice at home). Understanding why the Vietnamese, particularly those in its urban center, are more prone to EAS participation could inform public health workers in places with a similar background.

2. Literature Review

The benefits of EAS have been examined by a large range of studies. Not only do EAS help maintain the body's fitness as well as physical health, but they also improve mood, self-esteem, and social skills [15,16]. The activities are proven to have preventive effects among healthy individuals and treatment effects among patients of various illnesses [17–19]. EAS are beneficial to those with hypertension; they reduce the risk of obesity, heart disease, diabetes, and colon cancer; they lower premature mortality rates; and they enhance osteoarthritis function in older people [18,20–22]. Moreover, regular engagement in EAS is also related to improved respiratory function, is helpful in cases of chronic kidney disease or osteoporotic fractures, and leads to a possible reduction in inflammatory biomarkers [19,23].

This section provides an overview of the scholarship on the two groups of factors, namely physiological (sex, BMI) and external (education, health communication, and home medicine), and their association with regularity in physical exercise.

Sex differences in EAS participation happen as a result of the changing body size and composition between male and female from late childhood, through puberty, and into adolescence [16]. Particularly, as the endocrine changes with development, girls would accumulate more fat than boys, while boys would see their fat-free mass climb at a much higher rate than girls [16]. Studies have confirmed that not only do boys and girls not vary much regarding body size and composition until puberty, but with training, both sexes experience similar changes in body composition, "as determined by total energy expenditure during training" [16]. Yet, it is clear that while both sexes enjoy taking part in calisthenics, cycling, swimming, and bowling, males tend to prefer weightlifting, golf, volleyball, soccer, and handball, and females are more attracted to walking, aerobics, and dancing [16,24,25]. The choices are attributable to other factors, such as parental behaviors, muscle structure, lung size, respiratory mechanisms, and fat rates specific to the body of each gender [23,24]. Indeed, even when researchers found no comparable differences in sedentary behaviors between male and female adults, there remained differences in terms of changes in the physical activity behavior over time. For instance, a study on the elderly Swedish population noted that men decreased their total physical activity, but women increased their time in moderate- or higher-intensity physical activity [26]. For the purpose of quantitative analysis, the sex differences in EAS are often examined through the BMI figure, which is linked to the fat rate and thus indicates the body's level of obesity [25]. BMI is calculated using the formula BMI = weight/(height × height).

BMI, apart from varying by sex and ethnicity, also changes according to physical training and educational background [27–29]. Studies on the association between BMI and educational attainment, though they appear to be outdated, did point out the general influence of educational level on the BMI of males; for females, the only lower educational level is shown to be related to higher BMI [30]. The higher educated women seem to exercise more regularly, so they have stronger muscles compared with the less educated [30–32].

Health communication is another factor that could influence EAS regularity, because not only does health information changes people's behaviors, it also changes in line with sex and educational background [33]. In practice, it is difficult to separate the influence of sex and gender on human behaviors in healthcare. For instance, sex can modify testosterone, to the case of aggressive behavior being associated with risk-seeking and neglecting personal health, while gender-behavior such as lifestyle choices, exposure to stress, and environmental toxins, can have a certain impact on biological factors [34]. Concerning gender, studies over the years have often shown men to be unwilling and uninterested in seeking out health-related information both in times of stressful life events and generally in everyday life [35–38]. A Finnish study in 2013 on how gender affects health information behavior in people aged 18–65 years found that, compared with men, women paid more attention to health-related information and potential worldwide pandemics, as well as to how the purchase of daily goods affects their health [38]. The study noted that Finnish women also reported receiving far more informal health-related information from close family members, other kin, and friends/workmates than men did. Other studies did confirm that family members and friends are factors positively associated with people's healthcare [39,40].

As for the association between medical practice at home and EAS regularity, there has been no study explicitly linking the two. By medical practice at home, this study means simple health checkup such as measuring eyesight, weight, height, blood pressure, and using the common first aid kit.

Based on the above findings, we evaluate the reality of engagement in EAS in the Vietnamese population. The levels of EAS regularity are analyzed in relation to sex, educational background, BMI, health communication quality, and regular health check-ups at home.

3. Materials and Methods

3.1. Materials

The data of this study was collected as part of an interview-based survey of behavior and attitudes toward general health examinations (GHEs) in Hanoi and Hung Yen, Vietnam. The area has about 10 million people and is about 4300 km^2; the data were collected from the more urban places in this area. The data resulting from this study were deposited in the Open Science Framework [41] and

Harvard Dataverse [42], according to the principle of open data and FAIRsharing [43,44]. The details of how the survey was carried out and how the variables are coded can be viewed in the work of [45].

The survey was executed adhering to ethical standards under the license of V&A/07/2016 (15 September 2016). It was conducted in places such as schools, hospitals (Hospital 125 Thai Thinh in Dong Da District, Hanoi, and Vietnam–Germany Hospital in Hoan Kiem District, Hanoi), companies, government organizations, and randomly selected households in Hanoi. All residents in survey locations were invited to answer the questionnaire; the participants were randomly approached. The interviewers were required to wear an identification badge and had to give the participants information about the organizations responsible for the research, as well as the aims and methods of the research, and obtain a written agreement from the participants before starting the interview.

Overall, the study approached 2479 people; an average of one out of every six people invited to the interview refused to answer. Participants took roughly 10–15 min to complete the questionnaire. In the end, the final sample size was 2068 observations.

3.2. Methods

Specifically, this study examines and computes the probabilities of different levels of physical exercise in relation to gender, BMI, educational background, medical practice in the family, and perception of health communication quality. These variables are explained below:

"EvalExer" is the dependent variable, and stands for the level of EAS regularity. The participants were asked, "How much time do you spend on sports and physical exercise?" To which there were four options: "Comsuff" (completely sufficient), "Relsuff" (relatively sufficient), "Little" (do exercise but little), and "Trivial" (rarely do exercise). Thus, this variable is essentially about the self-reports of people on whether they feel their level of EAS is regular or not.

The predictors are:

- "Sex" includes two categories, "Male" and "Female."
- "Edu" is short for educational background, which includes two groups: "Highschool" (the people with high-school education or less) and "Graduate" (the people with a university education or higher).
- "BMI", or body mass index, has five categories: <18.5 (Underweight), 18.5–22.99 (Normal), 23–24.99 (Pre-obese), 25–29.99 (Obese level I), and >=30 (Obese level II). During the survey, the subjects were asked to provide their most recent measurements of height (in cm) and weight (in kg), based on which their BMI was calculated using the following formula: BMI = weight/(height × height).
- "ExamTools" is short for habitually checking health status in the family with common medical tools. The question was, "Does your family regularly take simple medical measurements (blood pressure, eyesight, weight, etc.)?" There were two options, "Yes" and "No."
- "HealthCom" is short for the perception of the participants towards the quality of mass communication on periodic GHEs; it is rated in a scale from 1 to 5, with 1 being the lowest and 5 being the highest.

The data are then structured in a CSV file and processed in R (3.1.1). The estimations are computed using the baseline category logit model (BCL), according to the work of [46]. The general equation of the BCL model is as follows:

$$\ln \frac{\pi_j(\mathbf{x})}{\pi_J(\mathbf{x})} = \alpha_j + \beta_j^T \mathbf{x}, \ j = 1, \ldots, J-1$$

where $\mathbf{x}$ is the independent variable, and $\pi_j(\mathbf{x}) = P(Y = j|\mathbf{x})$ is its probability. Thus, $\pi_j = P(Y_{ij} = 1)$, with Y being the dependent variable.

The estimated coefficients attained in multivariable logistic models are used to calculate the empirical probabilities according to the following formula:

$$\pi_j(\mathbf{x}) = \frac{\exp\left(\alpha_j + \boldsymbol{\beta}_j^T \mathbf{x}\right)}{1 + \sum_{h=1}^{J-1} \exp(\alpha_h + \boldsymbol{\beta}_h^T \mathbf{x})}$$

where $\sum_j \pi_j(\mathbf{x}) = 1$; and there are n observations in the sample, j represents the categorical values of an observation i, and h is a row in the matrix $\mathbf{X}_i$. Estimated probabilities can be used to predict the possibilities of Y under different conditions of $\mathbf{X}_i$ [42,45,47]. The statistical significance of independent variables in the model is determined based on z-value and p-value; with $p < 0.05$ being the conventional level of statistical significance required for a positive result.

4. Results

This section is divided by subheadings. It provides a concise and precise description of the experimental results, their interpretation, as well as the experimental conclusions that can be drawn.

4.1. Descriptive Statistics

Out of a total of 2068 observations obtained in the final sample, the majority of participants were young people (<30 years old) (63.15%), with the proportion of middle-aged and elderly participants (>= 50 years old) only accounting for 5.76% (Table 1). More females than males took part in the survey; females accounted for 64.08%.

Table 1. Descriptive statistics of the sample. BMI—body mass index.

Characteristics	N	Percentage (%)
Age		
<30	1306	63.15
30–49	643	31.09
≥50	119	5.76
Sex		
Male	728	35.20
Female	1340	64.80
Educational background		
High school or less	558	26.98
University or above	1.510	73.02
BMI		
<18.5 (Underweight)	408	19.73
18.5–22.99 (Normal)	1242	60.06
23–24.99 (Pre-obese)	279	13.49
25–29.99 (Obese level I)	128	6.19
>=30 (Obese level II)	11	0.53
Checking up health at home regularly (blood pressure, weight, eyesight, etc.)		
Yes	1242	60.06
No	826	39.94
The level of exercise and sports regularity		
Completely sufficient	132	6.38
Relatively sufficient	591	28.58
Little	863	41.73
Trivial	482	23.31

It can be seen from Table 1 that the majority of respondents are highly educated, with nearly three-quarters of participants having a university education or a higher degree (73.02%).

Concerning BMI, about 60% the participants are within the normal range, and the rest are distributed evenly between being thin or overweight. The average BMI is also in the normal range, at 20.85 (95% CI: 20.73–20.97) (Table 2). Most participants (60.06%) habitually receive simple health checks at home, including measurements of blood pressure, height, weight, and eyesight, as well as tracking of symptoms.

The level of participation in exercise and sports can be observed in Table 1 and Figure 1. Most survey participants self-reported that they did not regularly engage in physical activities. Those who felt they had a completely sufficient level of EAS represented the smallest group, with under 6%. The largest proportion (41.73%) claimed they did a little exercise, while those who felt their exercise and sports level are relatively sufficient and trivial accounted for 28.58% and 23.31%, respectively.

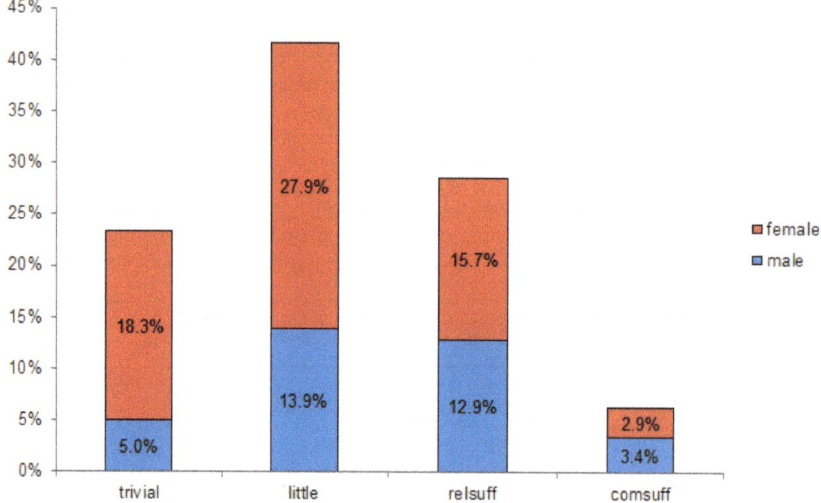

Figure 1. Distribution of respondents towards the level of exercise and sports (EAS) regularity, and by sex.

Figure 1 shows that the number of males and females is distributed unevenly at different activity levels. While more males claim to exercise at a completely sufficient level than females (3.4% versus 2.9%, respectively), females represented a higher proportion in all other levels of EAS regularity.

Also, the perception toward the quality of mass communications on healthcare also plays an important role. In the questionnaire, the study divided this factor into five levels of quality, which corresponds to a scale of 1 to 5, with 1 being the lowest and 5 the highest. The collected data showed that the participants perceived that the healthcare communication they received was only of average quality (2.83 points, 95% CI: 2.79–2.87) (see Table 2).

Table 2. Descriptive statistics for continuous variables.

Characteristics	Min	Max	Average	SD	CI
Age	18	83	29.17	10.09	28.73–29.60
BMI	14.48	37.20	20.85	2.69	20.73–20.96
Health communication quality perception	1	5	2.83	1.170	2.79–2.87

4.2. EAS Regularity Associated with Sex, Educational Background, and BMI

Firstly, the probability of sex and education associated with EAS regularity was considered. The regression model was constructed with the dependent variable being "EvalExer" (the level of EAS regularity), classified into four levels: "Comsuff" (completely sufficient), "Relsuff" (relatively sufficient), "Little" (do exercise but little), and "Trivial" (rarely do exercise); and two predictor variables were "Sex" and "Edu" (educational background). "Sex" includes "Male" and "Female", while "Edu" has two categories, "Highschool" (the people with high-school education or less) and "Graduate" (the people with a university education or higher). The estimation results follow in Table 3/subTable 3a.

Table 3. Exercise and sports (EAS) regularity associated with sex, educational background, and BMI.

(3a)	Intercept	"Sex" "Male"	"Edu" "Highschool"
	β_0	β_1	β_2
logit(trivial | comsuff)	1.846 *** [12.065]	−1.437 *** [−6.926]	−0.071 [−0.338]
logit(little | comsuff)	2.387 *** [16.134]	−0.808 *** [−4.256]	−0.536 ** [−2.686]
logit(relsuff | comsuff)	1.805 *** [11.818]	−0.315 [−1.623]	−0.491 * [−2.394]

Significant codes: 0 '***' 0.001 '**' 0.01 '*' 0.05 '.' 0.1 ' ' 1; z−value in square brackets; baseline category for "Sex" = "Female" and "Edu" = "Graduate". Log-likelihood: −36.94 with 3 degrees of freedom. Residual deviance: 4.17 with 3 degrees of freedom.

(3b)	Intercept	"Edu" "Highschool"	"BMI"
	β_0	β_1	β_2
logit(trivial | comsuff)	4.006 *** [5.297]	−0.14 [−0.677]	−0.127 *** [−3.586]
logit(little | comsuff)	4.158 *** [5.837]	−0.568 ** [−2.860]	−0.100 ** [−3.025]
logit(relsuff | comsuff)	1.919 ** [2.658]	−0.514 * [−2.510]	−0.012 [−0.366]

Significant codes: 0 '***' 0.001 '**' 0.01 '*' 0.05 '.' 0.1 ' ' 1; z−value in square brackets; baseline category for "Edu" = "Graduate". Log-likelihood: −2533.25 with 6195 degrees of freedom. Residual deviance: 5066.50 with 6195 degrees of freedom

(3c)	Intercept	"ExamTools" "Yes"	"HealthCom"
	β_0	β_1	β_2
logit(trivial | comsuff)	2.563 *** [7.566]	−0.622 ** [−2.867]	−0.297 ** [−2.976]
logit(little | comsuff)	2.973 *** [9.144]	−0.616 ** [−2.960]	−0.236 * [−2.497]
logit(relsuff | comsuff)	2.205 *** [6.600]	−0.464 * [−2.171]	−0.132 [−1.358]

Significant codes: 0 '***' 0.001 '**' 0.01 '*' 0.05 '.' 0.1 ' ' 1; z−value in square brackets; baseline category for "ExamTools" = "No". Log-likelihood: −2546.62 with 6195 degrees of freedom. Residual deviance: 5093.25 with 6195 degrees of freedom.

At $p < 0.05$, most of the estimated coefficients are statistically significant. The estimation equations representing the correlations are presented as follows:

$$\ln \frac{\pi_{trivial}}{\pi_{comsuff}} = 1.846 - 1.437 \times MaleSex - 0.071 \times HighschoolEdu \qquad (1)$$

$$\ln \frac{\pi_{little}}{\pi_{comsuff}} = 2.387 - 0.808 \times MaleSex - 0.536 \times HighschoolEdu \qquad (2)$$

$$\ln \frac{\pi_{relsuff}}{\pi_{comsuff}} = 1.805 - 0.315 \times MaleSex - 0.491 \times HighschoolEdu \qquad (3)$$

From that, the probability of a man with a high-school education or lower that reports exercising relatively sufficiently is as follows:

$$\pi_{relsuff} = \frac{e^{1.805-0.315-0.491}}{e^{1.805-0.315-0.491} + e^{2.387-0.808-0.536} + e^{1.846-1.437-0.071} + 1} = 0.341$$

Likewise, the remaining probabilities can also be calculated.

Next, the association of BMI with EAS levels was considered. In this BCL estimation, the dependent variable is still "EvalExer", and the predictors are "Edu" and "BMI." The results are reported in Table 3b. From the results, it can be concluded that a relationship between these factors exists. The estimation equations are displayed in Equations (4)–(6).

$$\ln \frac{\pi_{trivial}}{\pi_{comsuff}} = 4.006 - 0.140 \times HighschoolEdu - 0.127 \times BMI \qquad (4)$$

$$\ln \frac{\pi_{little}}{\pi_{comsuff}} = 4.158 - 0.568 \times HighschoolEdu - 0.100 \times BMI \qquad (5)$$

$$\ln \frac{\pi_{relsuff}}{\pi_{comsuff}} = 1.919 - 0.514 \times HighschoolEdu - 0.012 \times BMI \qquad (6)$$

4.3. EAS regularity Associated with Perception on Health Communication Quality and Habitual Health Checks at Home

The physiological factors have been examined above. Now, some other external factors, including perception on healthcare communication about periodic GHEs and habitual health checks at home, are taken into account. Again, the response variable is "EvalExer", and the two predictors are "ExamTools" (habitual health checks at home with common medical tools), including two options, "Yes" and "No"; and "HealthCom" (perception on the quality of health communication about periodic GHEs), scored from 1 to 5, with 1 being the lowest and 5 the highest. The estimation results are given in Table 3/subTable 3c.

At $p < 0.05$, the correlations between the above variables are confirmed, with eight out of nine of the estimated coefficients being statistically significant. The empirical relationships are presented in Equations (7)–(9).

$$\ln \frac{\pi_{trivial}}{\pi_{abssuff}} = 2.563 - 0.622 \times YesExamTools - 0.297 \times HealthCom \qquad (7)$$

$$\ln \frac{\pi_{little}}{\pi_{abssuff}} = 2.973 - 0.616 \times YesExamTools - 0.236 \times HealthCom \qquad (8)$$

$$\ln \frac{\pi_{relsuff}}{\pi_{abssuff}} = 2.205 - 0.464 \times YesExamTools - 0.132 \times HealthCom \qquad (9)$$

4.4. Interpretation of Estimation Results

The regression results partly show preliminary assessments about the association of the variables and people's EAS levels. The following discussion will give more details about both the degree and tendency of each factor. The figures were built using conditional probabilities (see Appendix A).

4.4.1. Physiological Factors

Figure 2a depicts the EAS tendency between males and females with high school education or less. It can be seen that for females, the probability of EAS at the trivial or little level is above 70%, and it drops dramatically to below 30% when associated with relatively or completely sufficient level of physical exercise. In contrast, for males, the probability of EAS at the trivial or little level is just above 50%, but it drops slightly to just slightly below 50%. The different slopes of the two lines demonstrate this tendency. These analytical results show that males tend to be more active than females in both groups of educational background, with the difference amounting to as much as 18.9% (Figure 2a). This is easily explained by the fact that males are generally conceived as the strong genus, as tending to prefer physical activities to females, and as having to do hard work more often. On the other hand, women might think that they often do housework, shopping, and taking care of children, which already require a significant amount of mobilization, so they do not necessarily participate in additional pure sports activities [15]. Moreover, the majority of female participants in the survey said they did not have enough time for themselves, as their official work and housework took up all their time.

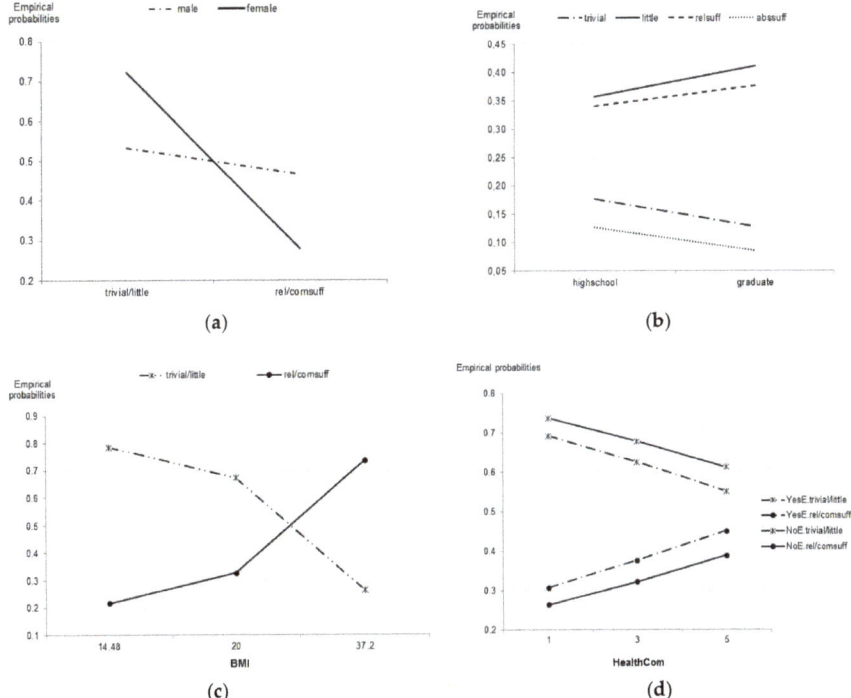

Figure 2. Probability lines represent EAS regularity levels towards physiological and external factors: (**a**) between males and females; (**b**) differences of intensivity levels between people with different education backgrounds; (**c**) activity levels against BMI; and, (**d**) association of perceived health communication value and exercise activity.

Meanwhile, Figure 2c helps clarify the trends of changes in activity levels in association with BMI. From this, it can be seen that when BMI increases from 18 to 23 (within the normal range), the "trivial/little" line (the probability of not exercising or training at negligible level) goes down, and the "rel/comsuff" (the probability of exercising relatively and absolutely sufficiently) goes up. This shows that people with a larger physique tend to exercise more. In particular, those with the largest BMI (BMI = 37.2) have a likelihood of exercising regularly as high as 74%, whereas this figure for the thinnest person (BMI = 14.48) is only slightly above 21% (Figure 2c). This can be explained by the fact that those who are overweight tend to choose exercise and sports as an effective and safe method to lose weight. Also, in the case of Vietnam, the higher average BMI of males compared with females could also be an explanation. The relationship between BMI and sex leads to the correlation between BMI, sex, and activity levels.

4.4.2. External Factors

Concerning the lines showing EAS level changes in relation to educational background, in Figure 2b, it can be observed that the lines of "trivial" and "comsuff" have the same downward trend, moving from the association with "highschool" to "graduate". Meanwhile, in contrast, the "little" and the "relsuff" lines both go up. An interpretation here is that Hanoi people with a university education or higher tend to feel they spend relatively sufficient or little time doing exercise. In contrast, Figure 2b also showed that those with a low level of education had two distinct trends, either reporting to engage in much more or much less exercise compared with those with higher levels of education.

Previous studies have shown the influence of the media on health care quality assessment, as well as on medical care [33,44]. This paper continues to show the media's association with EAS regularity. The evidence suggests that the "trivial_little" line goes down and the "rel/comsuff" goes up when the communication quality scored from 1 to 5 (Figure 2d). In other words, those who assess health communication quality as being at the highest level are 12% more likely to exercise frequently than those who assess it as being at the lowest. This means that when the communication quality is improved, people are more conscious about sports training, and this figure can be up to 45% (in the case of the regular check-ups at home being "yes"). The reason for this is that keeping track of healthcare information may prompt people to worry more than usual, which means more attention will be paid to their health [21,22]. Such information helps people understand the importance and benefits of habitual physical exercise, and, as a result, they will engage in more EAS.

In a similar vein, the study revealed that those who examine their health frequently also tend to attend sports activities more regularly. The above position of the lines representing relatively and completely sufficient exercise of those who usually practice common health checks in their home ("YesE.rel/comsuff") compared with which of those who do not ("NoE.rel/comsuff") provides support for this argument.

5. Discussion

5.1. Policy Implications

By evaluating the association of the self-reported regularity of leisure time EAS with two group of factors: (i) physiological factors (sex, body mass index or BMI) and (ii) external factors (education, health communication, medical practice at home), this study has filled in the gap in the literature on EAS correlations in a developing country of the middle-income level. The new insights can be used for forming policy related to social health; this section will discuss the implications.

In October 2017, the ruling Communist Party of Vietnam issued Resolution 21 on population works in the new era, which sets the target of bringing up the average Vietnamese height by 4 cm by 2030, representing a major goal in improving social public health status. Particularly, a Vietnamese male aged 18 years should reach 168.5 cm and females 157.5 cm over the next decade [48]. By comparison with regional countries, the height of Vietnamese youth is on par with that of Indonesians and

Philippines, but is below that of Singaporeans, Japanese, Thai, and Malaysians [49]. By showing the connection between EAS regularity and certain groups of factors, this study is instrumental in helping policymakers realize the above goal.

For example, the study found that the probability of females with a university education or higher feeling that they spend little or insufficient time exercising is 70%. Public health workers could use this information to target and promote more EAS participation among this group. Regarding BMI, because people with a larger physique tend to report exercising more (Figure 2c), a policy promoting EAS should take into account the population with a leaner physique. Most importantly, the study found an association between positive perception of health communication and people's engagement in EAS. Thus, this result suggests campaigns aimed at better health information coverage could encourage more Vietnamese people to exercise more regularly.

Another implication is that as knowing the factors associated with physical inactivity, which are increasingly seen to be among the causes of non-communicable diseases (NCDs) in countries of low and middle income [4], could improve evidence-based planning of public health interventions for NCDs. This is especially important for Vietnam, where NCDs, principally cardiovascular disease, diabetes, cancers, and chronic respiratory diseases, cause 73% of all deaths (more than 379,000) each year, according to WHO data [50]. Therefore, although the dataset covers only one location of Vietnam, the analysis results are no doubt useful for policy interpretation in other developing countries.

5.2. Limitations

The study is not without limitations. First of all, as the survey is exclusively based in Hanoi and its nearby areas, it poses a major geographical limitation. In order to investigate regional differences as well as shifting in behaviors and attitudes, it is necessary to conduct a nationwide survey, which would require resources beyond our current capacity. Hence, the findings in the study cannot be generalized to other regions in Vietnam, especially the rural or mountainous areas. Future research could improve upon this limitation by increasing the diversity of socio-demographic factors.

Secondly, the study is limited to the subjective perception of participants on whether or not they feel the amount of time they spend exercising is sufficient. The data were collected on a self-report basis, and thus the results are prone to subjective interpretation. Future research directions could refine the questionnaire by explicitly defining the amount of time one exercises that is sufficient or insufficient.

6. Conclusions

Overall, the above analyses drew links between EAS regularity and two groups of factors, the physiological ones (sex, BMI) and the external ones (education, health communication, and health checkup at home). Particularly, people with higher BMI are more inclined to do more EAS, perhaps because they want to work out to get fitter. The findings also show that those with a low level of education show two distinct trends, either reporting to engage in much more or much less exercise compared with those with higher levels of education. On the contrary, the people with higher education tend to stick with what they feel is a relatively sufficient or little but non-trivial amount of time exercising.

Furthermore, for females, those who graduate from university or have a higher degree usually claimed to exercise less than those with lower education, perhaps because of their job's attributes and their different routines. The study also found an opposite propensity among males, even if the differences in both sexes are negligible.

As for people's perception of health communication quality, the study found that as this perception got better, people were also more likely to report spending relatively or completely sufficient time doing sports and physical exercise. It seems that better-perceived quality of health information tends to make people more aware of their health status, so they actively take measures to care for themselves. The findings also indicate that those who habitually conduct simple health checks at home tend to self-report to be more active. Also, when considering the impact of media quality and regular monitoring of health status in comparison, the latter seems to have a greater influence, with the absolute value of the estimated coefficients being significantly larger.

Finally, although this study could be improved through surveying a larger demographic and defining which level of exercise is sufficient, it has provided a perspective from a developing country, and the information obtained through the empirical analyses is shown to have valuable implications for policy-makers and public health workers.

Author Contributions: Conceptualization, methodology, and supervision, Q.-H.V.; data curation, validation, and computations, Q.-H.V., V.-P.L., and T.-T.V.; investigation, Q.-H.V., H.M.T., and A.-D.H.; writing—original draft preparation, T.-T.V.; writing—review and editing, M.-T.H. and H.K.T.N.; visualization, T.-T.V., M.-T.H., and H.K.T.N. All co-authors read and approved the manuscript.

Funding: The authors received no external funding for this research.

Acknowledgments: The authors would like to thank Vuong & Associates' research team for assisting in collecting the raw data and preparing the dataset for this study: Dam Thu Ha, Nghiem Phu Kien Cuong, and Do Thu Hang.

Conflicts of Interest: The authors declare no conflict of interest.

Appendix A

a. Probabilities of EAS regularity towards gender and education.								
"EvalExer"	"trivial"		"little"		"relsuff"		"abssuff"	
"Edu" | "Sex"	"male"	"female"	"male"	"female"	"male"	"female"	"male"	"female"
"highschool"	0.176	0.347	0.357	0.375	0.341	0.219	0.126	0.059
"graduate"	0.128	0.261	0.411	0.448	0.376	0.250	0.085	0.041

b. Probabilities of EAS regularity towards BMI.					
		"EvalExer"			
"bmi"	"edu"	"trivial"	"little"	"relsuff"	"abssuff"
14.48	"highschool"	0.370	0.415	0.167	0.049
	"graduate"	0.286	0.493	0.188	0.033
20	"highschool"	0.292	0.381	0.249	0.078
	"graduate"	0.224	0.447	0.277	0.052
37.20	"highschool"	0.086	0.179	0.531	0.204
	"graduate"	0.066	0.209	0.589	0.135

c. Probabilities of EAS regularity towards health communication quality and usual medical practice in the family.					
		"EvalExer"			
"HealthCom"	"Examtools"	"trivial"	"little"	"relsuff"	"abssuff"
1	Yes	0.265	0.427	0.256	0.051
	No	0.283	0.454	0.234	0.029
3	Yes	0.222	0.403	0.298	0.078
	No	0.241	0.437	0.277	0.045
5	Yes	0.180	0.370	0.336	0.114

References

1. Van Bui, T.; Blizzard, C.L.; Luong, K.N.; Le Van Truong, N.; Tran, B.Q.; Otahal, P.; Srikanth, V.; Nelson, M.R.; Au, T.B.; Ha, S.T. Physical activity in Vietnam: Estimates and measurement issues. *PLoS ONE* **2015**, *10*, e0140941.
2. Althoff, T.; Hicks, J.L.; King, A.C.; Delp, S.L.; Leskovec, J. Large-scale physical activity data reveal worldwide activity inequality. *Nature* **2017**, *547*, 336–339. [CrossRef] [PubMed]

3. Ha, P. Vietnamese People among the Most Sedentary in the World—Survey. Available online: https://e.vnexpress.net/news/business/data-speaks/vietnamese-people-among-the-most-sedentary-in-the-world-survey-3613038.html (accessed on 17 April 2018).
4. Tuan, N.; Tuong, P.; Popkin, B. Body mass index (BMI) dynamics in Vietnam. *Eur. J. Clin. Nutr.* **2008**, *62*, 78–86. [CrossRef] [PubMed]
5. Cuong, T.; Dibley, M.; Bowe, S.; Hanh, T.; Loan, T. Obesity in adults: An emerging problem in urban areas of Ho Chi Minh City, Vietnam. *Eur. J. Clin. Nutr.* **2007**, *61*, 673–681. [CrossRef] [PubMed]
6. Nguyen, M.D.; Beresford, S.A.; Drewnowski, A. Trends in overweight by socio-economic status in Vietnam: 1992 to 2002. *Public Health Nutr.* **2007**, *10*, 115–121. [CrossRef] [PubMed]
7. Craig, D. *Familiar Medicine: Everyday Health Knowledge and Practice in Today's Vietnam*; University of Hawaii Press: Honolulu, HI, USA, 2002.
8. Bauman, A.E.; Reis, R.S.; Sallis, J.F.; Wells, J.C.; Loos, R.J.; Martin, B.W.; Lancet Physical Activity Series Working Group. Correlates of physical activity: Why are some people physically active and others not? *Lancet* **2012**, *380*, 258–271. [CrossRef]
9. De Rezende, L.F.M.; Azeredo, C.M.; Canella, D.S.; Claro, R.M.; de Castro, I.R.R.; Levy, R.B.; do Carmo Luiz, O. Sociodemographic and behavioral factors associated with physical activity in Brazilian adolescents. *BMC Public Health* **2014**, *14*, 485. [CrossRef] [PubMed]
10. Heseltine, R.; Skelton, D.A.; Kendrick, D.; Morris, R.W.; Griffin, M.; Haworth, D.; Masud, T.; Iliffe, S. "Keeping Moving": Factors associated with sedentary behaviour among older people recruited to an exercise promotion trial in general practice. *BMC Fam. Pract.* **2015**, *16*, 67. [CrossRef] [PubMed]
11. Humpel, N.; Owen, N.; Leslie, E. Environmental factors associated with adults' participation in physical activity: A review. *Am. J. Prevent. Med.* **2002**, *22*, 188–199. [CrossRef]
12. Bonaiuto, M.; Aiello, A.; Perugini, M.; Bonnes, M.; Ercolani, A.P. Multidimensional perception of residential environment quality and neighbourhood attachment in the urban environment. *J. Environ. Psychol.* **1999**, *19*, 331–352. [CrossRef]
13. Minichilli, F.; Gorini, F.; Ascari, E.; Bianchi, F.; Coi, A.; Fredianelli, L.; Licitra, G.; Manzoli, F.; Mezzasalma, L.; Cori, L. Annoyance Judgment and Measurements of Environmental Noise: A Focus on Italian Secondary Schools. *Int. J. Environ. Res. Public Health* **2018**, *15*, 208. [CrossRef] [PubMed]
14. Cassina, L.; Fredianelli, L.; Menichini, I.; Chiari, C.; Licitra, G. Audio-Visual Preferences and Tranquillity Ratings in Urban Areas. *Environments* **2018**, *5*, 1. [CrossRef]
15. Wilson, M.G.; Ellison, G.M.; Cable, N.T. Basic science behind the cardiovascular benefits of exercise. *Br. J. Sports Med.* **2016**, *50*, 93–99. [CrossRef] [PubMed]
16. Kenney, W.L.; Wilmore, J.; Costill, D. *Physiology of Sport and Exercise*, 6th ed.; Human Kinetics: Champaign, IL, USA, 2015.
17. McNally, S. *Exercise: The Miracle Cure and the Role of the Doctor in Promoting It*; Academy of Medical Royal Colleges: London, UK, 2015.
18. Macera, C.A.; Jones, D.A.; Yore, M.; Ham, S.; Kohl, H.W.; Kimsey Jr, C.; Buchner, D. Prevalence of physical activity, including lifestyle activities among adults-United States, 2000–2001. *Morb. Mortality Wkly. Rep.* **2003**, *52*, 764–769.
19. Beck, B.R.; Daly, R.M.; Singh, M.A.F.; Taaffe, D.R. Exercise and Sports Science Australia (ESSA) position statement on exercise prescription for the prevention and management of osteoporosis. *J. Sci. Med. Sport* **2017**, *20*, 438–445. [CrossRef] [PubMed]
20. Sharman, J.E.; Stowasser, M. Australian association for exercise and sports science position statement on exercise and hypertension. *J. Sci. Med. Sport* **2009**, *12*, 252–257. [CrossRef] [PubMed]
21. Tiedemann, A.; Sherrington, C.; Close, J.C.; Lord, S.R. Exercise and Sports Science Australia position statement on exercise and falls prevention in older people. *J. Sci. Med. Sport* **2011**, *14*, 489–495. [CrossRef] [PubMed]
22. Valderrabano, V.; Steiger, C. Treatment and prevention of osteoarthritis through exercise and sports. *J. Aging Res.* **2011**, *2011*, 374653. [CrossRef] [PubMed]
23. Smart, N.A.; Williams, A.D.; Levinger, I.; Selig, S.; Howden, E.; Coombes, J.S.; Fassett, R.G. Exercise & Sports Science Australia (ESSA) position statement on exercise and chronic kidney disease. *J. Sci. Med. Sport* **2013**, *16*, 406–411. [PubMed]

24. Warner, S.; Dixon, M.A. Competition, gender, and the sport experience: An exploration among college athletes. *Sport Educ. Soc.* **2015**, *20*, 527–545. [CrossRef]
25. Sheel, A.W.; Richards, J.C.; Foster, G.E.; Guenette, J.A. Sex differences in respiratory exercise physiology. *Sports Med.* **2004**, *34*, 567–579. [CrossRef] [PubMed]
26. Hagströmer, M.; Kwak, L.; Oja, P.; Sjöström, M. A 6 year longitudinal study of accelerometer-measured physical activity and sedentary time in Swedish adults. *J. Sci. Med. Sport* **2015**, *18*, 553–557. [CrossRef] [PubMed]
27. Flegal, K.M.; Carroll, M.D.; Kit, B.K.; Ogden, C.L. Prevalence of obesity and trends in the distribution of body mass index among US adults, 1999-2010. *JAMA* **2012**, *307*, 491–497. [CrossRef] [PubMed]
28. Ho, A.J.; Raji, C.A.; Becker, J.T.; Lopez, O.L.; Kuller, L.H.; Hua, X.; Dinov, I.D.; Stein, J.L.; Rosano, C.; Toga, A.W. The effects of physical activity, education, and body mass index on the aging brain. *Hum. Brain Mapping* **2011**, *32*, 1371–1382. [CrossRef] [PubMed]
29. Jackson, A.; Stanforth, P.; Gagnon, J.; Rankinen, T.; Leon, A.; Rao, D.; Skinner, J.; Bouchard, C.; Wilmore, J. The effect of sex, age and race on estimating percentage body fat from body mass index: The Heritage Family Study. *Int. J. Obesity* **2002**, *26*, 789–796. [CrossRef] [PubMed]
30. Wang, J.; Thornton, J.C.; Russell, M.; Burastero, S.; Heymsfield, S.; Pierson Jr, R.N. Asians have lower body mass index (BMI) but higher percent body fat than do whites: Comparisons of anthropometric measurements. *Am. J. Clin. Nutr.* **1994**, *60*, 23–28. [CrossRef] [PubMed]
31. Sundquist, J.; Johansson, S.-E. The influence of socioeconomic status, ethnicity and lifestyle on body mass index in a longitudinal study. *Int. J. Epidemiol.* **1998**, *27*, 57–63. [CrossRef] [PubMed]
32. Rantanen, T.; Parkatti, T.; Heikkinen, E. Muscle strength according to level of physical exercise and educational background in middle-aged women in Finland. *Eur. J. Appl. Physiol. Occup. Physiol.* **1992**, *65*, 507–512. [CrossRef] [PubMed]
33. Keller, P.A.; Lehmann, D.R. Designing Effective Health Communications: A Meta-Analysis. *J. Public Policy Mark.* **2008**, *27*, 117–130. [CrossRef]
34. Regitz-Zagrosek, V. Sex and gender differences in health. *Sci. Soc. Ser. Sex Sci.* **2012**, *13*, 596–603. [CrossRef] [PubMed]
35. Mansfield, A.K.; Addis, M.E.; Mahalik, J.R. "Why won't he go to the doctor?": The psychology of men's help seeking. *Int. J. Men's Health* **2003**, *2*, 93. [CrossRef]
36. Wellstead, P. Information behaviour of Australian men experiencing stressful life events: The role of social networks and confidants. *Inf. Res.* **2011**, *16*, 12120429.
37. Block, L.G.; Keller, P.A. Effects of self-efficacy and vividness on the persuasiveness of health communications. *J. Consum. Psychol.* **1997**, *6*, 31–54. [CrossRef]
38. Ek, S. Gender differences in health information behaviour: A Finnish population-based survey. *Health Promot. Int.* **2015**, *30*, 736–745. [CrossRef] [PubMed]
39. Kreps, G.L.; Sivaram, R. Strategic health communication across the continuum of breast cancer care in limited-resource countries. *Cancer* **2008**, *113*, 2331–2337. [CrossRef] [PubMed]
40. Hiatt, R.; Pasick, R.; Stewart, S.; Bloom, J.; Davis, P.; Gardiner, P.; Johnston, M.; Luce, J.; Schorr, K.; Brunner, W.; et al. Community-based cancer screening for underserved women: Design and baseline findings from the Breast and Cervical Cancer Intervention Study. *Prev. Med.* **2001**, *33*, 190–203. [CrossRef] [PubMed]
41. Vuong, Q.H. Vietnam General Health Examinations Propensity Survey 2016. Available online: https://osf.io/afz2w/ (accessed on 23 October 2018).
42. Vuong, Q.H.; Ho, T.M.; Nguyen, H.K.; Vuong, T.T. Healthcare consumers' sensitivity to costs: A reflection on behavioural economics from an emerging market. *Palgrave Commun.* **2018**, *4*, 70. [CrossRef]
43. Vuong, Q.-H.; La, V.-P.; Vuong, T.-T.; Ho, M.-T.; Nguyen, H.-K.T.; Nguyen, V.-H.; Pham, H.-H.; Ho, M.-T. An open database of productivity in Vietnam's social sciences and humanities for public use. *Sci. Data* **2018**, *5*, 180188. [CrossRef] [PubMed]
44. Wilkinson, M.D.; Dumontier, M.; Aalbersberg, I.J.; Appleton, G.; Axton, M.; Baak, A.; Blomberg, N.; Boiten, J.-W.; da Silva Santos, L.B.; Bourne, P.E. The FAIR Guiding Principles for scientific data management and stewardship. *Sci. Data* **2016**, *3*, 160018. [CrossRef] [PubMed]
45. Vuong, Q.H. Survey data on Vietnamese propensity to attend periodic general health examinations. *Scientific Data* **2017**, *4*, 170142. [CrossRef] [PubMed]

46. Agresti, A. *Categorical Data Analysis*; John Wiley & Sons: Hoboken, NJ, USA, 2003.
47. Vuong, Q.H.; Vuong, T.T.; Ho, T.M.; Nguyen, H.V. Psychological and socio-economic factors affecting social sustainability through impacts on perceived health care quality and public health: The case of Vietnam. *Sustainability* **2017**, *9*, 1456. [CrossRef]
48. State Audit of Vietnam. Nghi Quyet 21 NQ-TW cua Ban Chap Hanh Trung Uong Dang Ve Cong Tac Dan So Trong Tinh Hinh Doi Moi [Resolution 21 of Central Steering Committee on Population Works in a New era]. Available online: http://vanban.sav.gov.vn/2072-1-ddt/nghi-quyet-21nqtw-ngay-25102017-cua-ban-chap-hanh-trung-uong-ve-cong-tac-dan-so-trong-tinh-hinh-moi.sav (accessed on 17 April 2018).
49. Duy Tien. Vietnamese among the Shortest, Research Reveals. Available online: http://en.cand.com.vn/Law-Society/Vietnamese-among-the-shortest-research-reveals-459912/ (accessed on 3 October 2018).
50. World Health Organization. UN Interagency Task Force on NCDs Joint Country Mission to Viet Nam. Available online: http://www.who.int/ncds/un-task-force/vietnam-mission-september-2016/en/ (accessed on 17 April 2018).

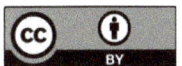

© 2018 by the authors. Licensee MDPI, Basel, Switzerland. This article is an open access article distributed under the terms and conditions of the Creative Commons Attribution (CC BY) license (http://creativecommons.org/licenses/by/4.0/).

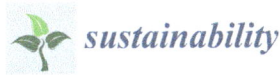

Article

Does Mobile Phone Penetration Affect Divorce Rate? Evidence from China

Jiaping Zhang [1], Mingwang Cheng [1,*], Xinyu Wei [1] and Xiaomei Gong [2]

1   School of Economics and Management, Tongji University, Shanghai 200092, China; 1710232@tongji.edu.cn (J.Z.); weixinyu@tongji.edu.cn (X.W.)
2   College of Economics and Trade, Hunan University of Commerce, Changsha 410205, China; gongxiaomeixisu@sina.com
*   Correspondence: 07099@tongji.edu.cn; Tel.: +86-21-65982272

Received: 12 September 2018; Accepted: 11 October 2018; Published: 15 October 2018

Abstract: Marital happiness is an important symbol of social harmony and can help promote sustainable economic and social development. In recent years, the rapid rise of the divorce rate in China, a country where the divorce rate had previously been low, has attracted wide attention. However, few articles have focused on the popularization of information and communication technology's impact on China's rising divorce rate in recent years. As a first attempt, the provincial panel data during the period 2001–2016 is applied to study quantitatively the relationship between mobile phone penetration and the divorce rate. In order to get more reliable estimation results, this paper uses two indicators to measure the divorce rate, and quantile regression is applied for further analysis. Additionally, one-year to five-year lag times of the mobile phone penetration are used as the core explanatory variables in order to analyse the lagging effect of mobile phone penetration on divorce rate. The result shows that the correlation between the mobile phone penetration and the divorce rate was statistically positive significant in China during the period 2001–2016. Furthermore, the paper also finds that mobile phone penetration had the greatest impact on divorce rate in central China, followed by eastern China, but it was not obvious in western China during this period. From a technological perspective, this paper provides some possible explanations for the rising divorce rate in China in recent years, and further enriches the relevant research on the impact of the development of information and communication technology on societal changes.

Keywords: mobile phone penetration; divorce rate; marital happiness; well-being

1. Introduction

The quality of marriage is an important guarantee of well-being [1–5]. In China's traditional marriage culture, "a woman follows her husband no matter what his lot is" is a commonly held belief, and divorce is often seen as a stigma [6]. However, China's divorce rates have appreciably risen in the 21st century. As shown in Figure 1, since 2001 the crude divorce rate (the number of divorces per 1000 population) increased from 0.98‰ to 3.02‰ in 2016 [7]. The increasing divorce rate in China, a country that has been heavily influenced by traditional marriage concepts, has attracted extensive attention from scholars in recent years [8–10].

Some scholars attribute the rising divorce rate in China to the rapid urbanization, marketization, industrialization, modern education development, and economic growth, etc., during the past 40 years, and those factors may contribute to changes in people's attitudes and beliefs, which can lead to shifts in family structure, functioning, and relationships [11,12]. However, these factors do not explain why China's divorce rate remained low and did not change much in the 1990s (as shown in the Figure 1).

Sustainability **2018**, *10*, 3701; doi:10.3390/su10103701   www.mdpi.com/journal/sustainability

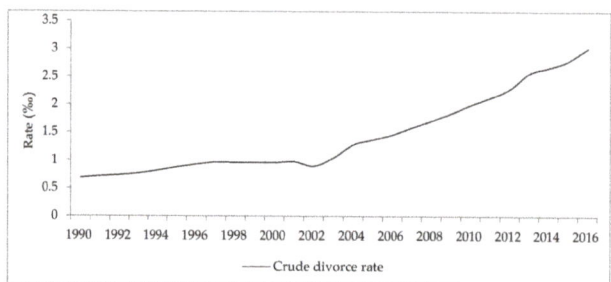

Figure 1. The crude divorce rate in China between 1990 and 2016. Data sources: China National Bureau of Statistics.

The main purpose of this paper is to explain the rising divorce rate in China from the perspective of the increasing mobile phone penetration in recent years. With the development of information and communication technology (ICT) in recent decades, the mobile phone has become a major communication tool [13]. Since 2005, the global mobile-cellular telephone penetration grew from 33.9% to 103.5% in 2017 [14]. The rapid spread of mobile phones has brought the world into a digital era, which has had a profound impact on economy, culture, and politics [15,16], and has greatly expanded the scope of interpersonal communication [17]. The rise in the mobile phone penetration may have the following effects on China's divorce rate:

(1) The popularity of mobile phone, whether for unmarried or married people, can greatly reduce the cost of searching for romantic partners. With the development of smart phones, mobile phone functions have become more and more diverse, which has had a significant impact on people's dating behaviours. Various social platforms and mobile phone applications, such as WeChat (Tencent, Shenzhen, China) and QQ (Tencent, Shenzhen, China), can closely connect individuals with common interests, offer a convenient condition for extramarital affairs, and increase the possibility of divorce. (2) The popularity of mobile phones has affected people's interpersonal relationships and the relationship between couples. (3) The spread of mobile phones has accelerated the spread of modern marriage concepts in China. Nowadays, especially for young people, mobile phones have become one of the most important tools for connecting to the Internet in order to find whatever information is needed. More and more people use mobile Internet to search for laws and regulations related to marriage, especially for couples experiencing marriage crises who may use mobile Internet to communicate with more people in common situations. As a result, people may be more daring to say goodbye to a failed marriage than to think that divorce is a shameful act.

The main contribution of this paper is embodied in the following three aspects. First of all, previous studies have tended to ignore the impact of advances in information technology on divorce rate, and the few relevant studies that have previously been published have mainly been based in developed countries. As a first attempt, this paper examines the explicit relationship between mobile phone penetration and divorce rate based on China's macro data at the provincial level, thus expanding on previous established research. Secondly, China is committed to the construction of a "harmonious society", and marital happiness is considered to be an important embodiment of a "harmonious society". Simultaneously, divorce may potentially result in negative effects on both health and well-being [18]. Therefore, this paper has many implications for Chinese public policy in the future. Furthermore, many countries in the world regard ICT as an important driving force for the promotion of the sustainable development of economy and society and the improvement of people's welfare [19]. Given the increasingly prominent role of mobile phones in people's daily lives, understanding their influence on individuals and families is crucial [20–22]. Thirdly, in this paper, the robustness and endogeneity of the model are considered rigorously and fully, which makes the conclusion more reliable.

The remainder of this paper is organised as follows. Section 2 briefly reviews the existing theory and literature. Section 3 presents the econometric model and data description. Section 4 provides the empirical results and relevant discussions. Finally, the Section 5 summarizes the conclusions drawn from this research.

2. Brief Review of the Literature and Theoretical Analysis

2.1. Theory Related to Marriage and Divorce

Unlike traditional marriages, divorce rates are high in modern marriages [23], which has led many scholars to become interested in the reasons why people choose to divorce after a period of marriage. Becker [24] was an early researcher on marriage and family behaviour. In considering mainly an economics perspective, Becker thought that each person tries to find the best mate available to them in the marriage market. Becker believed that when the expected utility of marriage is greater than that of being single, people will get married. When the expected utility of being single or remarrying is greater than the loss of utility from divorcing (including the separation from family, the separation of family property, legal expenses, and other losses), the married person will terminate their marriage. Similar to this theory, Weiss and Willis [25] considered that a marriage would end when the other partner meets a better match, whereafter Becker et al. [26] stressed the important role of "search costs" both before and after the marriage. In this theory, the individual selects firstly or sets the retention value (or threshold value, which is a minimum acceptable quality level) for a future matcher, and then restores the search within the accessible crowd. When an individual finds an individual that exceeds the retention value, she or he will get married. When the search cost is high, the retention value of the individual will generally be lower. Otherwise, the individual will give up the benefit of marriage for an unacceptably long period.

Many other studies also focused on the explanation factors for divorce from other perspectives. Societal transition was widely regarded as an important factor for the rise of divorce rates. Over the past two decades, egalitarian beliefs have been spread worldwide, which has profoundly influenced the nature of family relationships. Especially with the improvement of the status for women and children, the traditional patriarchal system based on blood and hierarchy has been greatly challenged, and family relations are constantly changing [27–30].

Economic factors are also cited as important reasons for divorce. Amato and Beattie [31] studied how unemployment affects divorce rates by studying data from the United States during the period from 1960 to 2005. They found that the relationships between unemployment rate and divorce rate changed over time. Rainer and Smith [32], Battu et al. [33], and Klein [34] all found a close relationship between house prices and divorce rate.

The social-economic growth hypothesis theory emphasizes that urban society will first exhibit low marital stability, such as that commonly observed in the middle class, which typically lives in a more affluent environment [35–38]. For example, Sandström [39] found that the divorce rate in rural, single-provider family, low-income households was significantly lower than that in urban, dual-provider family, high-income households through an analysis of the divorce behaviour in Swedish from 1911 to 1974.

Some scholars have begun to pay attention to the impact of population mobility on marriage. Glenn and Supancic [40], Landale and Ogena [41], Frank and Wildsmith [42], and Gautier et al. [43] all found that the divorce rate is usually high in areas with high migratory and floating populations. Caarls and Mazzucato [44] found that the likelihood of divorcing is higher when a wife (without her husband's escort) works abroad, but lower when the husband (without his wife's escort) works abroad.

2.2. Mobile Phone and Mobile Internet

With the rapid development of mobile communication, especially smartphones, and Internet technology, the number of mobile Internet (MI) users has increased rapidly [45]. In the past, the main function of mobile phones was communication (i.e., voice calls and text messages). However, more and more mobile phone users have conducted information searches, online shopping, social entertainment, and other activities through the mobile Internet in the last few years [46]. According to the 41st China Internet Development Statistics Report, as of December 2017, the number of mobile Internet users in China reached 753 million, and the proportion of netizens using mobile phones to surf the Internet increased from 95.1% in 2016 to 97.5% [47]. Mobile phones have become the main channel for residents to access the Internet. The tremendous impact of mobile phones and mobile Internet on people's life has attracted wide attention from scholars [48]. On the one hand, the relevant studies examine the impact of mobile phones and/or mobile Internet on the economy or personal income and employment from both micro and macro perspectives. For example, at the micro level, Bertschek and Niebel [49] analysed date from a German firm and found that mobile Internet access was able to significantly improve labour productivity. Islam et al. [22] found that mobile phone use had a significant promoting effect on performance of a microenterprises in Bangladesh. At the macro level, there is a broad range of literature showing a significant positive relationship between mobile phone and/or mobile Internet use and the economic growth in a region or country [50–53].

On the other hand, the impact of mobile phones or mobile Internet on social development or individual well-being has also received extensive attention from scholars [19]. There is quite an extensive amount of literature showing that mobile phone and/or mobile Internet use can reduce corruption [54,55], improve institutional quality [56], affect individual social networks [57], increase search convenience [46,58], etc. However, other studies have also found that excessive use of mobile phones can cause "technostress", which has negative effects on users' mental and physical health and work efficiency [59–61].

As can be seen from the above literature review, although existing literature has conducted research on the impact of mobile phones and mobile Internet on economic growth and social development, there is a lack of studies that discuss the impact of mobile phone penetration on family interpersonal relationships, such as marriage stability. However, from the perspective of personal well-being, sustainable economic development, and social harmony, it is of great practical significance to discuss the impact of mobile phone penetration on divorce rate. This article attempts to fill this gap.

2.3. Theoretical Analysis of the Possible Impact of the Mobile Phone Penetration on the Divorce Rate in China

In traditional Chinese society, marriage usually follows the principle of "arrange a match by parents' order and on the matchmaker's word". The right of young men and women to freely choose their spouses is greatly restricted. Freedom to marry or divorce between men and women was frowned upon by public opinion. Moreover, in traditional Chinese society, interpersonal communication is often based on blood relationship, which greatly reduces the chance of finding a suitable partner for both men and women. Although China has achieved great economic and social development in recent decades, the traditional marriage concept still has far-reaching influence, which is an important reason why the divorce rate in China has remained low [6].

However, the emergence of new media tools, such as the Internet and mobile phones, are changing the way that people produce and live, and people's attitudes and beliefs are changing drastically. These changes can also affect the traditional forms of interpersonal communication between men and women, and people's social networks, all of which can ultimately affect the stability of marriage. Scholars and institutions have previously considered the impact of new media on marital stability. Merkle and Richardson [62] and Rosen et al. [63] all found that online dating is a unique way to pursue romance. Valenzuela et al. [64] found that the use of social networks sites has negative effects on marriage quality, and is positively associated with individuals thinking about divorce. The spread of mobile phones may have a positive effect on divorce rate for the following reasons:

Firstly, mobile phone use can affect people's social networks [65] and reduce the cost of a married person searching for a "third party" after marriage [6]. Nowadays, social media networks or apps, such as WeChat (Tencent, Shenzhen, China), QQ (Tencent, Shenzhen, China), and Microblog (Sina,

Beijing, China), have become the main ways for Chinese residents to engage in social activities [63]. The use of mobile phones can reduce the cost of searching for partners, expand the range of people seeking the opposite sex, and increase the substitution of spouses [57,66–69], all of which can reduce the stability of marriage [70]. Furthermore, if a married person thinks that it will be easy to find a more suitable partner after marriage, he or she may reduce his/her investment in his/her existing marriage, such as by choosing to not have children [71], which may ultimately increase the divorce rate.

Secondly, the use of mobile phones can affect people's interpersonal relationships [72]. There is a broad range of literature indicating that the excessive use of mobile phones can lead to "dependency", "compulsion", and "mobile phone addiction", all of which may have negative effects on the health, psychology, study, and work of individuals [73–75]. Furthermore, for young people today, mobile phones represent the most common way to access the Internet. However, the "digital world" has created a virtual environment that may cause couples to distrust each other, thereby potentially undermining the quality and stability of their marriages. Both of these can ultimately have negative effects on the relationships of married couples [76–82]. Clayton et al. [83] found that people who regularly use Facebook are more likely to have negative interpersonal relationship outcomes such as breakups, divorces, or romantic cheating.

Thirdly, according to the societal transition theory, the increase in the mobile phone penetration has promoted the spread of democracy and freedom ideology [20,84], which could accelerate the spread of modern marriage concepts and affect the stability of family and marriage. In addition, the spread of mobile phones and mobile Internet has also accelerated the spread and improvement of modern marriage laws and regulations [6]. As a result, more and more Chinese are daring to say goodbye to failed marriages for the pursuit of happiness. Last but not least, the use of social media tools, such as mobile phones and the internet, has boosted women's access to the labour market, raising the status of women in their families [85–87]. The studies of Spitze and South [88] and Kalmijn and Poortman [89] found that women's participation in the labour market increased divorce rates.

From the above analysis, mobile phones reduce the cost of searching for romantic partners, change people's marriage concepts, and deeply affect people's interpersonal communications. Therefore, there may be a significant positive relationship between mobile phone penetration and divorce rate in China. Consequently, the Chinese provincial panel data has been used to examine potential relationships between mobile phone penetration rates and divorce rates for the rest of this paper.

3. Research Methods and Data

3.1. Estimation Model and Methods

In previous studies on divorce, scholars mostly used individual micro data. However, individual data are prone to problems in that certain (or unobservable) characteristics of a spouse can affect both divorce and mobile phone use simultaneously. Fortunately, China's provincial panel data can solve this problem by adding the provincial fixed effects to control other unobservable variables that may affect divorce rate. From a few relevant studies using macro panel data, scholars usually use regression analysis [31,71]. Likewise, this study uses econometric regression models to examine the explicit relationship between mobile phone penetration and divorce rate. Since data for mobile phone use at the provincial level in China started in 2001, the dataset uses 496 observations from China's 31 mainland provinces between 2001 and 2016.

In order to examine the impact of China's mobile phone penetration on divorce rate, this paper uses a province effects panel model, which controls for the unobserved heterogeneity among provinces. Specifically, this research study formulates the following regression model:

$$\text{Divorce}_{it} = a_0 + a_1 \text{Mobile}_{it} + CX_{it} + \lambda_i + \varepsilon_{it} \tag{1}$$

where the subscripts i = 1,2,...,31 index each of the 31 provinces; the subscripts t = 1,2,...,16 index each of the specific year during the sample period from 2001–2016; and Divorce_{it} is the dependent variable in province i in year t. Among the regressions, Moblile$_{it}$ is the core explanatory variable of province i in the year t. The vector X is defined as a set of controls commonly used in divorce rate literature. λ_i represents province dummies, and the ε_{it} represents the error term.

3.2. Variable Settings and Data Source Description

Considering the purpose of this paper is to analyse the impacts of mobile phone penetration on divorce rate, the dependent variable is the divorce rate, and this study uses the mobile phone penetration rate as the core explanatory variable. Additionally, the control variables X mainly include: the urbanization level, the average educational year, the total of elderly adult and child dependency ratio, and a policy dummy variable. More specifically, all the above variables are set as follows:

The divorce rate is denoted by "Divorce". For ease of calculation, scholars generally use crude divorce rates to measure divorce rate levels [31]. This paper also adopts this index; the calculation method is as follows:

$$\text{Divorce} = \frac{\text{The number of divorces in a given year}}{\text{The total population}} \times 1000 \quad (2)$$

For more supplementary analyses (discussed later), this study uses another index to measure the divorce rate (denoted by Divorce1), which uses the following formula:

$$\text{Divorce1} = \frac{\text{The number of divorces in a given year}}{\text{The total population between 15 and 64 years old}} \times 1000 \quad (3)$$

This index can accurately measure the divorce rate for marriage-age populations.

The mobile phone penetration is denoted by "Mobile". This paper uses the number of mobile phone users per 100 people to measure the mobile phone penetration rate level. The corresponding calculation formula is as follows:

$$\text{Moblie} = \frac{\text{The number of mobile phone users}}{\text{The total population}} \times 100 \quad (4)$$

The urbanization level is denoted by "Urban". In accordance with a large number of previous studies, urbanization level has an important relationship with divorce rate. Urbanization is a trend that accompanies economic and social development, frequent population movements, and advanced human civilization. Urban areas, where modern industrial agglomeration occurs and industrial civilizations are developed, may have higher divorce rates than rural areas [8,43,90]. Therefore, it is necessary to add urbanization level as a control variable for the divorce rate in China. For ease of calculation, this study used the proportion of urban residents within the total population to measure the level of urbanization.

The average educational year is denoted by "Education". With the improvement of human civilization, people have more freedom to pursue a high quality marriage or dissolve their marriage, especially women [91,92]. Many previous studies have found that education has a positive relationship with divorce rates [93]. In this paper, education level is measured by education years per capita for people six years old or above. The formula is: Education = (population for primary school education × 6 + population for junior high school education × 9 + population for high school education × 12 + population for college degree or above × 16)/population for age 6 or above.

The total dependency ratio is denoted by "Dependency". The age structure of a population has an important influence on its divorce rate [94,95]. In recent years, China has fully liberalized the two-child policy, and China's aging population has become an increasingly serious issue. Therefore demographic changes may have had an important impact on the divorce rate. In order to measure the dependency ratio, the population below the age of 14 and over the age of 65 was divided by the population between age 15 to 64.

The policy dummy variable is denoted by "Policy". The "Marriage Registration Ordinance" of China, amended in 2003, simplifies marriage and divorce proceedings and may also have an important impact on the divorce rate [96,97]. For this reason, this paper sets up a dummy variable for marriage policy. Therefore, the policy dummy variable is measured as follows:

$$\text{Policy} = \begin{cases} 0 \text{ if year} < 2003 \\ 1 \text{ if year} \geq 2003 \end{cases} \quad (5)$$

China's provincial panel data during the period between 2001 and 2016 is utilized in this study. The data for divorce rate and the mobile phone penetration rate were cited from China Statistical Yearbooks. The data for the control variables, including Urban, Education, and Dependency, were all collected from China Demographic Yearbooks.

3.3. Trends for Core Variables

Figure 2 depicts the changes to the crude divorce rate in 31 provinces. The figure reveals two major outliers. On the one hand, the crude divorce rate in Xinjiang province was extremely high during the period from 2001 to 2010 and then it had small drops in the substantially years. On the other hand, the crude divorce rate in the Tibet was the lowest during the whole period. The religious beliefs common to these areas can clearly explain the two outliers. The Tibetan area is mainly affected by Buddhist culture, which does not advocate divorce. The people of Xinjiang Uygur have long been deeply influenced by Islamic culture, which allows polygamy, and where men typically have absolute control over marriage. Due to the atypical pattern in Tibet and Xinjiang, this paper also carried out regression estimation on the samples excluding Xinjiang and Tibet. However, it found that the removal of Xinjiang and Tibet had no obvious influence on the estimation results, which may be due to our datasets being weighted by province population, as both Tibet and Xinjiang are underpopulated. The following regression results are based on samples including Xinjiang and Tibet. Obviously, the divorce rates in the remaining 29 provinces showed a highly consistent trend. While divorce rates vary widely among the 29 provinces, almost all provinces follow a similar trend, with divorce rates rising across all provinces from 2001 to 2016.

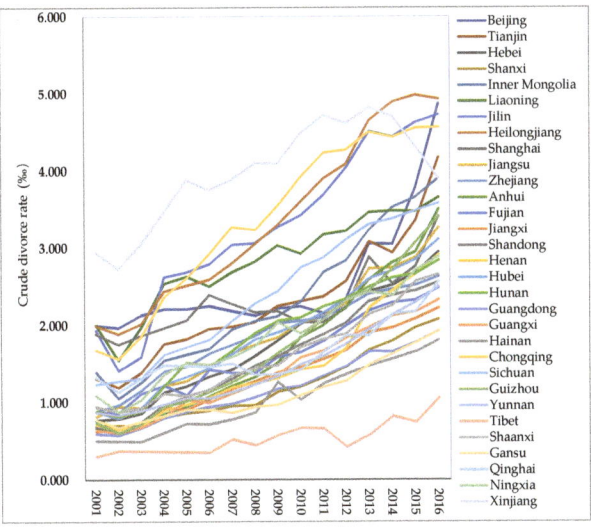

Figure 2. The crude divorce rates for 31 provinces of China: 2001–2016.

Figure 3 provides a scatter diagram between crude divorce rate and mobile phone penetration, demonstrating a significant positive correlation between the two factors. However, because other factors have not been considered, the relationship between divorce rate and mobile phone penetration needs to be further examination.

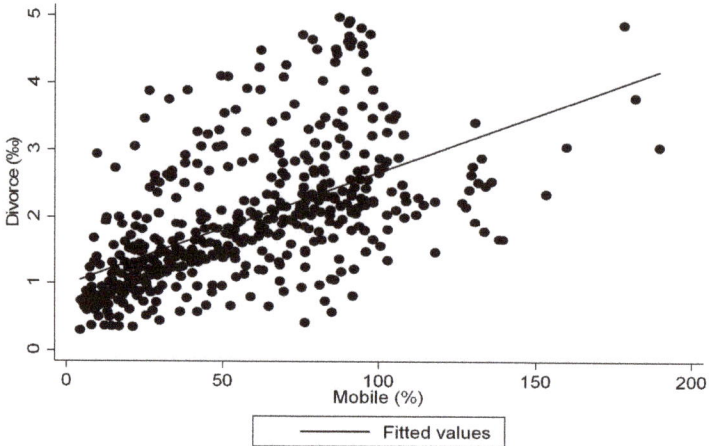

Figure 3. A scatter diagram of crude divorce rate against mobile phone penetration.

4. Empirical Results and Discussions

4.1. Statistical Analysis of Variables

In summary, the mean, standard deviation, maximum, and minimum values of key variables are shown in Table 1. Furthermore, this paper conducted multiple collinear tests on the main explanatory variables before the empirical analysis, and the highest variance inflation factor (VIF) is 4.73. Experience shows that when VIF is less than 10, multiple collinearity does not have much effect on regression analysis [98].

Table 1. Summary statistics of the key variables.

Variables	N	Mean	Standard Deviation	Min	Max	Unit
Divorce	496	1.937	1.017	0.303	4.979	‰
Mobile	496	56.660	34.746	4.280	189.424	%
Urban	496	49.194	15.528	19.392	89.600	%
Education	496	8.423	1.239	3.738	12.546	Years/per capita
Dependency	496	37.441	7.029	19.267	57.579	%
Policy	496	0.875	0.331	0	1	–

4.2. Estimation Results of the Benchmark Model

Generally speaking, panel data estimation models include the ordinary least squares (OLS), fixed effects model (FE), and random effects model (RE); F test and the Hausman test were conducted to select the most appropriate model. Considering the possible heteroscedasticity and the autocorrelation of the panel model, this paper used the clustering robust standard deviation in all results. The regression results of the benchmark model are shown in Table 2.

Table 2. Regression results of the effect of mobile phone penetration on divorce rate.

Variables	Dependent Variable: Divorce					
	(1)	(2)	(3)	(4)	(5)	(6)
Mobile		0.020 *** (0.001)	0.011 *** (0.004)	0.009 ** (0.004)	0.011 *** (0.004)	0.011 *** (0.004)
Urban	0.054 *** (0.011)		0.050 *** (0.016)	0.045 *** (0.016)	0.036 ** (0.014)	0.033 ** (0.015)
Education	0.666 *** (0.149)			0.187 * (0.099)	0.356 *** (0.095)	0.371 *** (0.094)
Dependency	0.042 *** (0.010)				0.043 *** (0.008)	0.048 *** (0.009)
Policy	0.158 ** (0.074)					0.133 ** (0.059)
Constant	−8.036 *** (1.128)	0.815 *** (0.099)	−1.170 * (0.611)	−2.344 ** (0.968)	−5.080 *** (0.953)	−5.321 *** (0.910)
F	105.630	86.760	103.720	93.250	112.040	113.000
Hausman	52.750 (0.000)	2.120 (0.347)	22.360 (0.000)	24.950 (0.000)	24.720 (0.000)	22.630 (0.000)
Observations	496	496	496	496	496	496
Provinces	31	31	31	31	31	31
R^2	0.817	0.772	0.807	0.811	0.840	0.842
Model	FE	RE	FE	FE	FE	FE

Note: *, **, and *** represent 10%, 5%, and 1% levels of statistical significance, respectively. Robust standard errors are reported in parentheses. The p values shown are according to the Hausman test. FE stands for fixed effects model, RE stands for random effects model.

As shown in Table 2, Model (1) only considers the influence of control variables on the divorce rate. Model (2) simply investigates the direct relationship between mobile phone penetration and divorce rate. Models (3)–(6) add the control variables successively on the basis of Model (2). From the R^2 value of each model, Models (2)–(6) increase by degrees. At the same time, The R^2 value of Model (6) is also larger than that in Model (1), indicating that it is necessary to add the control variables and that the model is set appropriately. According to the estimation results, it can be seen that:

According to Model (2), the direct influence coefficient of mobile phone penetration on the divorce rate is 0.02 and is significant at the 1% level. This indicates that a 1% increase in the mobile phone penetration rate was associated with a 0.02‰ increase in the divorce rate. The regression coefficient for the mobile phone penetration in Model (6) reduces, but it is still statistically significant at 1% level. The result shows that a 1% increase in the mobile phone penetration rate was associated with a 0.011‰ increase in the divorce rate during this period. As shown in Figure 3, there was a significant positive correlation between mobile phone penetration and divorce rate.

For the control variables, Model (6) shows that both the urbanization level and the human capital level have significantly positive coefficients. This indicates that improvements to urbanization and education levels were important contributing factors for the increase in China's divorce rate in this period. As the largest developing country and the most populous country, China has seen rapid economic development since the late 1970s. However, China has not completed the urbanization process. China's urbanization rate was just 57.3% in 2016 according to China's National Bureau of Statistics (NBS). Therefore, with the advancement of China's urbanization process, China's public policy should pay more attention to the influence of the rising urbanization level on the concept of marriage across Chinese society. Additionally, the estimation results revealed that there was a significant positive correlation between dependency ratio and divorce rate. Perhaps the reason is that the growth of the dependency ratio significantly increased the cost of living and the stress of life, which have an impact on marriage. Furthermore, the policy change on divorce had an important effect on divorce rate, which means that China's "Marriage Registration Ordinance", amended in 2003, contributed to the increase in divorce rate.

4.3. Mobile Phone Penetration and Divorce Rate: Regional Differences

Considering the big differences for divorce rates and mobile telephone penetrations among the 31 provinces in China, this study further divided the sample into three parts: the eastern, central, and western regions of China according to the usual methods. As shown in Table 3, Models (1) and (2) show the results of the eastern provinces. Models (3) and (4) show the results for the central provinces. Finally, Models (5) and (6) show the results for the western provinces.

Table 3. The effect of mobile phone penetration on divorce rate: regional differences.

Variables	Dependent Variable: Divorce					
	Eastern China		Central China		Western China	
	(1)	(2)	(3)	(4)	(5)	(6)
Mobile	0.016 *** (0.001)	0.006 * (0.003)	0.029 *** (0.003)	0.030 *** (0.005)	0.020 *** (0.003)	0.001 (0.004)
Constant	0.707 *** (0.133)	−6.554 *** (1.699)	0.703 *** (0.135)	−3.673 (2.110)	0.973 *** (0.207)	−3.289 ** (1.651)
F	52.180	76.480	108.910	82.240	119.010	137.020
Hausman	0.640 (0.724)	60.220 (0.000)	1.170 (0.557)	44.750 (0.000)	0.800 (0.670)	2.270 (0.810)
Control variables	NO	YES	NO	YES	NO	YES
Observations	176	176	128	128	192	192
Provinces	11	11	8	8	12	12
R^2	0.781	0.883	0.882	0.917	0.768	0.880
Model	RE	FE	RE	FE	RE	RE

Note: *, **, and *** represent 10%, 5%, and 1% levels of statistical significance, respectively. Robust standard errors are reported in parentheses. The p values shown are according to the Hausman test. FE stands for fixed effects model, RE stands for random effects model. Eastern China has 11 provinces, central China has 8 provinces, and western China has 12 provinces.

Specifically, from a regional perspective: Model (1) and Model (2) show that the association between the mobile phone penetration rate and divorce rate was positive and significant for eastern provinces. According to Model (2), a 1% increase in the mobile phone penetration rate was associated with a 0.006‰ increase in the divorce rate during this period. Model (3) and Model (4) reveal that the association between the mobile phone penetration rate and divorce rate was also positive and significant for central provinces, with a 1% increase in the mobile phone penetration rate associated with a 0.030‰ increase in the divorce rate. For the western region, the influence coefficient of mobile phone penetration on the divorce rate in Model (5) is significantly positive. However, after controlling for other variables, Model (6) shows that there is no direct relationship between mobile phone penetration and divorce rate.

By comparison, mobile phone penetration had the largest effect on the divorce rate in central China, followed by eastern China, but it was not obvious in western China during this period. Compared with the central and western regions of China, the eastern region of China has experienced a relatively fast economic development, a high degree of marketability, and higher average human capital. Therefore, the modern marriage concept is more popular and deeply ingrained in society. As a result, despite the high prevalence of mobile phones, the modern concept of marriage has not been impacted much. In the central regions, the economic development has been relatively slow, the industrialization degree is low, and the traditional culture and religious culture have a higher influence on marriage. Therefore, with the popularization of new media tools such as mobile phones, greater effects on traditional concepts of marriage and interpersonal communication may be experienced in the central regions. For western China, there was no direct link between mobile phone penetration and divorce rates. That may be because, on the one hand, the mobile penetration in western China was still low. On the other hand, especially for the vast rural areas in western China, traditional marriage concepts still have a deep impact.

4.4. Robust Analysis

Additional analyses were conducted to assess the stability of our research conclusions. As discussed above, this paper used the Divorce1 variable (divorce rate for the marriage-age population) to replace the Divorce variable (crude divorce rate) for additional analyses. The results are shown in Table 4. It can be observed that the results are substantively identical to the results shown in Tables 2 and 3, which supports the conclusion that there was significant positive correlation between the mobile phone penetration rate and the divorce rate during the period 2001–2016. Furthermore, the mobile phone penetration rate had the largest effect on the divorce rate in central China, followed by eastern China, but it was not obvious in western China during this period.

Moreover, considering our sample contains provinces with different levels of divorce rate, mobile phone penetration, urbanization, education, and economic development, this paper uses quantile regression to further test the reliability of benchmark model at the national level. Compared with the traditional method, which just examines the effect of the independent variable on the conditional expectation of the dependent variable, the advantage of quantile regression is that it can provide comprehensive information about the conditional distribution of the dependent variable [99]. In this paper, quantile regression was mainly used to investigate the effect of mobile phone penetration on divorce rate at five points including: 0.1, 0.25, 0.5, 0.75, and 0.9. The estimation results are shown in Table 5, and Figure 4 shows the variation in the mobile phone penetration coefficient over the conditional quantiles.

Table 4. Robust analysis using Divorce1 as the dependent variable.

Variables	Dependent Variable: Divorce1							
	Whole Nation		Eastern China		Central China		Western China	
	(1)	(2)	(3)	(4)	(5)	(6)	(7)	(8)
Mobile	0.026 *** (0.002)	0.013 *** (0.005)	0.021 *** (0.002)	0.008 * (0.004)	0.038 *** (0.004)	0.037 *** (0.006)	0.026 *** (0.004)	0.0004 (0.005)
Constant	1.161 *** (0.138)	−7.861 *** (1.189)	0.989 *** (0.172)	−9.297 *** (2.124)	0.971 *** (0.162)	−6.134 * (2.776)	1.427 *** (0.295)	−5.222 ** (2.211)
F	80.490	123.530	40.190	78.740	86.450	78.60	117.960	148.750
Hausman	3.350 (0.187)	26.650 (0.000)	1.240 (0.539)	67.390 (0.000)	0.650 (0.721)	41.130 (0.000)	0.540 (0.765)	2.430 (0.787)
Control variables	NO	YES	NO	YES	NO	YES	NO	YES
Observations	496	496	176	176	128	128	192	192
Provinces	31	31	11	11	8	8	12	12
R^2	0.747	0.846	0.741	0.878	0.881	0.919	0.745	0.880
Model	RE	FE	RE	FE	RE	FE	RE	RE

Note: *, **, and *** represent 10%, 5%, and 1% levels of statistical significance, respectively. Robust standard errors are reported in parentheses. The *p* values shown are according to the Hausman test. FE stands for fixed effects model, RE stands for random effects model.

Table 5. Robust analysis: quantile regression.

Variables	Dependent Variable: Divorce				
	0.1	0.25	0.5	0.75	0.9
	(1)	(2)	(3)	(4)	(5)
Mobile	0.004 ***	0.009 ***	0.012 ***	0.011 ***	0.017 ***
	(0.001)	(0.002)	(0.002)	(0.003)	(0.006)
Control variables	YES	YES	YES	YES	YES
Observations	496	496	496	496	496
Provinces	31	31	31	31	31

Note: *** represents 1% levels of statistical significance. Standard errors are reported in parentheses. The bootstrap value was set to 300.

According to the results in Table 5 and Figure 4, the mobile phone penetration has a significantly positive effect on divorce rate for all quantiles, which is consistent with the benchmark model estimation results in Table 2. In summary, the above analysis shows that the estimation results are robust and reliable in this paper.

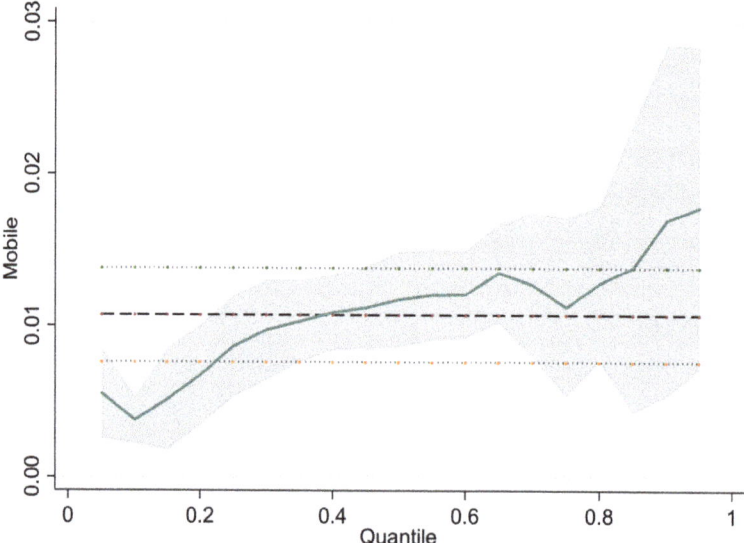

Figure 4. Variation in the mobile phone penetration coefficient over the conditional quantiles. Confidence intervals extend to 95% confidence intervals in both directions. Horizontal bold dotted lines represent ordinary least squares (OLS) estimates with 95% confidence intervals.

4.5. The Lagged Effect of Mobile Phone Penetration on Divorce Rate

Measurement errors, omitted variables, and mutual causal relationships among the independent variable with the dependent variables may all lead to endogenous problems. In this paper, a mutual relationship between the mobile phone penetration rate and the divorce rate may exist. With the increase in divorce rates, the dating behaviour of people (e.g., using mobile phones to meet people) and the holding rate of mobile phones may possibly change. Generally, two approaches are used to solve endogenous problems. One way is to use instrumental variables that are highly relevant to mobile phone penetration rate but do not have direct relationships with divorce rate. Another method is to add the lag term of endogenous variables. However, it is difficult to find an appropriate instrumental variable for mobile phone penetration. As such, this paper adopts the latter method of applying the lag term of mobile phone penetration. The main logic is that the divorce rate in the current period has no effect on the lag of the mobile phone penetration rate. In addition, theoretically, there is a time lag between residents' use of mobile phones and the possible impact on divorce rates. This paper successively added the one-year to five-year lag times of the mobile phone penetration; the estimation results are shown in Table 6. Furthermore, adding different lag terms of mobile phone penetrations is valuable in order to observe the dynamic impact of mobile phone penetration on divorce rate. Since the adoption of the lag term of mobile phone penetration would reduce the sample size, this paper conducts the analysis only at the national level.

Models (1)–(5) are the estimation results with the crude divorce rate as the dependent variable, and Models (6)–(10) are the estimation results with divorce rate for the marriage-age population as the dependent variable. As shown in Table 6, there was still significant positive relationships between the lag term of mobile phone penetration and divorce rate, which is consistent with the process of "Mobile phone use → Making friends → Having an affair → Having family conflict → Divorce" [100]. It was shown that the mobile phone penetration had a dynamic impact process on the divorce rate. In addition, according to the R^2 value and the mobile phone penetration coefficient of each model, the mobile phone penetration rate with one lag period has the greatest impact and predictive ability on the divorce rate.

Table 6. The lagged effect of mobile phone penetration on divorce rate.

Variables	Dependent Variable: Divorce					Dependent Variable: Divorce1				
	(1)	(2)	(3)	(4)	(5)	(6)	(7)	(8)	(9)	(10)
L1.Mobile	0.010 *** (0.001)					0.012 *** (0.002)				
L2.Mobile		0.009 *** (0.001)					0.011 *** (0.002)			
L3.Mobile			0.007 *** (0.001)					0.009 *** (0.002)		
L4.Mobile				0.008 *** (0.001)					0.009 *** (0.002)	
L5.Mobile					0.009 *** (0.002)					0.010 *** (0.002)
Constant	−4.923 *** (0.563)	−4.660 *** (0.584)	−5.275 *** (0.600)	−5.216 *** (0.652)	−5.269 *** (0.661)	−7.411 *** (0.742)	−7.069 *** (0.772)	−7.920 *** (0.794)	−7.939 *** (0.862)	−8.046 *** (0.874)
Control variables	YES	YES	YES	YES	YES	YES	YES	YES	YES	YES
Observations	465	434	403	372	341	465	434	403	372	341
R^2	0.839	0.835	0.833	0.825	0.811	0.843	0.839	0.838	0.830	0.820
Model	FE	FE	FE	FE	FE	FE	FE	FE	FE	FE

Note: *** represents 1% levels of statistical significance. Robust standard errors are reported in parentheses. FE stands for fixed effects model, RE stands for random effects model. L represents the lag term. Because of multicollinearity, policy variable is removed in Models (2)–(5) and Models (7)–(10).

5. Discussion

Marital happiness is of great practical significance to China's social stability and economic sustainable development in the future. In traditional Chinese society, interpersonal communication is often based on blood ties, and men and women are limited in their choice of partners. Furthermore, traditional Chinese societal values typically look unfavourably upon, which still has a profound impact on the marriage concepts of modern Chinese residents. However, since the beginning of the 21st century, the divorce rate in China has risen rapidly compared with that before the 21st century, which has attracted wide attention from various social institutions. Previous literature has explained the rising divorce rate in China from various aspects, such as economic development and social reform, but few studies have paid attention to the possible significant impact of the popularization of mobile phones on China's divorce rate. Moreover, this is of great value in explaining why the divorce rate in China has changed so much since the beginning of the 21st century.

Therefore, this paper attempts to study the relationship between the mobile phone penetration and the divorce rate in China based on province-level data during the period 2001–2016. The most striking conclusion of this study is that there was a significant positive correlation between the mobile phone penetration and the divorce rate in China during the period 2001–2016. Furthermore, mobile phone penetration had the largest effect on the divorce rate in central China, followed by eastern China, but it was not obvious in western China during this period.

In order to get a more robust conclusion, this paper further conducts the robustness test through two steps. Firstly, two indexes of divorce rate are adopted as the dependent variables. Secondly, this paper uses quantile regression to further test the reliability of the benchmark model at the national level. Although no suitable instrumental variables were found to deal with the possible endogenous problem caused by mobile phone penetration, the one-year to five-year lag times of mobile phone penetrations are used as the core explanatory variable to deal with endogeneity problem and to analyse the possible delayed impact of mobile phone penetration on divorce rate. Through the above tests, the main conclusions of this paper are still reliable and robust.

China is vigorously promoting the construction of a digital economy and trying to promote the sustainable development of the Chinese economy through information technology. Information technology has had a profound impact on Chinese society. Although for a long time, the relationship between social media tools, such as the Internet and mobile phones, and the divorce rate was recognized by scholars, little research has been done to explain the rising divorce rate in China in recent years from the perspective of the spread of mobile phones.

In the theoretical analysis part of this paper, three reasons are provided for the mobile phone penetration contributing to the rising divorce rate in China. First, the spread of mobile phones has affected people's social networks and greatly reduced the cost of searching for partners for both men and women. Secondly, the use of mobile phones can affect people's interpersonal communication, thus affecting the relationships between couples. Finally, the popularization of mobile phones promotes the spread of modern marriage concepts, democracy concepts, and equality concepts.

Why does mobile phone penetration have the largest effect on the divorce rate in central China, followed by eastern China, but not have an obvious effect in western China during this period? This paper argues that, compared with central and western of China, the eastern part of China has experienced a relatively fast economic development, a high degree of marketability, and a higher average human capital. Therefore, the modern marriage concept is more popular and deeply ingrained in society. As a result, despite the high prevalence of mobile phones, the modern concept of marriage has not been impacted much. In the central regions, the economic development has been relatively slow, the industrialization degree is low, and the traditional culture and religious culture have a higher influence on marriage. Therefore, with the popularization of new media tools such as mobile phones, greater effects on traditional concepts of marriage may be experienced in the central regions. For western China, there is no direct link between mobile phone penetration and divorce rates. That may be because, on the one hand, mobile penetration in western China is still low. On the other hand, especially for the vast rural areas in western China, the traditional marriage concept still has a deep impact on the values and beliefs of residents.

The results are consistent with Valenzuela et al. [64] in that the use of social media tools (mobile phones in this study) is positively correlated with experiencing a troubled relationship and thinking about divorce. These findings shall inspire China and other countries in the future. The quality of marriage is an important guarantee for a happy life and harmonious society. With the development of the economy in developing countries, ICT will be further popularized and applied. Thus, public policy formulation should consider the potential impact of ICT on marriage stability in the future. Deciding how to guide and standardize the behaviour of citizens using mobile phones is an important issue to be considered in public policy. This paper also further enriches relevant studies on the impact of ICT on social development.

There are still many aspects that can be further explored in the future. Firstly, future research may use smaller geographical units (such as cities) and family or individual data, which will be better able to investigate the relationship between mobile phone use and the risk of divorce for particular couples. Secondly, a common issue involving endogenous problems was encountered in this study due to the lack of suitable tool variables for mobile phone penetration. As such, endogenous problems are not solved perfectly in this paper. However, future research can address this problem by other means, such as through approaches using Generalized Method of Moments (GMM) and propensity score matching (PSM). Finally, future studies can also empirically examine the mechanisms by which mobile phone penetration affects divorce rate.

Author Contributions: J.Z. conceived and designed the study and completed the paper in English; M.C. participated in drafting the article and provided critical revisions for important intellectual content; X.W. and X.G. provided research advice, revised the manuscript, and made comprehensive English revisions.

Funding: This research was funded by the National Natural Science Foundation of China (71373179, 71673200, 71173156, and 71873095), Major Projects in Philosophy and Social Science from the Ministry of Education of China (15JZD026), Shanghai Universities Distinguished Professor (Oriental Scholar) Position Plan (TP2015023), Shanghai Universities PuJiang Talent Program (15PJC087), and Shanghai Universities Program of Shuguang Scholars (15SG17).

Conflicts of Interest: The authors declare no conflicts of interest.

References

1. Zhang, S.; Liu, B.; Zhu, D.; Cheng, M. Explaining individual subjective well-being of urban China based on the four-capital model. *Sustainability* **2018**, *10*, 3480. [CrossRef]
2. Gove, W.R.; Hughes, M.; Style, C.B. Does marriage have positive effects on the psychological well-being of the individual? *J. Health Soc. Behav.* **1983**, *24*, 122–131. [CrossRef] [PubMed]
3. Acs, G. Can we promote child well-being by promoting marriage? *J. Marriage Fam.* **2007**, *69*, 1326–1344. [CrossRef]
4. Qari, S. Marriage, adaptation and happiness: Are there long-lasting gains to marriage? *J. Behav. Exp. Econ.* **2014**, *50*, 29–39. [CrossRef]
5. Guner, N.; Kulikova, Y.; Llull, J. Marriage and health: Selection, protection, and assortative mating. *Eur. Econ. Rev.* **2018**, *104*, 138–166. [CrossRef]
6. Zheng, S.; Duan, Y.; Ward, M.R. The effect of broadband internet on divorce in China. *Technol. Forecast. Soc. Chang* **2018**, in press. [CrossRef]
7. China National Bureau of Statistics. Crude divorce rate. 2018. Available online: http://data.stats.gov.cn/english/easyquery.htm?cn=C01 (accessed on 30 September 2018). (In Chinese)
8. Zhang, C.; Wang, X.; Zhang, D. Urbanization, unemployment rate and China' rising divorce rate. *Chin. J. Popul. Resour. Environ.* **2014**, *12*, 157–164. [CrossRef]
9. Su, L.; Liu, Y.; Peng, X. Spatial aggregation and spatial-temporal pattern of provincial divorce rate in China. *Popul. Res.* **2015**, *6*, 74–84.
10. Su, L.; Liang, C.; Yang, X.; Liu, Y. Influence factors analysis of provincial divorce rate spatial distribution in China. *Discret. Dyn. Nat. Soc.* **2018**. [CrossRef]
11. Wang, Q.; Zhou, Q. China's divorce and remarriage rates: Trends and regional disparities. *J. Divorce Remarriage* **2010**, *51*, 257–267. [CrossRef]
12. Mu, Z.; Xie, Y. Marital age homogamy in China: A reversal of trend in the reform era? *Soc. Sci. Res.* **2014**, *44*, 141–157. [CrossRef] [PubMed]
13. Petrovčič, A.; Fortunati, L.; Vehovar, V.; Kavčič, M.; Dolničar, V. Mobile phone communication in social support networks of older adults in Slovenia. *Telemat. Inform.* **2015**, *32*, 642–655. [CrossRef]
14. International Telecommunication Union (ITU). Mobile-cellular subscriptions. 2018. Available online: https://www.itu.int/en/ITU-D/Statistics/Pages/stat/default.aspx (accessed on 30 September 2018).
15. Wang, Y.; Li, J. ICT's effect on trade: Perspective of comparative advantage. *Econ. Lett.* **2017**, *155*, 96–99. [CrossRef]
16. Shi, J.; Si, H.; Wu, G.; Su, Y.; Lan, J. Critical factors to achieve dockless bike-sharing sustainability in China: A stakeholder-oriented network perspective. *Sustainability* **2018**, *10*, 2090. [CrossRef]
17. Hwang, Y. Is communication competence still good for interpersonal media?: Mobile phone and instant messenger. *Comput. Hum. Behav.* **2011**, *27*, 924–934. [CrossRef]

18. Vaus, D.D.; Gray, M.; Qu, L.; Stanton, D. The economic consequences of divorce in six OECD countries. *Aust. J. Soc. Issues* **2017**, *52*, 180–199. [CrossRef]
19. McDaniel, B.T.; Coyne, S.M. "Technoference": The interference of technology in couple relationships and implications for women's personal and relational well-being. *Psychol. Pop. Media Cult.* **2016**, *5*, 85–98. [CrossRef]
20. Katz, J.E.; Aspden, P. Theories, data, and potential impacts of mobile communications: A longitudinal analysis of U.S. national surveys. *Technol. Forecast. Soc. Chang.* **1998**, *57*, 133–156. [CrossRef]
21. De, G.C.; Truong, L.T.; Htt, N. Who's calling? Social networks and mobile phone use among motorcyclists. *Accid. Anal. Prev.* **2017**, *103*, 143–147.
22. Islam, M.M.; Habes, E.M.; Alam, M.M. The usage and social capital of mobile phones and their effect on the performance of microenterprise: An empirical study. *Technol. Forecast. Soc. Chang.* **2018**, *132*, 156–164. [CrossRef]
23. Marinescu, I. Divorce: What does learning have to do with it? *Labour Econ.* **2016**, *38*, 90–105. [CrossRef]
24. Becker, G.S. A theory of marriage. *J. Political Econ.* **1973**, *36*, 119–133.
25. Weiss, Y.; Willis, R.J. Match quality, new information, and marital dissolution. *J. Labor Econ.* **1997**, *15*, S293–S329. [CrossRef]
26. Becker, G.S.; Landes, E.M.; Michael, R.T. An economic analysis of marital instability. *J. Political Econ.* **1977**, *85*, 1141–1187. [CrossRef]
27. Hoffman, S.D.; Duncan, G.J. The effect of incomes, wages, and AFDC benefits on marital disruption. *J. Hum. Resour.* **1995**, *30*, 19–41. [CrossRef]
28. Smock, P.J.; Manning, W.D.; Gupta, S. The effect of marriage and divorce on women's economic well-being. *Am. Sociol. Rev.* **1999**, *64*, 794–812. [CrossRef]
29. Ressler, R.W.; Waters, M.S. Female earnings and the divorce rate: A simultaneous equations model. *Appl. Econ.* **2000**, *32*, 1889–1898. [CrossRef]
30. Han, S.H. Korean family litigation laws toward minor children of divorced families. *Korean Law J. Civ. Lawsuit* **2010**, *14*, 311–347.
31. Amato, P.R.; Beattie, B. Does the unemployment rate affect the divorce rate? An analysis of state data 1960–2005. *Soc. Sci. Res.* **2011**, *40*, 705–715. [CrossRef]
32. Rainer, H.; Smith, I. Staying together for the sake of the home?: House price shocks and partnership dissolution in the UK. *J. R. Stat. Soc.* **2010**, *173*, 557–574. [CrossRef]
33. Battu, H.; Brown, H.; Costagomes, M. *Not Always for Richer or Poorer: The Effects of Income Shocks and House Price Changes on Marital Dissolution*; ERSA Conference Papers; European Regional Science Association: Louvain-la-Neuve, Belgium, 2013.
34. Klein, J. House price shocks and individual divorce risk in the United States. *J. Fam. Econ. Issues* **2017**, *38*, 628–649. [CrossRef]
35. Goode, W.J. Economic factors and marital stability. *Am. Sociol. Rev.* **1951**, *16*, 802–812. [CrossRef]
36. South, S.J.; Trent, K.; Shen, Y. Changing partners: Toward a macrostructural-opportunity theory of marital dissolution. *J. Marriage Fam.* **2001**, *63*, 743–754. [CrossRef]
37. Ono, H. Husbands' and wives' education and divorce in the United States and Japan, 1946–2000. *J. Fam. Hist.* **2009**, *34*, 292–322. [CrossRef]
38. Sandström, G. Socio-economic determinants of divorce in early twentieth-century Sweden. *Hist. Fam.* **2011**, *16*, 292–307. [CrossRef]
39. Sandström, G. Time-space trends in Swedish divorce behaviour, 1911–1974. *Scand. J. Hist.* **2011**, *36*, 65–69. [CrossRef] [PubMed]
40. Glenn, N.D.; Supancic, M. The social and demographic correlates of divorce and separation in the United States: An update and reconsideration. *J. Marriage Fam.* **1984**, *46*, 563–575. [CrossRef]
41. Landale, N.S.; Ogena, N.B. Migration and union dissolution among Puerto Rican women. *Int. Migr. Rev.* **1995**, *29*, 671–692. [CrossRef]
42. Frank, R.; Wildsmith, E. The grass widows of Mexico: Migration and union dissolution in a binational context. *Soc. Forces* **2005**, *83*, 919–947. [CrossRef]
43. Gautier, P.A.; Svarer, M.; Teulings, C.N. Sin city? Why is the divorce rate higher in urban areas? *Scand. J. Econ.* **2009**, *111*, 439–456. [CrossRef]

44. Caarls, K.; Mazzucato, V. Does International Migration Lead to Divorce?: Ghanaian Couples in Ghana and Abroad. *Population* **2015**, *70*, 127–150.
45. Ramirez-Correa, P.E.; Rondan-Cataluña, F.J.; Arenas-Gaitán, J. Predicting behavioral intention of mobile internet usage. *Telemat. Inform.* **2015**, *32*, 834–841. [CrossRef]
46. Singh, S.; Swait, J. Channels for search and purchase: Does mobile Internet matter? *J. Retail. Consum. Serv.* **2017**, *39*, 123–134. [CrossRef]
47. China Internet Network Information Center (CNNIC). 41st China Internet Development Statistics Report. 2018. Available online: http://www.cnnic.net.cn/hlwfzyj/hlwxzbg/hlwtjbg/201803/t20180305_70249.htm (accessed on 28 September 2018). (In Chinese)
48. Puspitasari, L.; Ishii, K. Digital divides and mobile Internet in Indonesia: Impact of smartphones. *Telemat. Inform.* **2016**, *33*, 472–483. [CrossRef]
49. Bertschek, I.; Niebel, T. Mobile and more productive? Firm-level evidence on the productivity effects of mobile internet use. *Telecommun. Policy* **2016**, *40*, 888–898. [CrossRef]
50. Lee, S.H.; Levendis, J.; Gutierrez, L. Telecommunications and economic growth: An empirical analysis of sub-Saharan Africa. *Appl. Econ.* **2012**, *44*, 461–469. [CrossRef]
51. Chavula, H.K. Telecommunications development and economic growth in Africa. *Inf. Technol. Dev.* **2013**, *19*, 5–23. [CrossRef]
52. Donou-Adonsou, F.; Lim, S.; Mathey, S.A. Technological progress and economic growth in sub-saharan Africa: Evidence from telecommunications infrastructure. *Int. Adv. Econ. Res.* **2016**, *22*, 65–75. [CrossRef]
53. Njoh, A.J. The relationship between modern information and communications technologies (ICTs) and development in Africa. *Util. Policy* **2018**, *50*, 83–90. [CrossRef]
54. Kanyam, D.A.; Kostandini, G.; Ferreira, S. The mobile phone revolution: Have mobile phones and the internet reduced corruption in sub-saharan Africa? *World Dev.* **2017**, *99*, 271–284. [CrossRef]
55. Sassi, S.; Ali, M.S.B. Corruption in Africa: What role does ict diffusion play. *Telecommun. Policy* **2017**, *41*, 662–669. [CrossRef]
56. Asongu, S.A.; Nwachukwu, J.C.; Orim, S.-M.I. Mobile phones, institutional quality and entrepreneurship in sub-saharan Africa. *Technol. Forecast. Soc. Chang.* **2018**, *131*, 183–203. [CrossRef]
57. Kardos, P.; Unoka, Z.; Pléh, C.; Soltész, P. Your mobile phone indeed means your social network: Priming mobile phone activates relationship related concepts. *Comput. Hum. Behav.* **2018**, *88*, 84–88. [CrossRef]
58. Shimamoto, D.; Yamada, H.; Gummert, M. Mobile phones and market information: Evidence from rural Cambodia. *Food Policy* **2015**, *57*, 135–141. [CrossRef]
59. Seo, D.G.; Park, Y.; Kim, M.K.; Park, J. Mobile phone dependency and its impacts on adolescents' social and academic behaviors. *Comput. Hum. Behav.* **2016**, *63*, 282–292. [CrossRef]
60. Boonjing, V.; Chanvarasuth, P. Risk of overusing mobile phones: Technostress effect. *Procedia Comput. Sci.* **2017**, *111*, 196–202. [CrossRef]
61. Jiang, Z.; Zhao, X. Brain behavioral systems, self-control and problematic mobile phone use: The moderating role of gender and history of use. *Pers. Individ. Differ.* **2017**, *106*, 111–116. [CrossRef]
62. Merkle, E.R.; Richardson, R.A. Digital dating and virtual relating: Conceptualizing computer mediated romantic relationships. *Fam. Relat.* **2000**, *49*, 187–192. [CrossRef]
63. Rosen, L.D.; Cheever, N.A.; Cummings, C.; Felt, J. The impact of emotionality and self-disclosure on online dating versus traditional dating. *Comput. Hum. Behav.* **2008**, *24*, 2124–2157. [CrossRef]
64. Valenzuela, S.; Halpern, D.; Katz, J.E. Social network sites, marriage well-being and divorce: Survey and state-level evidence from the United States. *Comput. Hum. Behav.* **2014**, *36*, 94–101. [CrossRef]
65. Salehan, M.; Negahban, A. Social networking on smartphones: When mobile phones become addictive. *Comput. Hum. Behav.* **2013**, *29*, 2632–2639. [CrossRef]
66. Hjorth, L.; Qiu, J.; Zhou, B.; Ding, W. The social in the mobile: QQ as cross-generational media in China'. In *The Routledge Companion to Mobile Media*; Goggin, G., Hjorth, L., Eds.; Routledge: New York, NY, USA, 2014; pp. 291–299.
67. Kraut, R.; Kiesler, S.; Boneva, B.; Cummings, J.; Helgeson, V.; Crawford, A. Internet paradox revisited. *J. Soc. Issues* **2002**, *58*, 49–74. [CrossRef]
68. Wei, R.; Lo, V. Staying connected while on the move: Cell phone use and social connectedness. *New Media Soc.* **2006**, *8*, 53–72. [CrossRef]

69. Manago, A.M.; Taylor, T.; Greenfield, P.M. Me and my 400 friends: The anatomy of college students' facebook networks, their communication patterns, and well-being. *Dev. Psychol.* **2012**, *48*, 369–380. [CrossRef] [PubMed]
70. South, S.J.; Lloyd, K.M. Spousal alternatives and marital dissolution. *Am. Sociol. Rev.* **1995**, *60*, 21–35. [CrossRef]
71. Kendall, T.D. The relationship between internet access and divorce rate. *J. Fam. Econ. Issues* **2011**, *32*, 449–460. [CrossRef]
72. Chen, L.; Yan, Z.; Tang, W.; Yang, F.; Xie, X.; He, J. Mobile phone addiction levels and negative emotions among Chinese young adults: The mediating role of interpersonal problems. *Comput. Hum. Behav.* **2016**, *55*, 856–866. [CrossRef]
73. Raacke, J.; Bonds-Raacke, J. MySpace and Facebook: Applying the uses and gratifications theory to exploring friend-networking sites. *Cyberpsychol. Behav. Soc. Netw.* **2008**, *11*, 169–174. [CrossRef] [PubMed]
74. Kuss, D.J.; Griffiths, M.D. Online social networking and addiction: A review of the psychological literature. *Int. J. Environ. Res. Public Health* **2011**, *8*, 3528–3552. [CrossRef] [PubMed]
75. Lee, Z.W.; Cheung, C.M.; Thadani, D.R. An investigation into the problematic use of Facebook. In Proceedings of the 45th Hawaii International Conference on System Sciences (HICSS), Maui, HI, USA, 4–7 January 2012; pp. 1768–1776.
76. Patrick, K.; Griswold, W.G.; Raab, F.; Intille, S.S. Health and the mobile phone. *Am. J. Prev. Med.* **2008**, *35*, 177–181. [CrossRef] [PubMed]
77. Muise, A.; Christofides, E.; Desmarais, S. More information than you ever wanted: Does Facebook bring out the green-eyed monster of jealousy? *Cyberpsychol. Behav. Soc. Netw.* **2009**, *12*, 441–444. [CrossRef] [PubMed]
78. Karaiskos, D.; Tzavellas, E.; Balta, G.; Paparrigopoulos, T. P02-232-social network addiction: A new clinical disorder? *Eur. Psychiatry* **2010**, *25*, 855–855. [CrossRef]
79. Helsper, E.J.; Whitty, M.T. Netiquette within married couples: Agreement about acceptable online behavior and surveillance between partners. *Comput. Hum. Behav.* **2010**, *26*, 916–926. [CrossRef]
80. Lu, X.; Watanabe, J.; Liu, Q.; Uji, M.; Shono, M.; Kitamura, T. Internet and mobile phone text-messaging dependency: Factor structure and correlation with dysphoric mood among Japanese adults. *Comput. Hum. Behav.* **2011**, *27*, 1702–1709. [CrossRef]
81. Elphinston, R.A.; Noller, P. Time to face it! Facebook intrusion and the implications for romantic jealousy and relationship satisfaction. *Cyberpsychol. Behav. Soc. Netw.* **2011**, *14*, 631–635. [CrossRef] [PubMed]
82. Gao, T.; Li, J.; Zhang, H.; Gao, J.; Kong, Y.; Hu, Y.; Mei, S. The influence of alexithymia on mobile phone addiction: The role of depression, anxiety and stress. *J. Affect. Disord.* **2017**, *225*, 761–766. [CrossRef] [PubMed]
83. Clayton, R.B.; Nagurney, A.; Smith, J.R. Cheating, breakup, and divorce: Is facebook use to blame? *Cyberpsychol. Behav. Soc. Netw.* **2013**, *16*, 717–720. [CrossRef] [PubMed]
84. Lee, C.; Shin, J.; Hong, A. Does social media use really make people politically polarized? Direct and indirect effects of social media use on political polarization in South Korea. *Telemat. Inform.* **2017**, *35*, 245–254. [CrossRef]
85. Stevenson, B. *The Internet and Job Search*; NBER Working Paper; NBER: Cambridge, MA, USA, 2009.
86. Herr, J.L.; Wolfram, C.D. Work environment and opt-out rates at motherhood across high-education career paths. *Ind. Labor Relat. Rev.* **2012**, *65*, 928–950. [CrossRef]
87. Kuhn, P.; Mansour, H. Is internet job search still ineffective? *Econ. J.* **2014**, *124*, 1213–1233. [CrossRef]
88. Spitze, G.; South, S.J. Women's employment, time expenditure, and divorce. *J. Fam. Issues* **1985**, *6*, 307–329. [CrossRef]
89. Kalmijn, M.; Poortman, A.R. His or her divorce? The gendered nature of divorce and its determinants. *Eur. Sociol. Rev.* **2006**, *22*, 201–214. [CrossRef]
90. Namihira, I. Divorce question in Okinawa: Rasing an issue based on special urbanization processes of postwar cities of Okinawa. *Okinawa Int. Univ. J. Cult. Soc.* **2006**, *9*, 1–19.
91. Wagner, M.; Weiß, B. On the variation of divorce risks in Europe: Findings from a meta-analysis of European longitudinal studies. *Eur. Sociol. Rev.* **2006**, *22*, 483–500. [CrossRef]
92. Cherlin, A.J. *Public and Private Families: An Introduction*, 5th ed.; McGraw-Hill: Boston, MA, USA, 2008.
93. Sokoloff, L.; Kennedy, C. Marriage and divorce in Belgium. The influence of professional, educational and financial resources on the risk on marriage dissolution. *J. Divorce Remarriage* **2006**, *46*, 151–174.

94. South, S.J. Economic conditions and the divorce rate: A time-series analysis of the postwar United States. *J. Marriage Fam.* **1985**, *47*, 31–41. [CrossRef]
95. Shim, H.; Choi, I.; Ocker, B.L. Divorce in South Korea: An introduction to demographic trends, culture, and law. *Fam. Court Rev.* **2013**, *51*, 578–590. [CrossRef]
96. González, L.; Viitanen, T.K. The effect of divorce laws on divorce rates in Europe. *Eur. Econ. Rev.* **2009**, *53*, 127–138. [CrossRef]
97. Hiller, V.; Recoules, M. Changes in divorce patterns: Culture and the law. *Int. Rev. Law Econ.* **2013**, *34*, 77–87. [CrossRef]
98. Lee, S.; Nam, Y.; Lee, S.; Son, H. Determinants of ICT innovations: A cross-country empirical study. *Technol. Forecast. Soc. Chang.* **2016**, *110*, 71–77. [CrossRef]
99. Koenker, R.; Bassett, G. Regression quantiles. *Econometrica* **1978**, *46*, 33–50. [CrossRef]
100. Li, X. The effect of internet penetration on China's divorce rate. *Chin. J. Popul. Sci.* **2014**, *34*, 77–87. (In Chinese)

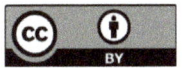

© 2018 by the authors. Licensee MDPI, Basel, Switzerland. This article is an open access article distributed under the terms and conditions of the Creative Commons Attribution (CC BY) license (http://creativecommons.org/licenses/by/4.0/).

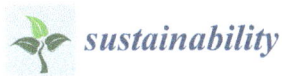

Article

Hospitals' Financial Health in Rural and Urban Areas in Poland: Does It Ensure Sustainability?

Agnieszka Bem [1], Rafał Siedlecki [1], Paweł Prędkiewicz [1], Patrizia Gazzola [2], Bożena Ryszawska [1] and Paulina Ucieklak-Jeż [3,*]

[1] Department of Corporate Finance and Public Finance, Wrocław University of Economics, 53-345 Wrocław, Poland; agnieszka.bem@ue.wroc.pl (A.B.); rafal.siedlecki@ue.wroc.pl (R.S.); pawel.predkiewicz@ue.wroc.pl (P.P.); bozena.ryszawska@ue.wroc.pl (B.R.)
[2] Department of Economics, Università degli Studi dell'Insubria, 21100 Varese, Italy; patrizia.gazzola@uninsubria.it
[3] Faculty of Philology and History, Jan Dlugosz University in Czestochowa, 42-200 Częstochowa, Poland
* Correspondence: p.ucieklak@o2.pl; Tel.: +48-502-296-808

Received: 16 February 2019; Accepted: 26 March 2019; Published: 1 April 2019

Abstract: Literature review suggests that rural hospitals are in the worst financial conditions due to several factors: They are smaller, located in remote areas, and they provide less specialized services due to their problems with employing well-qualified staff. We decided to check whether it is true in the case of Polish hospitals. Based on the literature review, we have assumed that rural hospitals have less favorable financial conditions. In order to verify this assumption, we use seven indicators of financial health as well as a synthetic measure of financial condition. We have found that, in fact, there is no difference in financial condition between rural and urban hospitals, or even that the financial health of rural hospitals is better if we employ the synthetic measure. Additionally, we have found that the form of activity can be a crucial driver of better financial performance. The concept of rural sustainability is supported by good financial conditions of rural hospitals, which helps to provide better access to medical services for inhabitants of rural areas.

Keywords: hospital; rural and urban hospitals; healthcare; sustainable rural health; the financial condition

1. Introduction

Sustainability is a model of an economy based on increased social and environmental responsibility [1]. The environmental dimension means introducing low-carbon green economy, which decouples economic growth from consumption of natural resources and energy, at the same time reducing the pressure on the planet by lower emission of CO_2 and energy, and resource efficiency. The social dimension supports the idea of responsible consumption, social justice, and equality (both inter- and intra-generational). Transition to sustainability is a long-term, multi-level, complex, and holistic process which involves many actors/stakeholders. The concept of sustainability is tightly bound with technology changes, innovations, and the general digital revolution. Sustainability transition is creating an alternative model of the economy, setting new priorities in social development, and inspiring radical change of attitude towards natural environment, climate, and energy issues [2].

There is a growing recognition that achieving sustainability rests almost entirely on achieving the balance between economic, social, and environmental aspects of development. It also emphasizes the crucial role of the social aspect. It is a large-scale societal transition made by many factors as an agent of change, and the specificity of the concept is associated with public involvement, activism, participation, and has a holistic character [3]. This is interesting from the point of view of policymakers because they have to deal with many dimensions of the crisis and the idea of sustainable development is offering the path to transform the economy, but also to support citizens and the environment [4] to achieve a higher quality of life [5]. The problems associated with achieving sustainability of the system affect particularly rural areas, which are struggling with deficits in almost every area [6].

While health is one of the most important fields of social and environmental change, fair access to health benefits is one of the most important goals of the health system. According to that, Fineberg [7] suggests new additional attributes which should characterize a sustainable healthcare system: Affordability, acceptability, and adaptability. It is relatively difficult to ensure, mostly due to high information asymmetry [8] and fast technological progress [9,10], or an innovative approach to health care services [11]. The other hidden factor is health communication, which has the strongest impact on people's positive perceptions about healthcare quality [12,13]. Regardless of the above factors, rural areas, by nature, are less equipped with the health care infrastructure, which is the result of sparser population density. This means reduced potential access to benefits—patients living in rural areas, economically more fragile than residents of urban areas, must usually overcome a longer distance to a doctor or a hospital, which requires transportation as well as engages time and financial resources. Hence, the closure of rural healthcare providers deteriorates the availability of benefits.

In this study we focus on the hospital sector due to several reasons: It consumes an important part of financial resources, offers life-saving benefits, and is characterized by high fixed costs. We make an assumption, that a better financial condition is crucial from the point of view of the continued existence of a hospital, as well as the quality of provided services. Poor financial conditions force a change of scope of a hospital's activity, its commercialization, or even closure. According to that, the aim of our research is to assess and compare the financial conditions of rural and urban hospitals in order to examine whether rural hospitals are at higher risk of financial distress. We take into account the fact that the consequences of a rural hospital's closure are more severe than in the case of hospitals located in large cities. A weaker financial condition of rural hospitals might potentially, not only decrease the access to health benefits, but also lower the quality of the provided services. Due to that, sustainable development of rural areas requires actions which would strengthen rural entities. Based on the literature review and previous studies, we propose the following research hypothesis *(H1): Rural hospitals are characterized by poorer financial conditions than urban entities*. We assume that an acceptable level of financial performance can maintain the existence of rural hospital infrastructure. If in fact, rural hospitals are at higher risk of financial distress, then they should be a subject of a policy aimed to strengthen their potency to survive.

The paper is organized as follows: After the introduction (Section 1), we briefly present a health care system in Poland, then (Section 2) we describe the role of rural hospitals as an essential part of sustainable rural development. Based on the review of the literature, we indicate factors which cause the poor financial condition of rural hospitals. In Section 3, we describe the design of the presented study. Next sections are devoted to the description of the data (Section 4) and the methodology (Section 5). In Section 6, we present results and discussion which are followed by the conclusions (Section 7).

The data has been obtained from the Emerging Markets Information System (EMIS) Database, covering the years 2012–2016 and our analysis is supported by Statistica 13.1 and Gretl.

2. Health Care System in Poland—Brief Description

Health care in Poland is organized on the basis of a system of universal health insurance. Insurance premiums are discharged from all categories of income and the system does not allow the possibility to substitute the mandatory public insurance with a private one. Financial resources are collected and distributed by the monopolist payer—National Health Fund (Narodowy Fundusz Zdrowia, NFZ). One of the main problems is the low level of funding—the current expenditure on health is just 6.52% (last available data for 2016) of GDP (Gross Domestic Product) and 4.55% GDP comes from public sources (generally the public insurance scheme). Patients significantly participate in the financing of health—the out-of-pocket spending is 23% of current healthcare expenditure. The private sector is strong in the area of outpatient care—a large part of the providers, particularly in primary health care are non-public actors. The hospital care sector is dominated by public entities—hospitals are mainly owned by local government entities for which providing access to inpatient care is one of the statutory tasks.

Hospitals operate in two basic forms—Independent Public Health Care Institution (SPZOZ) or companies; regardless of the form of the activity, all hospitals owned by the public sector are non-profit. Purely private hospitals play a marginal role from the point of view of access to benefits and, as the for the public ones, they are dependent on public funds. The contracts between hospitals and the National Health Fund specify a range of benefits and the amount of them. The healthcare services provided above the predetermined limit are remunerated only partially or not at all, which is often a source of financial distress. From the year 2018, the network of hospital providers was launched, under which hospitals are paid a flat rate. There are two main differences between SPZOZ and companies: Hospitals operating in the form of a company must keep the financial discipline due to the risk of bankruptcy, but on the other hand, they can benefit from additional sources of income by selling services within supplementary private insurance schemes or out-of-pocket spending. Hospitals operating as SPZOZ cannot effectively go bankrupt, but they are forbidden to privately sell the same services like the ones provided within contracts with the public payer.

Most of the hospitals in Poland struggle with financial difficulties. This applies both to the large hospitals in cities as well as to small hospitals located in rural areas. However, while large urban hospitals are supported by wealthier urban local governments, which, as the owners, finance their investments or supplement the shortage of financial resources, the hospitals in rural areas cannot benefit from such support. Poorer local governments do not have the ability to finance such hospitals and are not able to bear the financial responsibility for the debts of their medical entities (due to the public debt limits). As a result, such local governments seek the possibilities of commercializing or even privatizing their hospitals to get rid of this responsibility.

3. Rural Hospitals as Part of a Sustainable Health System

Sustainable rural development is crucial to the economic, social, and environmental development of societies. The discussion on sustainable development emerged in the 1970s and 1980s because humanity became aware that production and consumption destroy the foundations of their life through the over-exploitation of natural resources [14]. The concept of sustainable development was used for the first time at the Stockholm Conference in 1972, in connection with the discussion of the tasks and goals of global environmental protection. The transfer of this concept to international documents took place at the UN Conference "Environment and Development" in Rio de Janeiro in June 1992. The famous Burtland World Commission on Environment and Development in 1987 defined sustainable development as development that meets the needs of the present without compromising the ability of future generations to meet their own needs [15]. Existing definitions emphasize three interconnected aspects of the concept: Environmental, social, and economic. Sustainable development means managing the use of natural environmental resources and the organization of social life, which will improve and then preserve a high quality of life [16] maximizing the net benefits of economic development in the long-term perspective [17]. Other authors note that sustainable development means the evolution of human society [18,19].

The idea of sustainable development became an important element of political debate and the priority of development strategies and sectorial policies. It combined the three main pillars of economic and social development with the protection of the environment and its resources. Sustainable development as an international political idea defined the concept of sustainable production and consumption, and sustainable transport. It also encouraged people to mitigate climate change and strongly emphasized the importance of the problems of poverty, inequality, social exclusion, and the public-health sector.

The current evolution of the sustainable development concept under the guidance of the United Nations leads us to the turning point. The United Nations (UN) Member States in 2015 adopted the 2030 Agenda for Sustainable Development with the 17 sustainable development goals (SDGs). As a result, a new systemic holistic definition of sustainable development was identified with the core principle of global cooperation and national development [20]. Agenda 2030 is a future, long-term social contract for the world. Recently, SDGs became a benchmark for countries, local communities, business, and NGOs, and they are present in many strategies and policies. The core part of the new approach is social sustainability (exclusion, poverty, inequalities) represented by the sentence "no one will be left behind". So, economic and environmental sustainability must be aligned with social sustainability [21].

The rural and urban areas are facing strong global challenges, especially those related to poverty, exclusion, lack of justice, inequality, climate, environmental damage, and peace. SDGs address these issues and formulate a new social, economic, and environmental vision. For example, goal 1: No poverty says that economic growth must be inclusive and promote equality. The next goal proposed is Zero Hunger and it emphasizes the role of rural areas and agriculture sector in providing food, stopping hunger, and eradicating poverty. Very important for quality of life goals 3 and 4 are good health and wellbeing, and quality education—ensuring healthy lives and wellbeing are essential to sustainable development, and obtaining a quality education is the foundation for improving people's lives and sustainable development. Next, the crucial goal for sustainability is to reduce inequalities (Goal 10). It means that policies should be universal in principle, paying attention to the needs of disadvantaged and marginalized populations [22]. The new, multidimensional, complex identification of sustainability is unique because, except all specific goals, it is underlining the importance of cooperation of everybody with the leading role of the government and its institutions in implementing just transition to sustainability [23]. The transformations require governance structures and capabilities, political action, and the formation of actors of change [24].

Therefore, coordinating rural development initiatives that contribute to sustainable social environment is critical. In different parts of rural Europe, a new paradigm of sustainable rural development has begun to take hold. There are several main reasons for the emerging new paradigm: (1) The 'squeeze' on European agriculture, (2) new sources of income, (3) changing role of rural areas from food production to multifunction, and (4) the aesthetic-consumptive functions of places [25]. The environmental aspects of the definition of traditional sustainability mean that agriculture is not only regarded as an economic sector and food-producing sector but also has to maintain multifunctional green space and landscape quality as well [26]. Farmers get direct payment to protect the environment and landscape and develop agro-tourism. On this basis, we define sustainable rural development as territorially based development that redefines nature by re-emphasizing food production and agro-ecology and that re-asserts the socio-environmental role of agriculture as a major agent in sustaining rural economies and cultures [27]. The 'new rural paradigm' (NRP) includes a new, multi-sector, place-based approach to rural development that claims the need for closer cooperation and synergy between the rural and urban economy, and towards rural development as a way to reduce exclusion, poverty, and inequalities on the regional and local level more generally [28]. It presents the emerging tendency of decentralization, re-localization, and self-organization, which is a new regional paradigm, resulting in new linkages among sectors, businesses, producers, consumers, and markets [29].

Sustainable development also means a new perspective on health issues, where sustainable development is perceived as a part of the wider concept consisting of health, wellbeing, economy, environment, and social justice [30]. According to the social pillar of the traditional definition of the sustainable development, one of the important roles of the rural hospital is to help the community. The existence of hospitals in rural areas improves access to health benefits so the rural hospitals' surviving is a key factor of sustainable rural health [31]. It is very important because rural inhabitants are less probable to benefit regularly from doctor's consultation and have weaker access to emergency services [32], which are usually situated in more urbanized areas. Rural hospitals can leverage their strong relationships with local communities and patients; they have also a significant positive influence on health of the population. When a hospital is closed, patients are forced to seek a new provider, which sometimes means a break in therapy [33]. A remote location also generates costs of transport, if it is available at all. This problem can be particularly important in the case of the elderly or persons suffering from chronic diseases [34]. This prolonged travel time to the hospital also increases mortality in cases of emergency [35].

According to the economic pillar of the traditional definition of the sustainable development, all hospitals operate using valuable and scarce resources and they have faced significant changes over recent decades [36]. Those changes of economic environment resulted in many countries in massive closures of rural hospitals due to their poor financial condition [37–39], so rural hospitals must adapt to reach the level of sustainability [31]. In most countries, hospitals located in rural areas are smaller and deliver less specialized services. Despite this smaller range of services, rural hospitals play an important role in satisfying the rural population's health needs [40–43] or just in being part of local health infrastructure [44], which is so crucial because barriers in access to hospital, or broadly speaking, health services, impacts rural population's health outcomes [45]. Furthermore, we consider health services higher than public and private services. Rural health services have infrastructure and people that are part of local communities. Health professionals are often important members of their communities and they are also actively engaged in the social life of the rural communities.

Rural hospitals impact economic rural development through their health care infrastructure, employment of doctors, dentists, nurses, the quality of medical and health services, and pharmacies. The localization of rural hospitals and medical services encourage localization of care centers for the elderly and influence the development of the silver economy. It means that there is the demand for supply of different services and goods for retired people. In the past two decades, consumer spending among those aged 60 and over increased 50% faster when compared to those under 30. Rural hospital infrastructure increases the attractiveness of a community for physicians as well as for retail business and manufacturing firms. Thus, it might indirectly affect the overall level of community economic activity [46]. Examples of sectors expected to benefit significantly from the silver economy are cosmetics and fashion, tourism, smart homes supporting independent living, service robotics, health (including medical devices, pharmaceuticals, and e-Health) and wellness, safety, culture, education and skills, entertainment, personal and autonomous transport, banking, and relevant financial products [47].

Finally, it increases the growth of sales, consumption, and taxes for local budget. Rural hospitals bring in money from the outside, for example from National Health Funds, and they positively support the prosperity of the local economy [48]. From the economic and social point of view of the traditional definition of sustainability, the health sector provides significant direct benefits through employment and growing incomes. The employment of one physician in a rural area can create an additional five jobs and have an impact on income, retail sales, and sales tax collections. The study concludes that a physician plays a vital role in the economy of the host community. Many researchers in the US confirmed that rural hospitals are the second largest employer in rural counties [46].

Based on the literature review, we can indicate factors contributing to rural hospitals' poor financial condition. They are:

(1) Smaller size [37,49–57], which seems to be the most important determinant of lower profitability and poor financial performance;
(2) Lower elasticity and higher sensitivity to changes [58,59];
(3) Lack of skilled professionals [34,44,60–62];
(4) Poor equipment [61];
(5) A small range of benefits [50,53,55,60,63];
(6) Lower bed occupancy [34,41] declining inpatient admissions [60], the lower economy of scale [57,61].

Those risk factors are generally the consequences of the remote location [41] and the small size of the population covered [54]. Among them, the smaller size seems to be the most important determinant—this is, at the same time, the consequence of the rural location and the main factor determining poor financial condition. Previous findings prove that a smaller hospital is heavily exposed to financial distress, regardless of the ownership or the aim of activity [51–54]. Bigger hospitals, despite their rural location, can achieve as good effectiveness as their urban counterparts [50]. So, to ensure the continuance of such economically sensitive hospitals [64], policymakers should employ a system of support [54], for example in the form of special rules of payment for the benefits that they provide [31,65]; this can also help to improve public perception of the organization [66].

Although the hospital's activity is very specific, however, in economic terms the enterprise and its financial condition strongly affect the quality of services [67]—higher direct costs are related to lower readmission rates [68]. Though hospitals in Poland are not-for-profit at the vast majority, they are obliged to keep the financial balance to continue their activity. This means there is a need to assess financial health on the basis of the indicators used in enterprises. Some of them are modified by introducing the specific values characterizing hospitals' activity, for example a number of beds. Usually, the following financial indicators are employed: (1) Profitability, (2) liquidity, (3) capital structure, (4) revenue indicators, (5) costs, and (6) utilization (bed occupancy) [57,68,69]. Most of the previous studies confirm rural hospitals' poor financial performance (based on indicators listed above) [37,69,70], while some results are inconsistent, suggesting that rural hospitals can be as profitable (or efficient) as their urban counterparts [58,71]. According to the pillars of the environment of the traditional definition of sustainable development, the efficiency of rural hospitals can help them use their resources in the best way and to direct them toward their missions of patient care. Due to the nature of the services they provide, health services use significant amounts of energy and water and generate large volumes of waste. Thus, their efficiency is fundamental.

4. Data

A major concern in the assessment of the financial conditions of rural hospitals is, in fact, the definition of rurality, which should take into account the specific character of a given country. In this study, we cannot directly adopt the definition proposed by the Polish Main Office, which defines rural areas, as "the areas situated outside the administrative boundaries of cities" (rural municipality, rural parts of the urban-rural municipalities) [72]. We cannot employ this definition in our study due to the fact that rural areas, based on this statistical spin, are strongly diversified and some of them have more urbanized character despite the low population density [73,74]. Due to the lack of a wider definition of a "rural hospital", we employ our own definition, assuming that a "rural hospital" fulfills contemporaneously the following criteria:

(1) Is located in a county town;
(2) The population of the county is lower than 100,000 people.

In practice, it means a rural area with one small urban center where a hospital is located. As a result, the hospital serves patients not only from the city center but also, and perhaps above all, from the surrounding villages; then, it can be assumed that the health service provider can be assessed as a "rural hospital". The definition of an urban hospital is similarly formulated. Only hospitals located in cities with a population exceeding 100,000 residents qualified for the analysis. Additionally, all hospitals located in "Katowice urban area" (highly urbanized part of Poland with population density above 1500/km^2) were qualified as urban hospitals. All hospitals owned by the regional authorities (NUTS 2), regardless of their real location, were included in the research sample as "urban hospitals". Such hospitals, due to their regional nature and more specialized services, usually serve very large populations.

The research data was collected by hand from the Emerging Markets Information Service [EMIS] Database, covering the years 2012–2017. Initially, we analyzed 1123 entities classified in the database as "hospitals" or "hospital and medical activity". First, 327 entities were excluded due to lack of all the required data. During the next stage of data construction, based on the detailed analysis of every entity, we excluded:

(a) Entities which provide mainly other services than stationary health care;
(b) Hospitals, which provide primarily long-term care (psychiatric hospitals, rehabilitation hospitals, sanatoriums) because of the specificity of the activities;
(c) Entities, providing mainly ambulatory care and "one-day procedures", classified in the database as "hospitals and medical activity";
(d) Hospitals providing services in only one specialization (for example cardiology or radiology) due to its specificity.

"Rural hospitals" characterized by annual income higher than 22 million euro and providing medical services for the regional population regardless of their location in rural areas have also been excluded from the research sample. "Urban hospitals" with annual income lower than 6 million euro have also been rejected, in order to exclude small urban hospitals providing a low range of services, especially "one-day" surgical procedures. Ultimately, the research sample consisted of 150–199 hospitals, depending on the year (Table 1). Whenever the wording "rural hospital" or "urban hospital" appears in this paper, it refers to the definitions of "rural hospital" and "urban hospital" adopted in this study.

Table 1. Number of observations.

Division	2012	2013	2014	2015	2016
Rural	80	80	80	76	98
Urban	70	70	70	85	101
Total	150	150	150	161	199

5. Methodology

According to the literature review, we analyzed four pillars of financial health: Profitability, liquidity, efficiency, and debt using 7 variables (Table 2) which were selected based on their descriptive statistics. Profitability seems to be, in the light of previous studies, the most important factor determining a hospital's financial health. It can be measured using several financial indicators, which were selected due to their importance to the assessment of its financial condition in the case of Polish hospitals. For example, Polish hospitals usually pursue to obtain a positive value of EBIDTA (Earnings before Interest, Taxes, Depreciation, and Amortization), while EBIT (Earnings before Interest and Taxes) remains negative. Indicators like ROS (Return on Sales) or total margin, which are the best synthetic indicators of the profitability on sales [75], could not be employed in this study, because the hospitals analyzed operate in different organizational forms (public entities, companies owned by public bodies, private companies) [76]. Additionally, we checked the differences in size (both in terms of assets and income) between rural and urban hospitals.

The differences between the values of financial indicators for rural and urban hospitals were tested using the non-parametric Mann–Whitney U test due to the abnormal distribution of all analyzed ratios.

In the second stage of research, in order to provide a more comprehensive assessment of the financial health, we employed a synthetic measure of a hospital financial condition (M2) created based on the gradient method. The gradient was based on the determination of taxonomic distances between examined objects and defined reference points (bottom, top) [77–79] (see also, Appendix A). The obtained values range is 0–1 [80,81]. In order to build this synthetic measure, we used the selected indicators of profitability, liquidity, debt, and efficiency employed in the first stage of the study (Table 3) [82–85].

Table 2. Financial indicators employed in the research.

Ratio	Formula	Character	Group
OPM	EBIT/Sales	stimulant	profitability
CR	Current Assets/Current liabilities	nominant	liquidity
D%	Total debt/Total Assets	destimulant	debt
CF/Debt	(Net Profit + Depreciation)/Total debt	stimulant	debt
TAT	Sales/Total Assets	stimulant	efficiency
CES	Employee benefit expense/Sales	destimulant	efficiency
ROCF	(Net Profit + Depreciation)/Total Assets	stimulant	profitability
ASSETS	Ln Total Assets	nominant	size
INCOME	Ln Revenue from sales	stimulant	size

Sales—the revenue from provided services, both from contracts with NFZ and private sources (only in the case of companies)

Table 3. Financial indicators chosen to construct the synthetic measure M2.

Ratio	Formula	Character	Group
OPM	EBIT/Sales	stimulant	profitability
CR	Current Assets/Current liabilities	nominant	liquidity
D%	Total debt/Total Assets	destimulant	debt
TAT	Sales/Total Assets	stimulant	efficiency
CES	Employee benefit expense/Sales	destimulant	efficiency

Where: Nominants and destimulants have been converted into stimulants respectively: nominants: $x\_ij := -|x\_ij - avarage(x\_i)|$, destimulants: $x\_ij := [\![-x\_ij]\!]$

We defined the minimum and maximum values in the sample for the years 2012–2014 using the following formula:

$$M2 = 0.29196 * OPM - 0.031242 * CR - 0.84 - 0.031112 * D\% + 0.017609 * TAT - 0.066345 * CES - 0.75344 \quad (1)$$

During the last stage, we estimated three random-effects models with time dummies where the independent variables were: Legal form (0—public entity, 1—company), size (ln revenue), and localization (0—urban, 1—rural), and the dependent variable was the M2 indicator. We estimated models for the whole group and for rural and urban hospitals separately.

6. Results and Discussion

In this study, we form the assumption that hospitals located in rural areas are smaller and characterized by more difficult financial situations than hospitals in urban areas. The literature review indicates that the source of this disadvantage may be a smaller size, which enables hospitals to benefit from the economy of scale, and/or less specialized range of services. Employed measures of the size better than a number of beds reflect the potential to generate cash flows. Additionally, the value of total assets approximates the size of a hospital, not only in the physical dimension, but it also reflects the value of the hospital's equipment (which also affects the volume of revenue). The operating revenue is strictly associated with both the volume of provided services and its level of specialization, assuming that more specialized health benefits are better compensated. Our study confirms that rural hospitals in Poland are in fact smaller—both in terms of operating revenue and the value of total assets—and these differences are statistically significant at the level of $\alpha = 1\%$ in all analyzed years (Table 4). This is generally consistent with the characteristics presented in the literature which confirms the smaller size of rural hospitals [37,41,49,86].

Table 4. Results of Mann-Whitney U test—differences between urban and rural hospitals.

2012			
Ratio	Rural	Urban	p-value
OPM	6149	5176	0.6827
CR	6239	5086	0.4546
D%	5596	5729	0.0948
CF/Debt	6439	4886	0.1333
TAT	6239	5086	0.4546
CES	5718	5607	0.2258
ROCF	6146	5179	0.6911
Ln(Assets)	4610	6716	0.0000
Ln(Sales)	4363	6962	0.0000
M2	6808	4517	0.0038

2013			
Ratio	Rural	Urban	p-value
OPM	5926	5399	0.4760
CR	6129	5196	0.9609
D%	5770	5555	0.1933
CF/Debt	6243	5082	0.6320
TAT	6539	4786	0.1107
CES	5725	5600	0.1414
ROCF	6021	5304	0.7230
Ln(Assets)	4529	6796	0.0000
Ln(Sales)	4435	6890	0.0000
M2	6763	4562	0.0147

2014			
Ratio	Rural	Urban	p-value
OPM	5868	5457	0.5182
CR	5862	5463	0.5037
D%	5700	5625	0.2009
CF/Debt	6272	5053	0.3832
TAT	6443	4882	0.1295
CES	5812	5513	0.3914
ROCF	5980	5345	0.8226
Ln(Assets)	4493	6832	0.0000
Ln(Sales)	4398	6927	0.0000
M2	6613	4712	0.0310

2015			
Ratio	Rural	Urban	p-value
OPM	6034	7007	0.6808
CR	6220	6821	0.8297
D%	6060	6981	0.7464
CF/Debt	5934	7107	0.4532
TAT	6727	6314	0.0534
CES	6290	6751	0.6512
ROCF	5945	7096	0.4760
Ln(Assets)	4502	8539	0.0000
Ln(Sales)	4416	8625	0.0000
M2	6695	6346	0.0682

2016			
Ratio	Rural	Urban	p-value
OPM	9659	10,241	0.7294
CR	9882	10,018	0.8410
D%	9673	10,227	0.7555
CF/Debt	9601	10,299	0.6250
TAT	10,695	9205	0.0276
CES	9863	10,037	0.8777
ROCF	9686	10,214	0.7799
Ln(Assets)	7387	12,513	0.0000
Ln(Sales)	7276	12,624	0.0000
M2	10,975	8925	0.0038

This difference should significantly influence the financial health of a hospital. Higher income means a higher scale of activity, but it can be also related to a higher intensity of care as a result of providing more specialized services. Regardless of the source of this difference, it may be associated with the ability to exploit economies of scale—the median value of assets for urban hospitals is EUR 11.45 million, whereas for rural hospitals it is EUR 4.53 million. The volume of assets translates partially into the ability to generate revenue—the median of revenue for hospitals located in urban areas is EUR 13.57 million whereas for rural hospitals it is EUR 6.38 million (data for 2016).

The main part of the research, which relates to the H1 hypothesis, consists of testing differences in the financial health for urban and rural hospitals. We cannot confirm the difference at the level of the individual indicators—these differences are not statistically significant—however, if we apply the synthetic measure of financial condition (M2), we can observe that the overall financial condition of rural hospitals is better than urban of the urban ones in every analyzed year and those differences are statistically significant for all years (except 2015) (Table 4).

The estimated models (Table 5) confirm that rural hospitals are characterized by better financial condition (the value of the variable "rural" is positive (0.023) and statistically significant). We also find that hospitals with higher revenue have better financial health (the variable "Ln Revenue" has a positive coefficient (0.015) and is statistically significant). Also, hospitals operating in the form of companies achieve better financial condition than those operating in the form of SPZO—the variable "Legal_form" has a positive coefficient (0.030) and is statistically significant. The same relationship can be observed at the level of the whole sample and in the case of urban hospitals, but the increase in revenue boost the financial condition of urban hospitals is slightly stronger than in the case of the whole sample.

Table 5. Regression results.

	Whole Sample		Urban Only		Rural Only	
	Coefficient	p-Value	Coefficient	p-Value	Coefficient	p-Value
Const	0.53791 (0.05824)	<0.0001	0.45424 (0.07920)	<0.0001	0.70449 (0.03730)	<0.0001
Legal_form	0.03073 (0.00503)	<0.0001	0.04280 (0.00763)	<0.0001	0.02180 (0.00541)	<0.0001
Ln Revenue	0.01571 (0.00588)	0.0076	0.02376 (0.00806)	0.0032	0.00034 (0.00406)	0.9315
dt_2	−0.00099 (0.00218)	0.65	−0.00269 (0.00389)	0.4894	−0.00032 (0.00163)	0.8424
dt_3	−0.00140 (0.00228)	0.5382	−0.00254 (0.00365)	0.4868	−0.00161 (0.00244)	0.5084
dt_4	−0.02517 (0.00904)	0.0054	−0.03622 (0.01338)	0.0068	−0.00656 (0.00636)	0.3019
dt_5	−0.02770 (0.00932)	0.003	−0.03935 (0.01362)	0.0039	−0.00741 (0.00673)	0.2706
Rural	0.0238431 (0.00673)	0.0004				
Mean dependent variable	0.708122		0.69962		0.716214	
Sum squared residuals	1.010879		0.625202		0.35885	
Log-likelihood	1558.576		713.1112		874.6649	
Schwarz criterion	−3063.576		−1384.370		−1707.132	
Rho	−0.271669		−0.313066		−0.216595	
S.D. dependent variable	0.040083		0.045105		0.032693	
S.E. of regression	0.035481		0.04009		0.029621	
Akaike criterion	−3101.153		−1412.222		−1735.330	
Hannan–Quinn	−3086.726		−1401.187		−1724.179	
Durbin–Watson	1.524023		1.627987		1.421658	

When we analyze the model estimated only for rural hospitals, a completely different pattern can be observed. In the case of these hospitals, only the legal form of activity is statistically significant. A positive coefficient (0.02) for the variable "Legal form" indicates that the form of a company has a positive effect on the financial health, although to a lesser extent than in the case of urban hospitals (0.04) or at the level of the whole sample (0.03). In the case of rural hospitals, the size does not matter—an increase in revenue does not improve the financial health.

Our hypothesis was constructed on the basis of a literature review. Surprisingly, the presented results do not expressly support this assumption. The analysis of financial indicators clearly shows that there are no statistically significant differences between rural and urban hospitals, or even that the financial health of rural hospitals is better when we employ the synthetic measure. These results are inconsistent with those obtained in previous studies [41,49,50,63,76,86,87].

It seems that a smaller size, which in previous studies was seen as a factor increasing the risk of financial distress [28,34,86], might be even a source of competitive advantage. Large hospitals located in cities usually have higher assets, which, apart from generating higher revenues, may be associated with higher costs. Another risk factor indicated in the literature is a smaller range of benefits [50,63,76,87,88]. A smaller range of benefits usually means less specialized procedures. Rural hospitals usually do not provide highly specialized life-saving procedures (invasive cardiology, transplants). Such highly specialized procedures are a source of higher income per bed, provided that they are well valued by the payer. Otherwise, they can lead to the deterioration of the financial situation.

The study identifies other important drivers of rural hospitals' financial health. We prove that the form of activity is very important, while it forces the hospital to maintain financial health. On the other hand, rural hospitals cannot improve their situation by seeking to increase the scale of medical activity, which can be a source of improvement in the case of urban entities.

7. Conclusions

We studied the economic situation of rural hospitals due to its importance for local communities. For the majority of the inhabitants of rural areas, the existence of a hospital in short means better access to benefits. Patients have a chance to maintain close contact with their families, which is especially important in the case of children and the elderly. However, the hospital is also an enterprise, though a very specific one. To be able to survive, it must keep financial condition sufficient to finance its current medical activity. The literature review presented in this research proves that rural hospitals are smaller and economically more sensitive, but those research results come generally from the American market. European studies on the financial health of rural hospitals are very few and, in the case of Poland, this is the first such study. Therefore, our results represent a very significant contribution to the science. Although our work is based on a relatively small research sample, we can conclude that rural hospitals, though smaller both in terms of income and assets, are at a lower risk of financial distress than their larger urban counterparts.

The result suggest that the size is not the main determinant of hospital financial performance. In the case of hospitals, the form of activity seems to play a crucial role—entities operating in the form of a company are forced to keep a greater financial discipline. This also explains the process of transformations into companies which can be observed in recent years. Paradoxically, the increasing scale of operations (increase in revenue) does not improve financial health—hospitals located in cities benefit more from such processes (the consolidation of hospitals). On the other hand, the fact that the level of revenue of rural hospitals does not affect the financial health suggests greater resistance to changes in the external environment.

This research is an important contribution to the discussion on the role and financial condition of rural hospitals. In all European countries, there are hospitals located in remote areas, distant from the large urban centers. As we have demonstrated, hospitals located in smaller centers, although smaller in terms of revenue and assets, are not characterized by a worse financial situation. Then, they are in line with the economic and environmental pillars of the sustainable development. Rural hospitals can use their economic and moral positions within their communities to help them achieve the two objectives of sustainable development goals related to health as well as sustainability and foster green economy. We can even hypothesize that smaller size is the source of their competitive advantage, just like the fact that they often operate as commercial law companies. It seems that our results might determine the new directions of changes for other European countries—creating networks of small, flexible hospital units, responsive to the needs of local communities, capable of providing equal and effective access to health services, in line with the social pillar and respect of rural communities.

The better, or just sufficient, financial condition of rural hospitals supports the concept of rural sustainability on many levels (Figure 1). The rural sustainability is focused on the local economic, social, and environmental development to create conditions for the elimination of poverty and better quality of life.

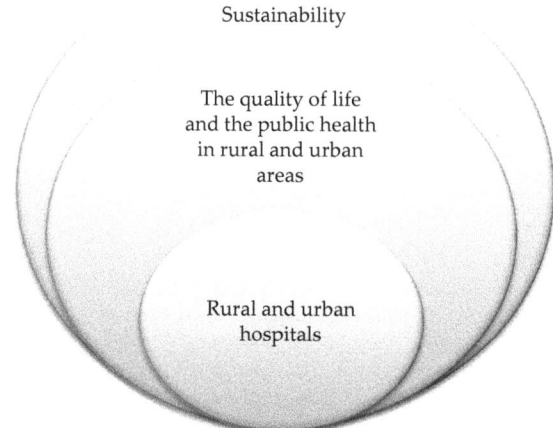

Figure 1. Impact of rural and urban hospitals on society and environment. Authors own elaboration.

The environmental protection and mitigation of climate change support the sustainable development of agriculture and better quality of food supply, which is important for public health. The rural health infrastructure and access to basic health services and education create opportunities for rural areas to develop, and it is critical for sustainability and national wellbeing. The general trend in the economy is orientated towards decentralization of production, which means also decentralization and democratization of social activities. Also, urban and local development is playing an important role in the decentralization process.

Sustainable rural development is also an answer to the crisis of conventional, industrial agriculture which is changing rural areas. A broader spectrum of risks emerged, especially health risks. The factors to increase health risk are environmental damage, pollution, soil erosion, and low quality of food. Redefinition of socio-environmental balance is necessary for better quality of living in the rural and urban areas. The good financial condition of rural hospitals can result in:

(1) Better access to health services;
(2) Reduction of health risks (climate, environmental, disabilities, aging);
(3) Elimination of poverty by dedicated actions for vulnerable households, in particular, the aged, persons with disabilities and the unemployed;
(4) Reducing costs of health services for citizens (better access, transport exclusion);
(5) According to the sustainable development goals, it can encourage rural communities, increase their participation in decision-making, and empower rural leadership;
(6) Reinforce environmental and social resilience in rural areas;
(7) As a result, public health and sustainability issues go together and try to establish a framework to face many challenges in rural and urban areas. The crucial part of the new approach is its long-term perspective, responsibility, and complexity. Public health must be aligned with sustainable development and climate change.

The primary weakness of the study is the relatively small research sample. We also adopt our own definition of "rurality", which can influence the obtained results. In further research, we plan to verify whether the change in criteria affects the results obtained.

Author Contributions: Conceptualization, A.B. and P.G.; methodology, R.S.; validation, A.B. and P.U.-J.; formal analysis, P.P.; investigation, A.B. and P.P.; data curation, R.S.; writing—original draft preparation, A.B.; writing—review and editing, P.U.-J.; supervision, B.R.

Funding: This research received no external funding.

Conflicts of Interest: The authors certify that they have no involvement in any organization or entity with any financial interest or non-financial interest in the subject matter or materials discussed in this manuscript.

Appendix A

A gradient method is a taxonomic tool based on determination of taxonomic distances of the examined objects from defined reference points [78,81]. This procedure allows construction of a synthetic indicator of different nature, by combining values of variables denominated in different units, including dummy ones. Variables might be of a financial and non-financial character but must be stimulant—nominant and destimulant variables should be transformed into stimulant ones.

The method assumes that the matrix X comprises financial ratio values (observations of the studied phenomenon) denoted as:xij, which can be converted into stimulants (Destimulants and nominants have to be converted into stimulants) x_{ij} where

i = 1,2,3, . . . , m, (a number of analyzed indicators—financial ratios);
j = 1,2,3, . . . , n, (a number of analyzed observations—hospitals);
and $x_{ij} \in R$.

In order to measure a taxonomic distance, two points must be determined:
Top: $P = [p_1, p_2, p_3, \ldots, p_m]$
Bottom: $Q = [q_1, q_2, q_3, \ldots, q_m]$
where $p_i = \max_j x_{i,j}$ and $q_i = \min_j x_{i,j}$

As the QP segment describes the axis of synthetic indicator, the PQ vector gradient takes a form of linear programming function:

$\Phi(X) = [P - Q]X^T$ and values of this function represent the value of the synthetic indicator, according to the formula:

$$\varphi = (p_i - q_i) * x_{i,j} \tag{A1}$$

The obtained values of specific indicators, due to their construction, might take potentially very dissimilar values. In this situation, some indicators would affect a synthetic measure more strongly than others. To avoid this effect, the obtained values are reduced to the range of 0–1, using the scaling method. Conversions should be made from matrix X to Z according to the following formula:

$$for\ every\ i\ z_{ij} = \frac{x_{ij} - \min(x_{ij})}{\max(x_{ij}) - \min(x_{ij})} \tag{A2}$$

As a result, points P and Q take the following form: $P = |1, \ldots 1|, Q = |0, \ldots 0|$:

$$\varphi = \sum_{i=1}^{m} z_{ij} \tag{A3}$$

and the measure of development M (M1 and M2) is defined as:

$$M = \frac{\varphi}{m} \tag{A4}$$

References

1. Papagiannis, F.; Gazzola, P.; Burak, O.; Pokutsa, I. Overhauls in water supply systems in Ukraine: A hydro-economic model of socially responsible planning and cost management. *J. Clean. Prod.* **2018**, *183*, 358–369. [CrossRef]
2. Siedlecki, R.; Papla, D.; Bem, A. A logistic law of growth as a base for methods of company's life cycle phases forecasting. *Proc. Roman. Acad. Ser. A* **2018**, *19*, 141–146.
3. Ocampo, J.A. The Macroeconomics of the Green Economy. The Transition to a Green Economy: Benefits, Challenges and Risks from a Sustainable Development Perspective, UNEP. Available online: http://wedocs.unep.org/handle/20.500.11822/9310 (accessed on 10 October 2018).
4. Saviano, M.; Barile, S.; Spohrer, J.C.; Caputo, F. A service research contribution to the global challenge of sustainability. *J. Serv. Theory Pract.* **2017**, *27*, 951–976. [CrossRef]
5. Gazzola, P.; Querci, E. The Connection Between the Quality of Life and Sustainable Ecological Development. *Eur. Sci. J. ESJ* **2017**, *13*. [CrossRef]
6. Farmer, J.; Prior, M.; Taylor, J. A theory of how rural health services contribute to community sustainability. *Soc. Sci. Med.* **2012**, *10*, 1903–1911. [CrossRef]
7. Fineberg, V.H. A Successful and Sustainable Health System—How to Get There from Here. *N. Engl. J. Med.* **2012**, *366*, 1020–1027. [CrossRef] [PubMed]
8. Barile, S.; Saviano, M.; Polese, F. Information asymmetry and co-creation in health care services. *Aust. Mark. J. AMJ* **2014**, *22*, 205–217.
9. Barile, S.; Polese, F.; Saviano, M.; Carrubbo, L. Service innovation in translational medicine. In *Innovating in Practice*; Springer: Cham, Switzerland, 2017; Volume 9, pp. 417–438.
10. Barile, S.; Polese, F.; Saviano, M.; Carrubbo, L.; Clarizia, F. Service Research Contribution for Health Networks' Understanding. In *Innovative Service Perspectives*; Mickelsson, J., Helkulla, A., Eds.; Hanken School of Economics: Helsinki, Finland, 2012; p. 71. Available online: https://ssrn.com/abstract=2121317 (accessed on 27 March 2019).
11. Polese, F.; Carrubbo, L.; Caputo, F.; Sarno, D. Managing Healthcare Service Ecosystems: Abstracting a Sustainability-Based View from Hospitalization at Home (HaH) Practices. *Sustainability* **2018**, *10*, 3951. [CrossRef]
12. Vuong, Q.H.; Ho, T.M.; Nguyen, H.K.; Vuong, T.T. Healthcare consumers' sensitivity to costs: A reflection on behavioural economics from an emerging market. *Palgrave Commun.* **2018**, *19*, 70. [CrossRef]
13. Paulina, U.-J. The macro-economic determinants of health inequalities. *Prace Naukowe Akademii im. Jana Długosza w Częstochowie. Pragmata tes Oikonomias* **2018**, *12*, 151–168.
14. Rogall, H. *Ekonomia zrównoważonego rozwoju. Teoria i praktyka*; Wydawnictwo Zysk i s-ka: Poznan, Poland, 2010.
15. Brundtland, G. *Our Common Future: The World Commission on Environment and Development*; Oxford University Press: Oxford, UK, 1987.
16. Borys, T. Sustainable Development—How to Recognize Integrated Order. *Probl. Sustain. Dev.* **2011**, *2*, 75–81.
17. Pearce, D.; Turner, R. *Economics of Natural Resources and the Environment*; Harvester Wheatsheaf: New York, NY, USA, 1990.
18. Glavic, P.; Lukman, R. Review of sustainability terms and their definitions. *J. Clean. Prod.* **2007**, *15*, 1875–1885. [CrossRef]
19. Meadowcroft, J. Sustainable development: A new(ish) idea for a new century? *Political Stud.* **2000**, *48*, 370–387. [CrossRef]
20. *Transforming Our World: The 2030 Agenda for Sustainable Development*; United Nations: New York, NY, USA, 2015.
21. Blakely, E. *Planning Local Economic Development: Theory and Practice*; Sage Library and Social Research: London, UK, 1989.
22. TWI2050. *The World in 2050. Transformations to Achieve the Sustainable Development Goals*; International Institute for Applied Systems Analysis: Laxenburg, Austria, 2018.
23. Loorbach, D. Transition management for sustainable development: A prescriptive, complexity-based governance framework. *Governance* **2010**, *23*, 161–183. [CrossRef]

24. Voss, J.; Bauknecht, D.; Kemp, R. *Reflexive Governance for Sustainable Development*; Edward Elgar Publishing: Cheltenham, UK, 2006.
25. Marsden, T.; Sonnino, R. Rural development and the regional state: Denying multifunctional agriculture in the UK. *J. Rural Stud.* **2008**, *24*, 422–431. [CrossRef]
26. Horlings, I.; Marsden, T. Towards the real green revolution? Exploring the conceptual dimensions of a new ecological modernization of agriculture that could 'feed the world'. *Glob. Environ. Chang.* **2011**, *21*, 441–452. [CrossRef]
27. Marsden, T. The condition of rural sustainability. In *European Perspectives on Rural Development*; Royal van Gorcum: Assen, The Netherlands, 2003; ISBN 978-9023238812.
28. OECD. *The New Rural Paradigm: Policies and Governance*; Organisation for Economic Cooperation and Development: Paris, France, 2006; ISBN 9264023917.
29. Horlings, I.; Marsden, T. Exploring the 'New Rural Paradigm' in Europe: Eco-economic strategies as a counterforce to the global competitiveness agenda. *Eur. Urban Reg. Stud.* **2014**, *21*, 4–20. [CrossRef]
30. Porritt, J. No sustainability without health equity. *Public Health* **2012**, *126*, S24–S26. [CrossRef]
31. Rutten, K. Making Rural Healthcare Sustainable. Ph.D. Thesis, The College of St. Scholastica, Manila, Philippines, 2018.
32. Arcury, T.A.; Preisser, J.S.; Gesler, W.M.; Powers, J.M. Access to transportation and health care utilization in a rural region. *J. Rural Health* **2005**, *21*, 31–38. [CrossRef] [PubMed]
33. Countouris, M.; Gilmore, S.; Yonas, M. Exploring the impact of a community hospital closure on older adults: A focus group study. *Health Place* **2014**, *26*, 143–148. [CrossRef]
34. Smith, J.G. Does Missed Care in Isolated Rural Hospitals Matter? *West. J. Nurs. Res.* **2018**, *6*, 775–778. [CrossRef]
35. Hunsaker, M.; Kantayya, V.S. Building a sustainable rural health system in the era of health reform. *Disease-a-month: DM* **2010**, *12*, 698–705. [CrossRef]
36. Watts, P.R.; Dinger, M.K.; Baldwin, K.A.; SiskBeth, R.J.; Brockschmidt, B.A.; McCubbin, J.E. Accessibility and Perceived Value of Health Services in Five Western Illinois Rural Communities. *J. Community Health* **1999**, *24*, 147. [CrossRef] [PubMed]
37. Garcia-Lacalle, J.; Martin, E. Rural vs urban hospital performance in a 'competitive' public health service. *Soc. Sci. Med.* **2010**, *71*, 1131–1140. [CrossRef] [PubMed]
38. Brozyna, E.; Michalski, G.; Soroczynska, J. E-commerce as a factor supporting the competitiveness of small and medium-sized manufacturing enterprises. In *Proceedings of the CEFE 2015—Central European Conference in Finance and Economics, Kosice, Slovakia, 30 September–1 October 2015*; Gavurová, B., Šolté, M., Eds.; Technical University of Košice: Kosice, Slovakia, 2015; Volume 1, pp. 80–90, ISBN 978-80-553-2467-8.
39. Michalski, G. Risk pressure and inventories levels. Influence of risk sensitivity on working capital levels. *Econ. Comput. Econ. Cybern. Stud. Res.* **2016**, *50*, 189–196.
40. Ucieklak-Jeż, P.; Bem, A. Dostępność opieki zdrowotnej na obszarach wiejskich w Polsce [Availability of health care in rural areas in Poland]. *Problemy Drobnych Gospodarstw Rolnych* **2017**, *4*, 117–131. [CrossRef]
41. Moscovice, I.; Stensland, J. Rural Hospitals: Trends, Challenges, and a Future Research and Policy Analysis Agenda. *J. Rural Health* **2002**, *9*, 197–210. [CrossRef]
42. Ona, L.; Davis, A. Economic Impact of the Critical Access Hospital Program on Kentucky's Communities. *J. Rural Health* **2011**, *27*, 21–28. [CrossRef]
43. Pink, G.H.; Holmes, G.M.; D'Alpe, C.; Strunk, L.A.; McGee, P.; Slifkin, R.T. Financial indicators for critical access hospitals. *J. Rural Health* **2006**, *3*, 229–236. [CrossRef] [PubMed]
44. Kenny, A.; Duckett, S. A question of place: Medical power in rural Australia. *Soc. Sci. Med.* **2004**, *58*, 1059–1073. [CrossRef]
45. Douthit, N.; Kiv, S.; Dwolatzky, T.; Biswas, S. Exposing some important barriers to health care access in the rural USA. *Public Health* **2015**, *6*, 611–620. [CrossRef] [PubMed]
46. Doeksen, G.A.; Johnson, T.; Willoughby, C. *Measuring the Economic Importance of the Health Sector on a Local Economy: A Brief Literature Review and Procedures to Measure Local Impacts*; Southern Rural Development Center: Starkville, MS, USA, 1997.
47. Doeksen, G.; Johnson, T.; Biard-Holmes, D.; Schott, V. A healthy health sector is crucial for community economic development. *J. Rural Health* **1998**, *14*, 66–72. [CrossRef]
48. European Commission. *Growing the European Silver Economy*; European Commision: Brussels, Belgium, 2015.

49. Barnett, R.; Barnett, P. If you want to sit on your butts you'll get nothing! Community activism in response to threats of rural hospital closure in southern New Zealand. *Health Place* **2003**, *9*, 59–71. [CrossRef]
50. McCue, M.J.A. Market, Operation and Missions Assessment of Large Rural for Profit Hospitals with Positive Cash Flow. *J. Rural Health* **2007**, *1*, 10–16. [CrossRef]
51. Augurzky, B.; Schmitz, H. Is There a Future for Small Hospitals in Germany? *Ruhr. Econ. Pap.* **2010**, *198*, 1–17. [CrossRef]
52. Prędkiewicz, P.; Prędkiewicz, K.; Węgrzyn, M. Rentowność szpitali samorządowych w Polsce. *Nauki o Finansach* **2014**, *3*, 28–43. [CrossRef]
53. Horwitz, J.R. Making Profits and Providing Care: Comparing Non-profit, For-Profit, And Government Hospitals. *Health Aff.* **2005**, *3*, 790–801. [CrossRef] [PubMed]
54. Bem, A.; Ucieklak-Jeż, P.; Prędkiewicz, P. Income per bed as a determinant of hospital's financial liquidity. *Probl. Manag. 21st Century* **2014**, *9*, 124–131.
55. Hajdikova, T.; Komarkova, L.; Pirozek, P. The Issue of Indebtedness of Czech Hospitals. In Proceedings of the 11th International Scientific Conference European Financial Systems, Lednice, Czech Republic, 12–13 June 2014; Deev, O., Kajurová, V., Krajíček, J., Eds.; Masarykova Univerzita: Brno, Czech Republic, 2014; pp. 230–235, ISBN 978-80-210-7153-7.
56. Tescher, P.; Chen, T.M. Emergency department performance at a small rural hospital: An independent in-depth review. *Aust. J. Rural Health* **2009**, *6*, 292–297. [CrossRef]
57. Kaufman, B.; Pink, G.; Holmes, M. *Prediction of Financial Distress among Rural Hospitals*; NC Rural Health Research Program Findings Brief: Chapel Hill, NC, USA, 2016; Volume 9, pp. 1665–1672.
58. Younis, M.Z. A comparison study of urban and small rural hospitals financial and economic performance. *Online J. Rural Nurs. Healthc.* **2012**, *1*, 38–48.
59. Rój, J. Efektywność usługowa jako kryterium wyboru mechanizmu finansowania szpitali. *Ruch Prawniczy, Ekonomiczny i Socjologiczny* **2003**, *4*, 153–171.
60. Rój, J. Forma organizacyjno-prawna a gospodarka finansowa szpitala. In *Komercjalizacja i prywatyzacja ZOZ: Kluczowe warunki osiągnięcia sukcesu*; Prace Naukowe Akademii Ekonomicznej we Wrocławiu; Akademii Ekonomicznej im. Oskara Langego we Wrocławiu: Wrocław, Poland, 2006; pp. 53–57.
61. Murphy, K.M.; Hughes, L.S.; Conway, P. A path to sustain rural hospitals. *JAMA* **2018**, *12*, 1193–1194. [CrossRef]
62. Martens, P.J.; Stewart, D.K.; Mitchell, L.; Black, C. Assessing the performance of rural hospitals. *Healthc. Manag. Forum* **2002**, *4*, 27–34. [CrossRef]
63. Doty, B.; Zuckerman, R.; Finlayson, S.; Jenkins, P.; Rieb, N.; Heneghan, S. General surgery at rural hospitals: A national survey of rural hospital administrators. *Surgery* **2008**, *5*, 599–606. [CrossRef]
64. Rechel, B.; Džakula, A.; Duran, A.; Fattore, G.; Edwards, N.; Grignon, M.; Ricciardi, W. Hospitals in rural or remote areas: An exploratory review of policies in 8 high-income countries. *Health Policy* **2016**, *7*, 758–769. [CrossRef] [PubMed]
65. Joynt, K.E.; Harris, Y.; Orav, E.J.; Jha, A.K. Quality of care and patient outcomes in critical access rural hospitals. *JAMA* **2011**, *306*, 45–52. [CrossRef] [PubMed]
66. Rosko, M.D.; Mutter, R.L. Inefficiency differences between Critical Access Hospitals and Prospectively Paid Rural Hospitals. *J. Health Politics Policy Law* **2010**, *35*, 95–126. [CrossRef] [PubMed]
67. Bazzoli, G.J.; Chen, H.F.; Zhao, M.; Lindrooth, R.C. Hospital financial condition and the quality of patient care. *Health Econ.* **2008**, *8*, 977–995. [CrossRef]
68. Bai, G.; Tim Xu, M.P.; Rogers, A.T.; Anderson, G.F. Hospitals with Higher Direct Cost Ratios Have Lower mission Rates. *J. Health Care Financ.* **2017**, *3*, 117–236.
69. Holmes, G.M.; Pink, G.H.; Friedman, S.A. The financial performance of rural hospitals and implications for elimination of the critical access hospital program. *J. Rural Health* **2013**, *2*, 140–149. [CrossRef]
70. Holmes, G.M.; Kaufman, B.G.; Pink, G.H. Predicting financial distress and closure in rural hospitals. *J. Rural Health* **2017**, *3*, 239–249. [CrossRef]
71. Holmes, M. Financially Fragile Rural Hospitals Mergers and Closures. *N. C. Med. J.* **2015**, *1*, 37–40.
72. Wang, B.B.; Wan, T.T.; Falk, J.A.; Goodwin, D. Management strategies and financial performance in rural and urban hospitals. *J. Med. Syst.* **20011**, *5*, 241–255.
73. Mijal, A. Uwarunkowania społeczno-ekonomiczne jako determinanta rozwoju obszarów wiejskich województwa opolskiego—Próba diagnozy. *J. Agrobusiness Rural Devel.* **2012**, *2*, 167–178.

74. Wilkin, J. Obszary wiejskie w warunkach dynamizacji zmian strukturalnych. In *Ekspertyzy do strategii rozwoju społeczno-gospodarczego Polski Wschodniej do roku 2020*; Ministerstwo Rozwoju Regionalnego: Warszawa, Poland, 2007; pp. 594–616.
75. Rakowska, J.; Wojewódzka-Wiewiórska, A. *Zróżnicowanie Przestrzenne Terenów Wiejskich w Polsce—Stan i Perspektywy Rozwoju w Kontekście Rozwiązań Strukturalnych*; Ekspertyza wykonana na zamówienie Ministerstwa Rozwoju Regionalnego; Ministerstwo Rozwoju Regionalnego: Warszawa, Poland, 2010.
76. Sinay, L. Hospital mergers and closures: Survival of rural hospitals. *J. Rural Health* **1998**, *14*, 357–365. [CrossRef] [PubMed]
77. Gapenski, L. *Healthcare Finance: An Introduction to Accounting and Financial Management*, 5th ed.; Health Administration Press: Chicago, CA, USA, 2012; ISBN 978-1567934250.
78. Bem, A.; Prędkiewicz, P.; Ucieklak-Jeż, P.; Siedlecki, R. Impact of hospital's profitability on structure of its liabilities. In Proceedings of the Strategica Local versus Global 2015 Proceedings, Bucharest, Romania, 29–30 October 2015; Brătianu, C., Zbuchea, A., Pînzaru, F., Vătămănescu, E.-M., Leon, R.D., Eds.; Tritonic: Newark, NJ, USA, 2015.
79. Bem, A.; Siedlecki, R.; Prędkiewicz, P.; Ucieklak-Jeż, P.; Hajdikova, T. Hospital's financial health assessment. Gradient method's application. In Proceedings of the 18 Annual International Conference on Enterprise and Competitive tive Environment, Brno, Czech Republic, 5–6 March 2015; Kapounek, S., Ed.; Mendel University in Brno: Brno, Czech Republic, 2015; pp. 76–85, ISBN 978-80-7509-342-4.
80. Siedlecki, R.; Bem, A.; Prędkiewicz, P.; Ucieklak-Jeż, P. Measures of hospital's financial condition—Empirical study. In Proceedings of the Strategica Local versus Global 2015 Proceedings, Bucharest, Romania, 29–30 October 2015; Brătianu, C., Zbuchea, A., Pînzaru, F., Vătămănescu, E.-M., Leon, R.D., Eds.; Tritonic: Newark, NJ, USA, 2015; pp. 666–676. ISBN 978-606-749-054-1.
81. Siedlecka, U.; Siedlecki, J. *Optymalizacja Taksonomiczna*; Wydawnictwo Akademii Ekonomicznej w Krakowie: Kraków, Poland, 1990.
82. Siedlecki, R. Forecasting Company Financial Distress Using the Gradient Measurement of Development and S-Curve. *Procedia Econ. Financ.* **2014**, *12*, 597–606. [CrossRef]
83. Bem, A.; Michalski, G. The financial health of hospitals. V4 countries case. In *Sociálna Ekonomika a Vzdelávanie*; Zborník vedeckých štúdií; Ľapinová, E., Gubalová, J., Eds.; Univerzita Mateja Bela v Banskej Bystrici: Banska Bystrica, Slovakia, 2014; Volume 1, pp. 1–10, ISBN 978-80-557-0623-8.
84. Bem, A.; Prędkiewicz, K.; Prędkiewicz, P.; Ucieklak-Jeż, P. Determinants of Hospital's Financial Liquidity. *Procedia Econ. Financ.* **2014**, *12*, 27–36. [CrossRef]
85. Bem, A.; Prędkiewicz, K.; Prędkiewicz, P.; Ucieklak-Jeż, P. Hospital's Size as the Determinant of Financial Liquidity. In Proceedings of the 11th International Scientific Conference European Financial Systems, Brno, Czech Republic, 27–28 June 2014; Deev, O., Kajurová, V., Krajíček, J., Eds.; Masarykova Univerzita: Brno, Czech Republic, 2014; pp. 41–48, ISBN 978-80-210-7153-7.
86. Bem, A.; Prędkiewicz, P.; Ucieklak-Jeż, P.; Siedlecki, R. Profitability versus Debt in Hospital Industry. In *European Financial Systems 2015, Proceedings of the 12th International Scientific Conference, Brno, Czech Republic, 18–19 June 2015*; Kajurová, V., Krajíček, J., Eds.; Masarykova Univerzita: Brno, Czech Republic, 2015; pp. 20–27, ISBN 978-80-210-7962-5.
87. Lubkowska, W.; Krzepota, J. Quality of life and health behaviours of patients with low back pain. *Phys. Act. Rev.* **2019**, *7*, 182–192.
88. Coburn, A.; Wakefield, M.; Casey, M.; Moscovice, I.; Payne, S.; Loux, S. Assuring rural hospital patient safety: What should be the priorities? *J. Rural Health* **2004**, *4*, 314–326. [CrossRef]

 © 2019 by the authors. Licensee MDPI, Basel, Switzerland. This article is an open access article distributed under the terms and conditions of the Creative Commons Attribution (CC BY) license (http://creativecommons.org/licenses/by/4.0/).

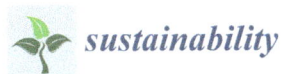

Article

The Role of Occupational Stress in the Association between Emotional Labor and Mental Health: A Moderated Mediation Model

Heyeon Park [1], Hyunjin Oh [2] and Sunjoo Boo [3],*

[1] Department of Public Health Medical Services, Seoul National University Bundang Hospital, Seoul 13620, Korea; ju-aa@hanmail.net
[2] College of Nursing, Gachon University, Seongnam-daero, Inchon 21936, Korea; hyunjino@gachon.ac.kr
[3] Research Institute of Nursing Science·College of Nursing, Ajou University, Gyeonggi-do, Suwon 16499, Korea
* Correspondence: sjboo@ajou.ac.kr

Received: 20 February 2019; Accepted: 24 March 2019; Published: 29 March 2019

Abstract: This study investigated whether occupational stress factors moderate the effect of emotional labor on psychological distress in call center employees. A cross-sectional and descriptive study using anonymous paper-based survey methods was conducted in a sample of 283 call center employees in South Korea. Participants completed the Emotional Labor Scale, the Depression Anxiety Stress Scale, and the Korean Occupational Stress Scale. Moderated mediation analyses were conducted using the PROCESS macro in order to investigate the relationship among variables. The results showed that the association between surface acting while having emotional labor and psychological distress was mediated by emotional dissonance. The mediated effect of emotional dissonance was moderated by discomfort in occupational climate, suggesting that improving the occupational environment can lessen the level of psychological distress among emotional workers, and that more attention should be devoted to the development of an intervention at the organizational level in order to prevent mental health problems in this population.

Keywords: emotional labor; surface acting; emotional dissonance; occupational stress; moderated mediation

1. Introduction

With the growth of the service industry, emotional labor and its consequences among front-line service employees have been receiving a lot of attention in the field of public mental health. Emotional labor is defined as the process by which workers have to control their feelings in accordance with the organizational demands and their occupational roles [1–3]. Emotional labor seems to play a critical role in the development of mental health problems. Previous studies have reported the association of emotional labor with depression, suicidal thoughts, anxiety disorder, and somatization [4–9]. Additionally, a recent study investigated the effect of emotional labor on the symptoms of post-traumatic stress disorders (PTSD) among firefighters and found that emotional damage from emotional labor while on duty had a moderating effect on the association between recent traumatic exposure and the level of PTSD symptoms [10].

There are two strategies of emotional labor: surface acting and deep acting. Deep acting indicates that employees try to create feeling that must be expressed, while surface acting refers to their merely putting on a mask [11,12]. When there was a discrepancy between felt emotions and displayed emotions, employees suffered from emotional dissonance, which is an important component of emotional labor [11]. The previous findings showed that emotional dissonance is associated with burnout and mediates between the association between emotional labor and employees' well-being [13,14]. Therefore, it is possible that emotional dissonance mediates the association of emotional labor with psychological distress.

The deleterious effect of emotional labor on mental health may be accelerated by work-related stress in an occupational environment. It has been known that work-related stress is an occupational hazard with a critical role in the development of mental disorder [15–18], as well as physical health problems [19–21]. In the field of research on occupational stress, the Job Demand-Control-Support (JDCS) model predicts that social support can moderate the negative effect of high-strain (high demand-low control) jobs on the well-being of employees [22]. According to the JDCS model, occupational support could moderate the association between emotional labor and mental health among employees who have to do high-strain emotional labor. In fact, previous research has reported that perceived organizational support influences employees' performances during emotional labor and moderates the association of emotional labor with job satisfaction, performance, and emotional exhaustion [23–26]. Besides organizational support, a variety of stress factors at work, such as the demands of the job, organizational injustice, and discomfort in the occupational climate, may influence the consequences of emotional labor. However, few investigations have assessed whether occupational stress factors affect the association between emotional labor and psychological distress, including depression and anxiety, or find how this correlation occurs.

The aim of the current study is to investigate whether various components of occupational stress moderate the effects of emotional labor on the psychological distress including depression, anxiety, and stress among employees in service work. Based on the findings of previous studies and theoretical background, we hypothesized that emotional dissonance mediates the association of surface acting while having emotional labor with psychological distress and that occupational stress factors moderates the mediating effect.

2. Methods

2.1. Study Design and Ethic

This was a cross-sectional study among employees recruited from a call center of a credit card company in South Korea, where about 1000 employees work. All participants gave their informed consent. Approval for the collection and analysis of the data was obtained from the Ethics Committee of a research institution (IRB #:1044396-201601-HR-005-01).

2.2. Study Population

The study involved a secondary analysis of quantitative data that originally were collected to investigate the mental health status of the employees of the call center. The initial finding from these data, which were published earlier [6], focused on the potential predictors of the status of mental health among the workers at the call center. These initial findings raised new questions concerning why some employees appeared to be mentally stable while others did not. Thus, we reinvestigated these data from the perspective of occupational stress since the environmentally-protective factors and the related stressors affected the employees in different ways. The ages of the participants in the study ranged from 18 to 55 (Mean = 36.05, SD = 8.17). The participants were 90.8% (n = 257) females and 9.2% (n = 26) males. High school graduates and those with less education were 33.6% (n = 95) of the total, 32.5% (n = 92) were junior college graduates, and 30.74% (n = 83) were college graduates (Table 1).

Table 1. Demographic characteristics of the sample (N = 283).

Characteristics	N (%) or M ± SD
Sex	
Male	26 (9.2)
Female	257 (90.8)
Age (year) (N = 278)	36.05 ± 8.17
Education (N = 270)	
High School graduation or less	95 (33.6)
Junior college graduation	92 (32.5)
College graduation or more	83 (30.74)

Note: N = total sample; M = mean; SD = standard deviation.

2.3. Instruments

2.3.1. The Korean Occupational Stress Scale

We used the culture-specific, 24-item, Korean Occupational Stress Scale (KOSS) to measure the participants' levels of occupational stress in the workplace [27]. The KOSS was developed and validated with a nationwide random sample of over 10,000 Korean employees to measure Korean-specific, job-related stress with seven subscales, i.e., job demands (4 items), insufficient job control (4 items), interpersonal conflict (3 items), job insecurity (2 items), organizational injustice (4 items), lack of rewards (3 items), and discomfort in occupational climate (4 items). Each item on the questionnaire was rated on a 4-point Likert scale from 1 (not at all) to 4 (very much). Scores for each subscale were calculated based on the scoring method provided by the developers. Possible ranges for each subscale was 0 to 100, with higher scores representing higher levels of job-related stress. The Cronbach's alpha values ranged from 0.51 (occupational climate) to 0.82 (organizational injustice) when they were determined for Korean employees nationwide [27]. Reliability coefficients in this study ranged from 0.60 to 0.86.

2.3.2. The Emotional Labor Scale

We used the Emotional Labor Scale (ELS) to measure participants' levels of emotional labor. The scale consists of nine items with three subscales, i.e., surface action, deep action, and emotional dissonance [12,28,29]. Each of the surface action and deep action subscales consisted of three items that asked participants to indicate how they managed their emotions to meet their job demands [28]. The emotional dissonance subscale (three items) measures the extent to which the participants feel apart from the emotions they express to their customers on the phone [12]; the response categories for all emotional labor items ranged from 1 to 5, i.e., "not at all" to "a lot." Summary scores and subscale scores were calculated by adding the scores for each item. Possible total score of the ELS ranged from 9 to 45, with higher scores indicating greater emotional labor. Cronbach's alpha for the ELS was found to be in the range of 0.85 (emotional dissonance) to 0.90 (deep action) for the employees of the call center [29]. In this study, the value of Cronbach's alpha for the total score of the ELS ranged from 0.86 to 0.89.

2.3.3. The Depression Anxiety Stress Scale (DASS)

The levels of psychological distress of call center employees in this study were assessed with the 21-item DASS [30], which measures levels of depression, anxiety, and stress. It consists of seven items in three different subdomains, each of which has self-rating statements of mental health on a 4-point severity/frequency Likert scale (0 = did not apply to me at all or never to 3 = applied to me very much or almost always). Based on the instructions in the scoring guidelines, the scores for the subdomains were calculated by adding the scores for relevant items and doubling those scores. Then, the scores of the three domains were combined to indicate an overall level of psychological distress.

The possible range for the total score on the DASS was 0 to 126. Higher scores represent higher levels of psychological distress. In this study, the Cronbach's alpha ranged from 0.88 to 0.89.

2.4. DATA Analyses

Descriptive statistics were used to evaluate sample characteristics and the distribution of main variables (psychological distress, emotional labor, and occupational stress factors). One-way analysis of variance, and an independent samples t-test were used to evaluate the differences in the psychological distress based on demographic variables. For the distribution of main variables, we examined mean with standard deviation, observed score range, skewness, and kurtosis. The analyses of the normality of the distribution of main variables were carried out using the Kolmogorow-Smirnow test. The distribution of measures of all scales differed from normal distribution. The correlations between the main variables were examined using Spearman correlation coefficients.

We performed the mediation analysis to investigate the association of psychological distress with two factors of emotional labor, surface acting, and emotional dissonance, which were significantly correlated with the DASS total score in the results of the correlation analysis. A simple mediation analysis proposed by Hayes [31] was conducted to examine mediating effects of emotional dissonance during emotional labor on the association between surface acting and psychological distress (Figure 1). We used 5000 bootstrap samples and determined the mediating effect of the 95% confident interval.

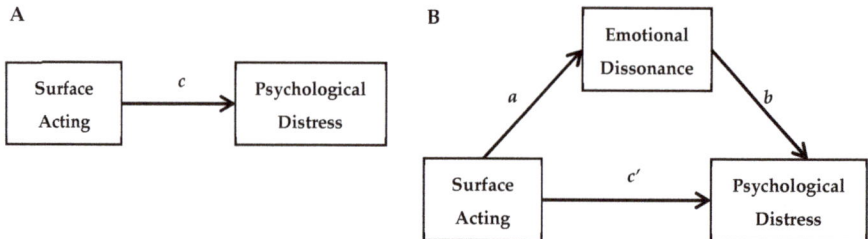

Figure 1. The mediation model. (**A**) depicts the direct effect of surface acting on psychological distress. (**B**) depicts that the effect of surface acting on psychological distress is mediated by emotional dissonance. Interaction indexes, *a* refers to the direct effect of the predictor on the mediator, *b* refers the direct effect of the mediator on the outcome variable, *c* refers to the direct effect of the predictor on the outcome, and *c'* refer to the direct effect of a predictor after controlling the indirect effect of predictor through the mediator on the outcome.

Next, moderated mediation analyses proposed by Hayes [31] were conducted to investigate whether occupational stress factors moderate the indirect effect of surface acting on psychological distress through emotional dissonance. Again, 5000 bootstrap samples and a confidence interval of 95% were selected. Once more, surface acting was entered as predictor, psychological distress as outcome, and emotional dissonance as mediator. In addition, each of four occupational stress factors, which were significantly related to psychological distress in the results of a preliminary correlation analysis, was added as a moderator. Figure 2 illustrates this moderated mediation model.

The data were analyzed using IBM SPSS statistics 22 software (SPSS, Inc., Chicago, IL, USA) and PROCESS macro v3.3 [31] for SPSS. Statistical significance was defined as a two-tailed *p*-value of < 0.01.

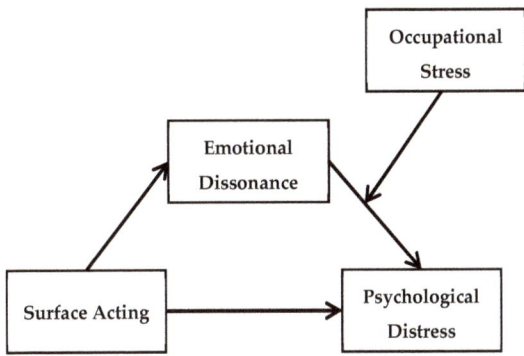

Figure 2. The moderated mediation model.

3. Results

3.1. Preliminary Analysis

The characteristics of the level of psychological distress, emotional labor, and occupational stress factors in the sample are presented in Table 2. There were no significant differences in the DASS scores based on demographic variables, such as gender and the level of education ($p > 0.05$).

Table 2. Descriptive statistics for the DASS, the ELS, and the KOSS-SF ($N = 283$).

Variables	M	SD	Min	Max	Skewness	Kurtosis
DASS total score	47.60	27.86	0	126	0.53	−0.30
ELS						
Surface acting	11.05	2.68	3	15	−0.48	−0.19
Deep acting	8.15	2.82	3	15	0.21	−0.18
Emotional dissonance	8.43	2.95	3	15	0.15	−0.66
KOSS-SF						
Job demand	62.60	19.93	25	100	0.02	−0.49
Insufficient job control	68.17	16.53	0	100	−0.20	−0.18
Interpersonal conflict	32.51	17.30	0	100	0.25	1.03
Job insecurity	48.65	20.94	0	100	0.13	−0.10
Organizational injustice	57.21	17.68	8.33	100	0.49	0.02
Lack of reward	59.60	18.52	0	100	0.15	−0.36
Discomfort in occupational climate	36.51	16.88	0	100	0.22	0.59

Note: M = mean; SD = standard deviation; DASS = Depression Anxiety Stress Scale; ELS = Emotional Labor Scale; KOSS-SF = Korean Occupational Stress Scale-Short Form.

Table 3 provides the Spearman correlation coefficients between the DASS total score with the KOSS-SF and the ELS scores. The DASS total scores had a positive correlation with the levels of surface acting and emotional dissonance due to emotional labor and the occupational stress factors, such as the demands of the job, job insecurity, organizational injustice, lack of rewards, and discomfort in the occupational climate ($p < 0.001$).

Table 3. Correlation between main variables (N = 283).

	1	2	3	4	5	6	7	8	9	10	11
1	1.000										
2	0.295 **	1.000									
3	0.113	0.253 **	1.000								
4	0.442 **	0.596 **	0.263 **	1.000							
5	0.395 **	0.431 **	0.225 **	0.424 **	1.000						
6	0.026	0.092	−0.254 *	0.027	0.008	1.000					
7	0.052	0.033	−0.097	0.083	0.192 *	0.276 **	1.000				
8	0.241 **	0.381 **	0.131	0.349 **	0.423 **	0.073	0.198 *	1.000			
9	0.318 *	0.236 **	0.011	0.228 **	0.417 **	0.279 **	0.436 **	0.392 **	1.000		
10	0.253 **	0.274 **	−0.151	0.218 **	0.320 **	0.423 **	0.344 **	0.304 **	0.646 **	1.000	
11	0.316 **	0.214 *	0.085	0.281 **	0.316 **	0.180 *	0.371 **	0.356 **	0.424 **	0.293 **	1.000

Note: 1 = DASS total score, 2 = Surface acting during emotional labor; 3 = Deep acting during emotional labor; 4 = emotional dissonance during emotional labor, 5 = job demand, 6 = insufficient job control, 7 = interpersonal conflict, 8 = job insecurity, 9 = organizational injustice; 10 = lack of rewards, 11 = discomfort in occupational climate; ** p < 0.001, * p < 0.01.

3.2. Mediation Model of the Association between Emotional Labor and Psychological Distress

The results of the mediation analysis are shown in Figure 3. The level of surface acting was positively related to emotional dissonance, and the emotional dissonance was positively associated with psychological distress. When statistically controlling for emotional distress, the level of surface acting was not significantly associated with psychological distress, which indicated that the direct effect of surface acting on psychological distress disappeared. The bootstrap confidence interval confirmed that the indirect effect of surface acting on psychological distress through emotional dissonance (Table 4). These results indicated that the relationship between surface acting and psychological distress was completely mediated by emotional dissonance.

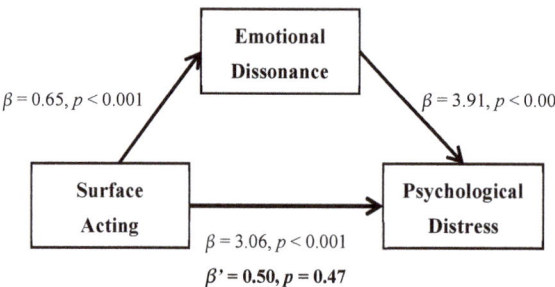

Figure 3. Mediation model showing that the effect of surface acting on psychological distress is mediated by emotional dissonance. Change in beta weight when the mediator is present is highlighted in bold.

Table 4. Bootstrap results for indirect effect.

Mediator	Effect	SE	LL 95% CI	UL 95% CI
Emotional dissonance	2.5569	0.4907	1.6455	3.5765

Notes: SE = standard error; LL95%CI = lower level of the 95% confidence interval; UL95%CI = upper level of the 95% confidence interval.

3.3. Moderated Mediation Models

Table 5 shows the results of the moderated mediation analyses treating emotional dissonance as the mediator when each of the four occupational stress factors was used as the moderator in the relationship between emotional dissonance and psychological distress: Job demand was a moderator in the model 1; job insecurity in the model 2; organizational injustice in the model 3; lack of reward in the model 4; and discomfort in occupational climate in the model 5. Emotional dissonance appeared to be significant mediators, which have already been reported in the previous paragraph.

Table 5. Moderated mediation analysis when assuming each of occupational stress factors as a mediator (outcome variable = psychological distress).

Variables	B	SE	t	p
Moderated mediation model 1 ($R^* = 0.249$)				
Surface acting	−0.17	0.70	−0.24	0.809
Emotional dissonance	3.22	0.64	5.05	<0.001
Job demand	0.36	0.08	4.32	<0.001
Job demand × Emotional dissonance	0.01	0.02	0.56	0.575
Moderated mediation mode 2 ($R^* = 0.204$)				
Surface acting	0.26	0.71	0.37	0.710
Emotional dissonance	3.72	0.64	5.80	<0.001
Insecurity	0.12	0.08	1.57	0.118
Insecurity × Emotional dissonance	0.01	0.02	0.33	0.743
Moderated mediation model 3 ($R^* = 0.261$)				
Surface acting	0.30	0.67	0.44	0.657
Emotional dissonance	3.42	0.61	5.54	<0.001
Injustice	0.36	0.08	4.29	<0.001
Injustice × Emotional dissonance	0.06	0.02	2.43	0.016
Moderated mediation model 4 ($R^* = 0.227$)				
Surface acting	0.19	0.69	0.28	0.781
Emotional dissonance	3.71	0.62	5.95	<0.001
Lack of reward	0.25	0.08	3.07	0.002
Lack of reward × Emotional dissonance	0.04	0.02	1.48	0.139
Moderated mediation model 5 ($R^* = 0.254$)				
Surface acting	0.57	0.68	0.85	0.397
Emotional dissonance	3.31	0.62	5.32	<0.001
Occupational climate	0.31	0.09	3.41	0.008
Occupational climate × Emotional dissonance	0.06	0.02	2.60	0.010

Notes: B = regression coefficient; SE = standard error of regression coefficient.

In the model 1, the main effect of job demand on psychological distress was significant ($p < 0.001$), but interaction between job demand and emotional dissonance was not significant ($p > 0.01$). In the model 2, job insecurity did not have significant main and moderating effects on psychological distress ($p > 0.01$). In the model 3, the main effect of organizational injustice was significant for psychological distress ($p < 0.001$), while moderating effect of organizational injustice was not significant ($p > 0.01$). In the model 4, the main effect of lack of reward was significant ($p < 0.001$), while moderating effect of lack of reward was not significant ($p > 0.01$). Finally, in the model 5, the main effect of discomfort in occupational climate was significant ($p < 0.008$) and the interaction between emotional dissonance and discomfort in occupational climate was significant in the model 5 ($p = 0.010$). Thus, these findings indicate that the mediation of emotional dissonance on the association between surface acting and psychological distress was moderated by discomfort in occupational climate.

The association between emotional dissonance and psychological distress was plotted when the levels of discomfort in the occupation climate was 1SD below and 1SD above the mean. This represents the simple effect of emotional labor at two levels of discomfort in the occupational climate (as a moderator) [32]. Figure 4 depicts emotional dissonance moderated by discomfort in occupational climate.

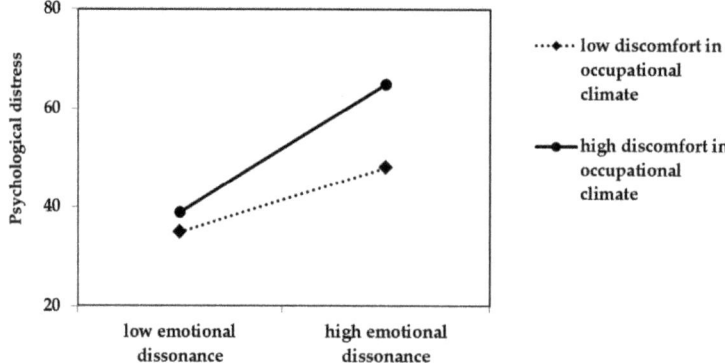

Figure 4. Moderating effect of the discomfort in occupational climate on the association between emotional labor and the severity of psychological distress.

To evaluate the conditional indirect effects of surface actin on psychological distress via emotional dissonance, as a function of different levels of the discomfort in the occupational climate, we used the bootstrap method for analysis. Indirect effects at three levels of the discomfort in the occupational climate (1SD above the mean, at the mean, and 1SD below the mean) were examined by using the 95% CIs of the bootstrap method. As shown in Table 6, the mediating effect of emotional dissonance changed according to the level of the discomfort in occupational climate and was weakest at 1SD below the mean of it. These indicate that emotional laborers suffering from emotional dissonance were susceptible to psychological distress when they felt discomfort in their occupational climate.

Table 6. Conditional indirect effect at specific levels of the moderator when treating emotional dissonance as a mediator.

Moderator: Discomfort in Occupational Climate	Effect	SE	LL 95% CI	UL 95% CI
1SD below the mean	1.45	0.54	0.44	2.58
Mean	2.17	0.47	1.28	3.13
1SD above the mean	2.89	0.53	1.89	3.96

Notes: SE = standard error; LL95%CI = lower level of the 95% confidence interval; UL95%CI = upper level of the 95% confidence interval.

4. Discussion

The current study investigated the relationship among emotional labor, occupational stress, and psychological distress using the moderated mediation analyses. The questions addressed by this study were whether emotional labor negatively influences mental health via emotional dissonance, and whether occupational stress factors moderates the negative effect of emotional labor on mental health. The main finding of the study was that emotional labor was related to psychological distress such as depression and anxiety when employees simulate emotions that are not actually felt (surface acting) and that the relationship was mediated by emotional dissonance which is the discrepancy between felt emotion and displayed emotion. Furthermore, we found that stress from an occupational environment moderated the mediating effect of emotional dissonance on the association between emotional labor and psychological distress. To the best of our knowledge, this is the first study to investigate the moderating role of occupational stress in the relationship between emotional labor and psychological distress among Korean service workers.

In this study, we obtained two findings about the association between emotional labor and psychological distress. First, surface acting was positively associated with psychological distress, while deep acting was not significantly related to psychological distress. Second, the effect of surface acting on psychological distress was mediated by emotional dissonance. It was repeatedly reported that there was the association of emotional labor with burnout and emotional exhaustion [28,33]. Moreover, a significant partial mediation role of emotional dissonance in the relationship between emotional labor and emotional exhaustion was revealed in a previous study [34]. Our results incorporate and confirm the previous findings, and also include new findings that emotional labor influences mental health through the mediation of emotional dissonance. Also, the finding that surface acting was negatively associated with mental health is consistent with previous findings that there are more negative outcome associated with surface acting such as turnover intentions, withdrawal, and job dissatisfaction in comparison to surface acting [35].

Furthermore, by using moderated mediation models, we found that the level of emotional labor has a positive association with the severity of psychological distress and that its effect on psychological distress varies according to the level of discomfort in the occupational climate. In KOSS-SF, which is the scale assessing occupational stress in this study, the discomfort in the occupational climate is defined as inconvenience caused by the degree of collectivism among workers, and it also may generate from dining out after work hours, inconsistency of job orders, an authoritarian culture, and gender discrimination [27,36]. Thus, the discomfort in occupational climate assessed in this study could be similar to the lack of organizational support which is perceived by employees in occupational environments. To our knowledge, our finding is the first to show the moderating effect of occupational stress on the negative association between emotional labor and mental health. This study suggests that alleviating discomfort in the occupational climate by constructing a less collectivistic work culture may make service workers less vulnerable to the psychological distress. Also, it suggests that the role of lower or middle managers in charge of these cultural factors seems to be important since subjective discomfort in the occupational climate may be different by the sub-cultures that make up the informal sector of the company.

In addition, we found that occupational stress factors such as high job demand, organizational injustice, lack of reward, as well as discomfort in organizational climate, were associated with mental health problems among call center employees. Occupational stress factors such as lack of support and discomfort in occupational stress have been found to be the risk factors for depression [36]. Also, job strain, organizational injustice, and the imbalance between effort and rewards were found to be related to suicidal ideation among workers [37]. According to the models for occupational stress factors, such as the demand-control-support model and the effort-reward imbalance model, high workload, lack of reward, and lack of organizational support could have a significant impact on psychological distress [38]. Considering the previous findings and hypothetical models of occupational stress, our finding of significant main effects of various occupational stress factors on psychological distress were expected.

Limitations should be considered when generalizing the results of this study. First, the cross-sectional design of the study limited our ability to infer causal relationships among emotional labor, occupational stress factors, and psychological distress. Future studies need to employ a longitudinal approach to investigate the causal relationships among the risk factors and psychological distress among emotional laborers. Second, this study collected data from self-report assessments, which could be consisted of response bias that affected the results. In future studies, conducting standardized interviews of employees to determine the states of their mental health and occupational stress would be better option to provide more accurate and detailed information regarding the mental health problem among emotional laborers. More than 90% of the workers who participated in this study were women, which was indicative of the fact that mainly women are working in the customer service industry in South Korea. The findings of this study cannot be generalized to call centers that have larger percentages of male employees.

5. Conclusions

In this study, we found that surface acting while having emotional labor was significantly associated with psychological distress via emotional dissonance. Furthermore, the discomfort in occupational climate turned out to be an important moderator of the association between surface acting and psychological distress. These findings suggest that improving the occupational environment can lessen the level of psychological distress among emotional workers, and that more attention should be devoted to the development of an intervention at the organizational level in order to prevent mental health problems in this population. Given the increases in the service industry and the accumulating findings of emotional labor as a risk factor of psychological distress, there is a need to investigate protective factors that can mitigate the negative effects of emotional labor on mental health problems in service workers.

Author Contributions: All authors contributed substantially to all aspects of this article.

Funding: This research received no external funding.

Acknowledgments: We express our sincere gratitude to the call center employees and managers who supported this study. We also thank Chulhang Lee for his cooperation and support with the data collection.

Conflicts of Interest: The authors declare no conflict of interest.

References

1. Grandey, A.A.; Gabriel, A.S. Emotional labor at a crossroads: Where do we go from here? *Annu. Rev. Organ. Psychol. Organ. Behav.* **2015**, *2*, 323–349. [CrossRef]
2. Hochschild, A. *The Managed Heart*; University of California Press: Berkeley, CA, USA, 1983.
3. Mann, S. Emotion at work: To what extent are we expressing, suppressing, or faking it? *Eur. J. Work Organ. Psychol.* **1999**, *8*, 347–369. [CrossRef]
4. Kim, I.-H.; Noh, S.; Muntaner, C. Emotional demands and the risks of depression among homecare workers in the USA. *Int. Arch. Occup. Environ. Health* **2013**, *86*, 635–644. [CrossRef] [PubMed]
5. Murcia, M.; Chastang, J.-F.; Niedhammer, I. Psychosocial work factors, major depressive and generalised anxiety disorders: Results from the French national SIP study. *J. Affect. Disord.* **2013**, *146*, 319–327. [CrossRef] [PubMed]
6. Oh, H.; Park, H.; Boo, S. Mental health status and its predictors among call center employees: A cross-sectional study. *Nurs. Health Sci.* **2017**, *19*, 228–236. [CrossRef] [PubMed]
7. Shin, M.-K.; Kang, H.-L. Effects of emotional labor and occupational stress on somatization in nurses. *J. Korean Acad. Nurs. Adm.* **2011**, *17*, 158–167. [CrossRef]
8. Wieclaw, J.; Agerbo, E.; Mortensen, P.B.; Burr, H.; Tuchsen, F.; Bonde, J.P. Psychosocial working conditions and the risk of depression and anxiety disorders in the Danish workforce. *BMC Public Health* **2008**, *8*, 280. [CrossRef] [PubMed]
9. Yoon, J.-H.; Jeung, D.; Chang, S.-J. Does high emotional demand with low job control relate to suicidal ideation among service and sales workers in Korea? *J. Korean Med. Sci.* **2016**, *31*, 1042–1048. [CrossRef]
10. Park, H.; Kim, J.I.; Oh, S.; Kim, J.-H. The impact of emotional labor on the severity of PTSD symptoms in firefighters. *Compr. Psychiatry* **2018**, *83*, 53–58. [CrossRef] [PubMed]
11. Grandey, A.A. When "the show must go on": Surface acting and deep acting as determinants of emotional exhaustion and peer-rated service delivery. *Acad. Manag. J.* **2003**, *46*, 86–96.
12. Morris, J.A.; Feldman, D.C. The dimensions, antecedents, and consequences of emotional labor. *Acad. Manag. Rev.* **1996**, *21*, 986–1010. [CrossRef]
13. Arshadi, N.; Piryaei, S. The mediating role of emotional dissonance in the relationship between teacher's emotional labor strategies and occupational well-being. *Int. J. Psychol.* **2016**, *10*, 15–33.
14. Pugh, S.D.; Groth, M.; Hennig-Thurau, T. Willing and able to fake emotions: A closer examination of the link between emotional dissonance and employee well-being. *J. Appl. Psychol.* **2011**, *96*, 377. [CrossRef] [PubMed]
15. Gallery, M.E.; Whitley, T.W.; Klonis, L.K.; Anzinger, R.K.; Revicki, D.A. A study of occupational stress and depression among emergency physicians. *Ann. Emerg. Med.* **1992**, *21*, 58–64. [CrossRef]

16. Melchior, M.; Caspi, A.; Milne, B.J.; Danese, A.; Poulton, R.; Moffitt, T.E. Work stress precipitates depression and anxiety in young, working women and men. *Psychol. Med.* **2007**, *37*, 1119–1129. [CrossRef] [PubMed]
17. Hwang, W.; Kim, J.; Rankin, S. Depressive symptom and related factors: A cross-sectional study of Korean female workers working at traditional markets. *Int. J. Environ. Res. Public Health* **2017**, *14*, 1465. [CrossRef]
18. Motowidlo, S.J.; Packard, J.S.; Manning, M.R. Occupational stress: Its causes and consequences for job performance. *J. Appl. Psychol.* **1986**, *71*, 618. [CrossRef] [PubMed]
19. Lecca, L.; Campagna, M.; Portoghese, I.; Galletta, M.; Mucci, N.; Meloni, M.; Cocco, P. Work Related Stress, Well-Being and Cardiovascular Risk among Flight Logistic Workers: An Observational Study. *Int. J. Environ. Res. Public Health* **2018**, *15*, 1952. [CrossRef]
20. Li, J.; Loerbroks, A.; Bosma, H.; Angerer, P. Work stress and cardiovascular disease: A life course perspective. *J. Occup. Health* **2016**, *58*, 216–219. [CrossRef]
21. Kivimäki, M.; Kawachi, I. Work stress as a risk factor for cardiovascular disease. *Curr. Cardiol. Rep.* **2015**, *17*, 74. [CrossRef]
22. Johnson, J.V.; Hall, E.M. Job strain, work place social support, and cardiovascular disease: A cross-sectional study of a random sample of the Swedish working population. *Am. J. Public Health* **1988**, *78*, 1336–1342. [CrossRef]
23. Hur, W.-M.; Won Moon, T.; Jun, J.-K. The role of perceived organizational support on emotional labor in the airline industry. *Int. J. Contemp. Hosp. Manag.* **2013**, *25*, 105–123. [CrossRef]
24. Kumar Mishra, S. Linking perceived organizational support to emotional labor. *Pers. Rev.* **2014**, *43*, 845–860. [CrossRef]
25. Duke, A.B.; Goodman, J.M.; Treadway, D.C.; Breland, J.W. Perceived organizational support as a moderator of emotional labor/outcomes relationships. *J. Appl. Soc. Psychol.* **2009**, *39*, 1013–1034. [CrossRef]
26. Nixon, A.E.; Yang, L.Q.; Spector, P.E.; Zhang, X. Emotional labor in China: Do perceived organizational support and gender moderate the process? *Stress Health* **2011**, *27*, 289–305. [CrossRef]
27. Chang, S.J.; Koh, S.B.; Kang, D.; Kim, S.A.; Kang, M.G.; Lee, C.G.; Chung, J.J.; Cho, J.J.; Son, M.; Chae, C.H. Developing an occupational stress scale for Korean employees. *Korean J. Occup. Environ. Med.* **2005**, *17*, 297–317.
28. Brotheridge, C.M.; Grandey, A.A. Emotional labor and burnout: Comparing two perspectives of "people work". *J. Vocat. Behav.* **2002**, *60*, 17–39. [CrossRef]
29. Jeong, K.; Choi, S.; Park, M.; Li, Y. The Effects of Customer Service Representatives' Emotional Labor by Emotional Display Rules on Emotional Dissonance, Emotional exhaustion and Turnover Intention in the Context of Call Centers. *Korean J. Bus. Adm.* **2015**, *28*, 529–551.
30. Lovibond, P.F.; Lovibond, S.H. The structure of negative emotional states: Comparison of the Depression Anxiety Stress Scales (DASS) with the Beck Depression and Anxiety Inventories. *Behav. Res. Ther.* **1995**, *33*, 335–343. [CrossRef]
31. Hayes, A.F. *Introduction to Mediation, Moderation, and Conditional Process Analysis: A Regression-Based Approach*; Guilford Publications: New York, NY, USA, 2017.
32. Aiken, L.S.; West, S.G.; Reno, R.R. *Multiple Regression: Testing and Interpreting Interactions*; Sage: Thousand oaks, CA, USA, 1991.
33. Grandey, A.A.; Kern, J.H.; Frone, M.R. Verbal abuse from outsiders versus insiders: Comparing frequency, impact on emotional exhaustion, and the role of emotional labor. *J. Occup. Health Psychol.* **2007**, *12*, 63. [CrossRef]
34. Van Dijk, P.A.; Brown, A.K. Emotional labour and negative job outcomes: An evaluation of the mediating role of emotional dissonance. *J. Manag. Organ.* **2006**, *12*, 101–115. [CrossRef]
35. Mesmer-Magnus, J.R.; DeChurch, L.A.; Wax, A. Moving emotional labor beyond surface and deep acting: A discordance–congruence perspective. *Organ. Psychol. Rev.* **2012**, *2*, 6–53. [CrossRef]
36. Cho, J.J.; Kim, J.Y.; Chang, S.J.; Fiedler, N.; Koh, S.B.; Crabtree, B.F.; Kang, D.M.; Kim, Y.K.; Choi, Y.H. Occupational stress and depression in Korean employees. *Int. Arch. Occup. Environ. Health* **2008**, *82*, 47–57. [CrossRef] [PubMed]

37. Loerbroks, A.; Cho, S.-I.; Dollard, M.F.; Zou, J.; Fischer, J.E.; Jiang, Y.; Angerer, P.; Herr, R.M.; Li, J. Associations between work stress and suicidal ideation: Individual-participant data from six cross-sectional studies. *J. Psychosom. Res.* **2016**, *90*, 62–69. [CrossRef] [PubMed]
38. Rydstedt, L.W.; Devereux, J.; Sverke, M. Comparing and combining the demand-control-support model and the effort reward imbalance model to predict long-term mental strain. *Eur. J. Work Organ. Psychol.* **2007**, *16*, 261–278. [CrossRef]

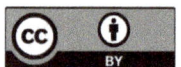

© 2019 by the authors. Licensee MDPI, Basel, Switzerland. This article is an open access article distributed under the terms and conditions of the Creative Commons Attribution (CC BY) license (http://creativecommons.org/licenses/by/4.0/).

MDPI
St. Alban-Anlage 66
4052 Basel
Switzerland
Tel. +41 61 683 77 34
Fax +41 61 302 89 18
www.mdpi.com

Sustainability Editorial Office
E-mail: sustainability@mdpi.com
www.mdpi.com/journal/sustainability

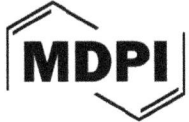

www.ingramcontent.com/pod-product-compliance
Lightning Source LLC
LaVergne TN
LVHW070051120526
838202LV00102B/2015